NATURAL WAYS TO DIGESTIVE HEALTH

- *Irritable Bowel Syndrome*
- *Heartburn*
- *Peptic Ulcer*
- *Dyspepsia and Stomach Upset*
- *Detoxification*
- *The Yeast Connection*
- *Friendly and Unfriendly Bacteria*
- *Diarrhea and Constipation*
- *Excessive Gas*
- *Enzyme Therapies*
- *Leaky Guts*
- *Probiotic Therapy*
- *Gallbladder Problems*

Also by Stephen Holt, M.D.

The Soy Revolution
Soya for Health
Miracle Herbs (with L. Comac)
The Power of Cartilage (with J. Barilla)
The Natural Way to a Healthy Heart
The Slim Chance
The Soy Lifestyle (with S. Granader)

NATURAL WAYS TO DIGESTIVE HEALTH

INTERFACES BETWEEN CONVENTIONAL AND ALTERNATIVE MEDICINE

Stephen Holt, M.D.

M. EVANS AND COMPANY, INC.
New York

DISCLAIMER

The ideas and advice in this book are based upon the experience and training of the author and the scientific information currently available. The suggestions in this book are definitely not meant to be a substitute for careful medical evalutation and treatment by a qualified, licensed health professional. The author and publisher do not recommend changing or adding medication or supplements without consulting your personal physician. They specifically disclaim any liability arising directly or indirectly from the use of this book.

M. Evans and Company, Inc.
216 East 49th Street
New York, New York 10017

Library of Congress Cataloging-in-Publication Data

Holt, Stephen, 1950–
    Natural ways to a digestive health : Interfaces between conventional and alternative medicine / Stephen Holt.
        p.   cm.
    ISBN 0-87131-909-8 (cloth)
    1. Indigestion—Popular works. 2. Indigestion—Alternative treatment.
    I. Title.
RC827.H65 2000
616.3'32—dc21   00-035329

Book design and typesetting by Rik Lain Schell

Printed in the United States of America

9   8   7   6   5   4   3   2   1

To George and Margaret, my parents, Karin, my wife, and Fraser, Stephanie, Andrew, Stephen, and ? on the way, my beloved children.

To God: Thank you for the gifts of life and thought, even though they sometimes come with discomfort.

ACKNOWLEDGMENTS

I thank Rik Schell for editorial work, my wife Karin Von Ah for typing with patience, and George de Kay for having confidence in me as an author.

CONTENTS

Diarrhea; Osmotic Diarrhea; Lactose Intolerance; The Origin of Lactose Intolerance; Drugs and Diarrhea; Pains in and Around the Anus; Serotonin; Use of Precursors of Neurotransmitters (Molecules of Emotion); Chapter Summary

Natural Ways to Digestive Health is a book that is brilliant and new, but it presents a quite controversial perspective on approaches to the management of certain gastrointestinal disorders. This book fills an important void in the practice of medicine for digestive health. Stephen Holt, M.D., navigates science and speculation in a clever manner with wit, eloquence, and novel thoughts. *Natural Ways to Digestive Health* takes a very interesting new look at digestive disorders, principally of functional cause, and provides great insight into what is known, while attempting to explain parts of the unknown.

A large percentage of healthcare seekers are self-medicating with over-the-counter drugs and dietary supplements—and some are even sharing prescription drugs with relatives or friends. Dr. Holt points out the problems that are inherent in self-diagnosis and self-treatment of gastrointestinal disorders. This work focuses on a forgotten area in conventional clinical gastroenterology that involves the use of natural remedies. Dr. Holt does not appear to embrace orthodox approaches entirely, and while he is supportive of alternative medicine, he is insightful of its short falls.

To Dr. Holt, terms like *alternative, conventional,* and *integrated medicine* possess disadvantages or limitations. He has preferred to talk about "pluralistic medicine"—a form of medicine that concentrates on "what works" regardless of its origins.

Dr. Holt is brave but cautious in his assertions so that controversial information is placed into perspective. The book illuminates some confusing concepts that continue to cause arguments and contention among rivals in conventional and alternative medicine.

Of particular importance are discussions about the ecology of the gut and its role in functional and organic digestive disorders. Dr. Holt proposes concepts that regard digestive disorders in a holistic and realistic way, without a misleading mix of science and wishful thinking—a phenomenon that has contaminated popular literature in alternative medicine.

This book is a quintessential example of lateral thought in medicine, and debate must ensue. The particular value of this work is to enlighten both the layperson and practicing physicians about emerging concepts in alternative medicine as applied to gastrointestinal disorders. Some patients self-medicate with natural remedies or engage in alternative treatments without discussing their activity with their own physicians. This book will help to break the ice on the subject and encourage greater dialogue between physician and patient.

The concentration of the book on functional gut disorders is appropriate, as these are the most common sources of digestive upset and reasons for self-treatment. They are also among the most common reasons for an individual to seek the services of a healthcare practitioner. Dr. Holt does not proselytize; he is very quick to point out the practice of "reinventing the wheel" in medicine, and he is unwilling to advise self-medication for serious disease without appropriate medical consultation.

Qualities like these make this book very desirable reading for patients and healthcare givers. In fact, it may help the practice of gastroenterology by breaking up the wall of division between orthodox and alternative medicine. It might also save consultation time for the specialist who cannot review all of the questions with his or her patients.

"Gut feelings" are only beginning to be understood, and nonconventional approaches may afford some solutions. It is refreshing that an expert gastroenterologist like Dr. Holt has tackled these difficult issues and produced a work that will find its place in the new type of eclectic medicine that is predicted to emerge in the twenty-first century.

Thomas V. Taylor, M.D.
Professor, Baylor College of Medicine, Houston, Texas

There is a hardcore group among the medical profession that worships at the shrine of the synthetic drug, rejects the importance of psychosocial issues in disease, and believes that alternative or complementary medicine is totally useless. This nebulous body of opinion is poorly counterbalanced by a small group of practitioners of alternative medicine that is unfamiliar with scientific peer-review and engages in mythical and magical thinking.

The groups espousing thse extremes of medical opinion are now, fortunately, diminishing in size. As the millennium turns, more physicians are prepared to consider pluralistic approaches to disease prevention and treatment.

In this book, I present thoughts about the guts that are in many cases neither novel nor new. My reliance on literature from the nineteenth century and early part of the twentieth century serves the purpose of showing how medical thought may have been quite slow on the uptake of important knowledge and its application in the management of common gut disorders. It could be argued that some of the treatment methods used in alternative and complementary medicine are antiquated. However, medical proposals that have been rejected in the name of modern medicine may have more benefit than hitherto supposed.

Modern research has shown us that there is a concept of the "bodymind," which could be segmented into the "gutmind," "stomachmind," "bowelmind," etc. The guts form a rich bed of receptors that respond to nervous impulses and hormonal agents. Like any organ in the body, the gut responds to the environment and occurrences that are global in origin. Many alternative interventions are holistic, and Gaia (oneness) is the quintessential concept behind this approach. The idea of the "Gaiagut" intrigues me—it could form a rational basis upon which some alternative medical interventions (or ancient treatment systems) could be effectively applied in modern therapeutics.

Medicine of the new millennium is increasingly pluralistic in its approach. Healthcare givers and recipients must have knowledge of all branches of medicine. Currently, modern medicine contains fragmented, eclectic approaches to diagnosis, treatment, and prevention. Treatment paradigms are shifting rapidly in many areas of medicine as remedies of natural origin become increasingly popular. Education in medicine is a key objective for public health. Knowledge of alternative medical practices and cooperation among the many disciplines of medical treatment can help solve the issues that surround the current status of "medicine at the crossroads."

A SPECIAL NOTE TO READERS

This book does not offer treatment advice. It is one of the first in-depth accounts of many issues in alternative medicine for the management of selected disorders of gastrointestinal function. The book warns about problems that are inherent in self-diagnosis and management of disease. Individuals with significant illnesses are encouraged not to self-medicate, they are consistently advised to seek the guidance of a healthcare practitioner of their choice.

Several concepts in this book cover areas of advanced biomedical research. In order to discuss these issues, topics are simplified with an attempt to maintain accuracy. In some cases, issues remain unresolved in the scientific literature, and opinions are divided. A growing number of physicians have incorporated nutritional, botanical, herbal, and other "alternative" approaches to disease management in their practices. Discussions of healthy bodily functions are incomplete without comments on disorders and disease. Dietary supplements, however, are not to be used to diagnose, prevent, or treat any disease—according to law in Western countries.

Patients are frequently known to use alternative medical interventions without informing their physicians. This is a dangerous practice. This book is designed to create open dialogue between patients and their physicians. Treatment decisions are a joint responsibility between patients and physicians.

If you like to read only medical information that you have a prearranged opinion about, then this book is not for you. I have been critical of some "conventional" medical approaches and some "alternative" medical interventions—in addition, I have on occasion endorsed both approaches. Failure on my part to embrace alternative or conventional medicine wholeheartedly could leave me "out in left field"—a lonely place that sees little action. Despite this obvious circumstance, I see the need to address the contention that has lead to a destructive dichotomy between alternative practice and orthodoxy, both of which figure strongly in medicine for the next millennium.

A lateral thinker on medicine (or science, religion, or politics) gathers few friends and even fewer brownie points. Lateral thoughts lead to new approaches and sometimes advances, but just as often they can be naïve proposals, though made in good faith, and they can readily evoke hostility from "hidebound" thinkers. As I like to say, "The individual who puts his head above the pulpit is likely to get hit with the Bible."

Some healthcare professionals read books as though they are gospel, with the sole intention of passing tests for higher education. This educational approach does not necessarily result in medical education. Selection processes for medical school have become automatically linked to academic performance—grades. No wonder we are struggling with attempts to blend old and new medicine and alternative and orthodox thinking.

Stephen Holt, M.D., FRCP(C), MRCP(UK), FACG, FACN, FACP

CHAPTER ONE

GETTING TO
KNOW THE
EMOTIONAL GUT

THE TWO PRIME PLEASURES OF LIFE

The acts of swallowing and defecating are regarded as the first two phases of childhood development, ingrained in Freudian theory. Philosophers and even politicians speak of the two prime pleasures, including the great British Prime Minister Winston Churchill, who was graphic in his descriptions of the gratification that can be achieved by swallowing and moving the bowels.

Sigmund Freud proposed his revolutionary theories at a time when few people would listen. In his theories, the two major phases in early life constitute the "oral" and "anal" stages of childhood development. It is believed by some that problems or "fixations" during the oral or anal stage of development of a child can create a legacy of medical and psychosocial problems throughout adult life. Many people subscribe to Freud's notions. Some believe that the mind and body are even more closely related.

Humankind has always seen regularity of bowel action as a sign of health. Who was lucky enough to have a grandma that did not browbeat every family member about a daily visit to the bowl? The obsession with moving bowels has enjoyed more periods of renaissance than any other physiological function. So important was the act of purging the bowel in healthcare that it became the primary therapeutic (treatment) intervention for almost every disease in Western medicine between the mid-seventeenth century and the early part of the twentieth century. The kings and queens of nations in the eighteenth and nineteenth centuries reveled in the delights of high colonic washouts, and physicians of the time carried a good "dose of salts" in their little black bags.

As we begin to better understand the negative health effects of stasis in the bowels, there has been a modern-day reactivation of interest in colon cleansing, sometimes referred to as an integral part of "total body detoxification." This rediscovered activity could make more sense than we may have hitherto supposed throughout the twentieth century, as we begin to understand the delicate balance between gut function, its contents, and general health. The gut has a host of friendly and unfriendly microorganisms (bacteria and yeasts), and it has transient contents of good and bad chemical compounds, or other components of the diet.

View the alimentary tract as a well-orchestrated organ that lives in harmony with its contents such as food, body secretions and bacteria. Its ecology includes the walls and surfaces of the guts. We know that life is obliterated by major changes in climate or the occurrence of disease. The balance of many factors in the guts determines healthy digestive function. We shall explore some of the conventional and alternative body of opinions about gut function, each of which can be sometimes quite nebulous.

EMOTIONAL GUTS

The importance of mind/body relationships has been popularized by the writings of "alternative" healers such as Deepak Chopra, M.D., and Andrew Weil, M.D. These authors present concepts of "Ageless Body, Timeless Mind" and "Spontaneous Healing," in their respective best-selling books. The alimentary tract and central nervous system are inextricably linked such that timeless stress can cause endless bellyache, and vice versa.

It is perfectly okay to give the guts an identity that can be expressed in terms of the moods of sadness and gladness. The balanced gut that receives good input will be glad if it is at peace with the mind and peaceful within itself. The sad gut is often a mere extension of a sad mind that is troubled by stress, anxiety, depression, adverse cultural influences, repressed conflicts, and other factors that are unrelated to the presence of readily identifiable disease. I want to reduce the inappropriate level of importance that is placed on a medical label (diagnosis) when the label falls far short of defining the disease or characterizing it in a useful manner.

The idea that guts can be glad or sad may seem curious. This concept is tenable in the face of the knowledge that the mind exerts control over the guts and the guts can often control the mind. This concept of a two-way street has been superseded by concepts of unity of function, for example, the "bodymind" or "mindbody." In fact, the mind and gut often function together (the mindgut) and the concept is even extended by the knowledge that the gut has its own brain (or many little brains). Implicit in the understanding of this situation is the fact that relations and connections between the brain (central nervous system) and the alimentary tract are very strong. So strong is this link that both physicians and lay people often talk about the "mind-gut interaction." The mind-gut interaction is so much a part of everyday life that we often forget this obvious link. If one feels emotion, one may inevitably have a reaction somewhere in the guts. We have all heard statements like: "My 'gut reaction' is to do it." Day-to-day living is accompanied by many "gut-wrenching" experiences. These are true "gut feelings."

THE CONCEPT OF "FUNCTIONAL"

Serious diseases (sometimes called organic disorders) of the alimentary tract must fit prominently into our thinking because colon cancer and inflammatory bowel disease are unfortunately common and increasing health problems. However, the most common disorders of the alimentary tract are not organic (disease related) in nature, but functional, such as functional bowel disease, functional dyspepsia, and the several functional disorders known as irritable bowel syndrome (we know that medicine is in trouble when multiple names are applied to the same thing).

While we cannot lose sight of the common occurrence of disease (organic disorders) in the gastrointestinal tract, it is important to reiterate that the majority of the disturbances in digestive function are not associated with organic disorders. Many gut disorders are examples of an imbalance in the mind-gut interaction, making them functional in nature. Unfortunately, some physicians, as well as sufferers, may not understand the mind-body link or its unity of function.

Table 1.1: A summary of the main functional gut disorders—not all-inclusive.

Region of Alimentary Tract	Disorder	Comment
Mouth	Bruxism	Teeth grinding usually in sleep associated with temporomandibular joint dysfunction.
	Rumination	Food regurgitated and rechewed is usually a sign of serious psychiatric problems—other tics.
Esophagus	Globus sensation	A lump in the throat sensation common in anxiety.
	Functional chest pain	Midline chest pain without anatomic cause often atypical for heart disease.
	Functional heartburn	Burning sensation, often behind breastbone in absence of detectable acid reflux.
	Functional dysphagia	Difficulty in swallowing without organic cause.
Gastroduodenum	Aerophagia	Swallowing air and belching.
	Nonulcer dyspepsia	Upper abdominal pain in the absence of organic cause that can be "ulcer-like" or atypical, including causes due to abnormal movements of stomach and duodenum.
Gallbladder	Motility upsets	Sphincter of Oddi dysfunction, etc.
Small Intestines	Irritable Bowel Syndrome	Altered bowel habit, abdominal pain.
Large Intestines	Irritable Bowel Syndrome	Diarrhea or constipation with or without excessive mucus, often aggravated by stress, pain, and altered bowel function.
Anus	Pelvic floor dysfunction	Anismus (obstructed defecation, anal sensations, others, e.g.,proctalgia fugax.

So far we have avoided the endless list of medical labels (diagnoses) that are attached to functional gastrointestinal complaints. I am referring to disorders that are not explained in terms of the presence of structural changes or disease of tissues in the gut, such as cancer or inflammation, which would be called organic disorders. When considering the label of *functional gastrointestinal disease*, the healer or diagnostician is often placed in the position where he or she must make a "diagnosis of exclusion," which is to say that the diagnosis of functional problems in the gut is often made by first excluding the possibility of organic problems. Table 1.1 gives a list of functional disorders of the gastrointestinal tract.

Diagnostic labels appease physicians and are necessary for them to select appropriate therapy and understand outcomes. Unfortunately, the appeasement of the physician with a label sometimes may not help the physician select therapy. Labels can sometimes stand in the way of appropriate interventions, the questioning of the physician by the patient, or good participation between physician and patient in the healing process, and this is wrong. However, some of these labels (diagnoses) are diagnostic dustbins that get filled with "diagnoses of the destitute."

It is clear that a diagnosis helps a patient only if it results in the selection of an effective treatment or intervention. As we shall learn in this book, not only are functional disorders of the digestive tract the most difficult to diagnose, they are often difficult to treat. These disorders are treated frequently by specialists with "refined" technical skills. This skill level is sometimes not portable or relevant to the need for the holistic care (treating the mind and body as a whole) that is required by the sufferer of functional gut disorders.

A BAD EMOTION OR A BAD MEAL?

The following dialogue is designed to help take the mystique out of one of the most common causes of human discomfort, namely, common digestive upset (the moaning, groaning, or grumbling of the stomach or guts). There are so many medical terms to describe this disturbance of mind-gut interaction that the situation becomes confusing for physicians, let alone patients! When it occurs in the absence of significant structural changes or diseases of the digestive tract, "grumbling guts" is due to an upset in the balance of digestive function, which is created by problems in one of three areas: the mind (a bad emotion), the gut (disturbed physiology), or by something taken into the body that upsets the balance between the two (or combinations of upset).

My feeling is that a bad emotion generally hangs around longer than a bad meal. There's a vast array of psychosocial factors that are associated with gut grumbling. Psychosocial factors refer to the mind, the environment, what we see, what occurs, what we feel, and how we react. People with irritable guts can sometimes have a psychological imbalance. This imbalance may not be obvious or it can be quite overt. At one end of the spectrum are individuals with a higher prevalence of neurosis, depression, and even suicide. In later parts of this book, we will examine in some detail this spectrum of the mind as it plays a causal role in the irritable gut.

On the other end of the spectrum are those with poor eating habits, gluttony, food allergy or intolerance, and starvation, which all have a major impact on the function of the guts. Logic dictates that a bad meal will produce only a transient upset—but if we keep dishing ourselves up bad meals, we can expect a long-term (chronic) complaint from the alimentary tract. The idea of the "bad meal" deserves some attention. On the one hand, it may be obvious when someone overeats, overdrinks or engages in dietary indiscretion. On the other hand, what may unwittingly be considered a good meal by an individual with lactose intolerance (inability to digest the milk sugar lactose) may actually be a bad meal that upsets the gut, for example. These individuals can fail to recognize that the colic, gas, and diarrhea are being induced by the sugar lactose (found in dairy products). It is amazing how commonly these simple factors are overlooked as causes of disabling gut symptoms.

"ALL GUTS ARE IRRITABLE"

Any part of the body can be irritated by influences from outside or inside the body. The guts are perhaps unique in their ability to be irritated from within by virtue of their highly intricate nerve supply. This highly developed network of nerves in the gut connects the alimentary tract to the master regulators, the brain, and ultimately the mind. The amount of nervous tissue found in the guts is staggering and has been calculated by researchers to be equivalent to the amount of nerve fibers and connections found in the entire spinal cord of the central nervous system. Nerve functions are so well developed in the gastrointestinal tract that it has been described as being the "second brain" of the body in a recent book by Michael D. Gershon, M.D.

The nervous connections between the brain and the gut are a vast network of nerve fibers of varying types that can respond to sensations in the gut, cause movements in the guts (motility), stop movement in the guts (hypomotility), or cause disorders of the movements of the guts (dysmotility). Since the guts are the receptacle of everything that passes our lips, there are many possible responses from the guts depending upon signals they receive or messages they send to the brain or create among their own network of nervous tissue.

It is not just nerve connections that affect the activity of the guts. The alimentary tract is regulated by a complex set of signals given by hormones that are released from many sites in the body, especially from the gastrointestinal tract itself. These hormones (chemicals or transmitter compounds) have been referred to by Dr. Candace B. Pert, Ph.D., as examples of the "Molecules of Emotion" in a book by the same title. Thus, our understanding of the workings of the gastrointestinal tract involve an understanding of nervous (nerves) and hormonal (hormones) control and these are conveniently lumped together in the complexities of the "neurohormonal" control of the guts—a function of our molecules of emotion.

IT WORKS BOTH WAYS

Two big words further explain the complexities of mind-body interactions. The first word, *psychosomatic*, means that a disorder of the mind (psycho) is often manifest in a disorder in the body (somatic). The second word, *somatopsychic* implies that a disorder in the body (somatic) may greatly impact the mind (psycho). Nowhere is this two-way street more apparent than in the coordinated responses of the alimentary tract and the brain.

That it works both ways between the guts and the brain is obvious in many circumstances. There is a vicious cycle that can be created for many individuals with gut disorders affecting the mind: More bellyache causes more stress and more stress causes more bellyache. As simple as this may seem, this is the reasoning that will contribute to a solution for common discomforts of the guts that may impact our quality of life.

Incidentally, the irritable gut has its own spectrum of disorders that can affect any part of the alimentary tract, from the mouth to the anus. The classic example of the irritable gut is the irritable bowel syndrome (IBS) that affects mainly the intestines, especially the colon. More simply stated, people with irritable bowels tend to have irritable stomachs or irritable gullets, etc.

THE TIP OF THE ICEBERG

The plot thickens when we have to acknowledge that there are events in the mind that might require expert attention from the mind doctor (psychiatrist) or events in the bowel that confront the doctor who deals with the gut (gastroenterologist). It is unfortunate that gastroenterologists are not often distinguished by their knowledge of psychological or social issues and few psychiatrists think about the anatomy of the guts! Neither of these valuable healthcare professionals can be blamed, but the winning manager of gut disease discounts neither the mind nor the body.

Several gastroenterologists have referred to the "iceberg" phenomenon in several gut disorders. The individuals with irritable guts that seek medical attention for severe and persistent grumbling are only the tip of the iceberg. The vast majority of suffering occurs below the visible level of the iceberg of grumbling guts; where many people have mild or moderate intermittent complaints in the abdomen.

Unfortunately, only the tip of the iceberg gets the attention of medicine. Those who suffer in silence are not just a forgotten few. They constitute a significant proportion of the population that cannot be accurately quantified. We know they exist because they gobble up billions of dollars of over-the-counter (OTC) drugs and digestive aids. Unfortunately, we have become increasingly aware that many medicines (drugs), including those used for digestive disorders, may cause a perverse array of side effects—including common side effects on the guts!

A SHOCKING STORY

I can relate a story that caused tragic problems. I was a bystander, a junior doctor, at the time. A senior academic of a major University in England, himself a physician, attended a senior gastroenterologist with "troublesome" bowels and hemorrhoids. This academic, at his own insistence, was reassured (a dangerous byproduct of "physician heal thyself!") and his hemorrhoids were removed surgically by an experienced, senior surgeon. Six months later, he returned to his surgeon and gastroenterologist with stubborn bowel trouble. The bowel problems proved to be due to colon cancer that had been overlooked! If this can happen among physicians, what can happen to the would-be self-healer or self-medicator?

Misdiagnosis or a delay in diagnosis can occur with many types of gastrointestinal disease. In many cases there are warning signs but the diagnosis is missed. On frequent occasions an individual will want to explain their symptoms in simple terms and deny or rationalize their ill health. Many people deal with the threat of ill health by an attempt to minimize its significance. This can be very dangerous and, at best, it results in delayed diagnosis. In 1998, several companies that issue malpractice insurance to physicians produced warnings to doctors about the escalating numbers of lawsuits that are being filed for the delayed diagnosis of colon cancer. Unfortunately, delayed diagnosis often means poor prognosis (outcome), especially in the case of cancer of the guts. Early diagnosis of gastrointestinal cancer really makes a difference in survival. Despite this circumstance, gastroenterologists have had to lobby and fight with the healthcare system in recent times to cover the cost of a decent service for early detection of colon cancer.

RED FLAGS!

In teaching documents for physicians, the American Gastro-enterological Association mentions "red flag" symptoms. The characteristics of these symptoms are such that they tend to be associated with severe diseases and they should precipitate a visit to a doctor. Therefore, a word of caution is required. It is not necessarily safe to conclude that symptoms originating in the alimentary system are of a functional (nonorganic, nondisease) origin. There has to be a balance in an individual's approach to self-diagnosis or attempts to self-medicate. In cases of even slight doubt about the origin of symptoms, an individual should seek medical advice. Table 1.2 should give you cues to discuss your digestive problems with a medical practitioner.

Table 1.2: Some symptoms, signs and findings that signal the likelihood of serious gut disease.

The "would be" self-diagnostician or healer must recognize these "red flags." This table is based in part on "Red Flags" listed in Unit 13 of the American Gastroenterological Association Clinical Teaching Project.

CONDITION	COMMENT
Difficulty in swallowing	Common first symptom of esophageal cancer in mature individuals.
Persistent, new abdominal pain	Anyone's guess! Can range from functional, to ulcer, to inflammation, to blockage, to cancer causes.
Family history of bowel cancer, inflammation, or polyps	Be aware that diseases run in families.
Blood in the stool or vomit	Cancers and ulcers bleed commonly, as well as hemorrhoids.
Change in digestive function in people over the age of 40 years	Most cancers in the gastrointestinal tract occur with advancing age.
Other general body upset	Weight loss, fever, joint disease added to grumbling guts often spells organic disease.

AGE AS A RISK FACTOR

In general, it is not acceptable to readily assume that persistent gastrointestinal upset in individuals over the age of forty years is due to functional disease. The occurrence of cancer of the digestive system rises with age in general. Everyone with a significant change of bowel habit who is over the age of forty years should be considered to be at risk of having colon cancer. Individuals with a family history of colon cancer, inflammatory bowel disease, (Crohn's disease or ulcerative colitis), or certain types of colon polyps are an at-risk group. There are several symptoms, including weight loss or disturbed sleep from gastrointestinal upset, that fall into the red-flag category (Table 1.2).

SELF-DIAGNOSIS IS
A RISKY BUSINESS

It is not possible to turn a layperson into an expert in self-diagnosis, and the whole concept of self-medication has worried the medical profession for years. There is a new self-reliance among individuals who'd like to involve themselves in their own medical therapy and this should be welcomed, as long as it results in prudent actions. The key issue that emerges in public health for the next millennium is consumer education. Education must occur from valid information sources. Bias in advertising and marketing of ethical drugs, OTC medications, and dietary supplements is rampant. A lot of highly effective remedies and drugs to suppress common gastrointestinal symptoms (like nausea, diarrhea, and heartburn) have emerged as OTC drugs or products. This presents problems in the face of the rising incidence of certain killer diseases such as colon cancer, where the person with early symptoms of cancer may delay a visit to the doctor in favor of self-medicating.

New cases of colon cancer will occur in about 140,000 Americans this year and many will present with altered bowel habit. Unfortunately, many OTC medicines (and dietary supplements) may *temporarily* improve altered bowel habits in patients with colon cancer (as they do in benign cases of altered bowel habit) and delayed diagnosis can result.

This is very alarming because we know that the prognosis from colon cancer is highly related to early diagnosis, frequently resulting in a cure (better than ten-year survival) in many cases.

These points are belabored because attention must be drawn to the red-flag symptoms of gastrointestinal disease. Delayed or misdiagnosis of gastrointestinal disease must be avoided where possible. Certain symptoms cannot be cast off as being of functional origin (nondisease) without careful evaluation (Table 1.2).

HAS MODERN MEDICINE IGNORED NATURE'S ROLE?

Conventional medicine has a great deal to offer and it is not my intention to represent alternative or complementary medicine as always the primary medical intervention of choice. Your doctor is acting in your best interests. I hope that he or she may show a willingness to discuss or even recommend natural therapies that form some of the contents of this book. The physician of the next millennium will select from all options, choose the best, and hopefully win the war against disease. This is what I have termed pluralistic medicine. However, your doctor may not have been exposed to some of the concepts or interventions discussed in this book, and he or she probably works in a practice or institutional system that may not even recognize the legitimacy of alternative healing.

Modern medicine is well equipped to deal with the intricacies of reengineering the gut by surgery or modifying its function by powerful synthetic drugs (e.g., suppressing secretions of stomach acid). I am not minimizing the importance of this approach for some diseases, which require these interventions. However, this focus of conventional medicine is generally applied in the treatment of advanced or well-delineated disease. This focus does not always serve the needs of millions of people who walk around with grumbling guts. These grumbles are of varying severity, often caused by imbalances in the interactions between the mind (CNS or gutmind) and the alimentary system.

I believe an important switch in thought is required as we recognize that the effects of mind-body interactions on the guts are often ignored. However, the mind-gut interaction is not the whole story of functional disease, in my opinion. It is important to realize that modern medicine may not have examined the disturbance of the "balance of nature" as a cause of many common diseases that have been labeled functional. For example, the role of the flora of the guts (microorganisms that normally live in the guts) in the maintenance of digestive health is recognized to be of great importance, but it receives little attention in conventional medicine as a focus of treatment for digestive upset or other disease states. There are many other examples where nature's balance is important in maintaining digestive health. These are key areas where alternative medicine has major roles to play.

THE NEW SELF-RELIANCE FOR THE NATURAL OPTION

The modern patient has knowledge and a new self-reliance to engage in his or her own healthcare decisions. I reiterate that patients are exhibiting a tendency to self-diagnose, self-medicate, and question or even "pester" their physician, especially about remedies of natural origin. The problem is that patients are questioning their physicians about natural remedies that are not part of the repertoire of conventional medicine. So great is the thirst for consumer information about natural remedies that a plethora of books on natural health care has invaded every bookstore in the realm.

I stress that I am acutely aware of the restraints that my colleagues in conventional medical practice face when they venture into remedies of natural origin. The "doctor watchers," including regulatory bodies and HMOs, will often clobber any physician who does not provide a treatment plan that matches a preconceived recipe for disease management. Practicing medicine by "disease state algorithms" (mandated recipes) may not be a bad idea if the limitation of the algorithm is appreciated. Unfortunately, many doctors are losing their ability to exercise their own discretion about treatment in the managed-care environment. Pressured by patients to provide natural therapies, the managed-care physician is in a Catch-22 situation.

I have known patients with gastrointestinal disease who require only one visit for a certain diagnosis, while other patients have required multiple visits and multiple testing for the same diagnosis. I believe that managed care and cost containment in healthcare is stripping the "art" out of the practice of medicine. This very situation prevents alternative practices that may afford a solution to patients who are stuck in a revolving door of no relief. Unfortunately, some conventional medical practitioners still show a complete unwilling-ness to address their patients' newfound needs and demands con-cerning natural healthcare. Some intransigent practitioners of con-ventional medicine will soon become devoid of patients unless they exert a new level of tolerance to alternative healing. Dr. Robert C. Atkins, M.D., a famous alternative thinking physician, has indicated that if a doctor will not discuss natural therapies with his or her patients these days, then the patient will "vote with their feet."

A ROUGH LESSON

We must recognize that the current problems we face in the direction of healthcare have been precipitated to a major degree by the patient's disenchantment with many conventional medical interven-tions. A good example in recent history is the early treatment pro-grams used to cure peptic ulcers between the 1940s and the 1960s. Over this twenty-year period, people with ulcer disease were assault-ed with tubes that were stuck through their nose into their stomach to remove acid or to deliver nauseating amounts of milk products. This treatment was often worse than the disease!

We may be fooling ourselves if we try to convince ourselves that we have universally pleasant, conventional treatments these days. Some of the earlier treatment combinations proposed in the 1980s to eradi-cate the bacterium *Helicobacter pylori* (the principal cause of peptic ulcer) involved the consumption of nauseating amounts of bismuth salts together with variable cocktails of antibiotics or antimicrobials. These treatments could often cause gut pain and rampant diarrhea. Having tried this regime myself to cure my own dyspepsia, I can attest to complete disenchantment. Fortunately, treatment has improved in the 1990s—but the *Helicobacter* is showing signs of resistance to antibi-otics. Nature often challenges modern medical interventions.

MIRACLE HERBS?

There are herbs on the horizon that may deal with certain illnesses that do not respond to conventional drug therapy. Even if herbs serve only the purpose of making the patient feel better with safety and tolerance, then there is some value. I would go further and state that I am aware of herbal compounds that seem to act in an additive manner with synthetic antiviral drugs, anti-inflammatory drugs and anti-cancer drugs. I am convinced that one day the medical profession will use this knowledge increasingly in the fight against chronic disorders and viral diseases that threaten entire communities in certain countries. Examples of these viral diseases are Hepatitis B and C virus infection and the scourge of AIDS (HIV infection).

GASTROQUACKERY

The term *gastroquackery* was coined by Dr. Stephen Barrett, M.D., an eminent psychiatrist from Pennsylvania who has contributed greatly to uncovering health schemes and scams. I believe that peer review is extremely important in medicine, but polar opinions in medicine create confrontations. To use the word *quackery* is to imply that a healthcare giver knowingly applies an ineffective form of treatment. The motive of personal gain is also often implied with this term.

Scoundrels and scalawags exist in all professions, but there is a tendency to believe that practitioners of alternative medicine are overrepresented by such miscreants. While an opinion prevails that alternative therapies have not withstood or been subjected to the kind of rigorous scientific scrutiny that may have been applied to many conventional approaches, there is a major problem with a lack of economic, political, and professional incentives to study alternative therapies or remedies of natural origin.

A number of alternative and complementary therapies have been labeled as examples of gastroquackery (Table 1.3). Though some of these therapies legitimately have limitations or drawbacks, in many circumstances they have not been investigated in detail. I intend to discuss a number of these issues in this book. I am convinced that some of these interventions deserve much further study, especially in the face of common failures of some conventional medical treatments for diseases of the gut. After all, if existing therapies worked consistently, there would be no need to seek an alternative. I support Dr. Barrett in his work and feel that much more research is required before all aspects of alternative medicine can be embraced. Nevertheless, conventional and alternative medicine are not perfect treatment domains. Each has something to offer when applied with a pluralistic approach.

I believe that medicine in the twenty-first century will be more about healthcare than care of the sick. Care of the diseased person in

Table 1.3: Some examples of alternative medicine practices labeled by some as quackery.

INTERVENTION	COMMENT
Purging for health	Controversy exists about the phenomenon of autointoxication due to stasis and fermentation of food and associated with a lack of regular bowel habit. Insufficient contemporary studies. Body detoxification is a very popular practice with a real need for outcome research.
Special food combinations	Many nonsensical ideas exist about food-food interactions but food selection and health is an exploding field with great promise. The idea of a diet for a certain genetic makeup lacks scientific proof—as yet!
Probiotic therapy	Encouraging the colonization of the bowel with friendly microorganisms is a very underexplored therapy for a variety of diseases.
Remedies of natural origin	Specific nutrients, botanicals, and herbs are grossly underexplored in modern medicine.
Mind-body medicine	Probably the most important, underexplored option to explain the cause of and manage the expressions of functional gut disease.

modern medicine involves the use of chemicals (drugs), and corrective surgical "cures" of variable efficacy. Healthcare may be more ideal in some circumstances with the addition of more natural approaches that are applied in a preventive manner with an emphasis on gentle and holistic care.

THE SOLUTION AT HAND

I believe that there should be a preoccupation with what works rather than what is more palatable to a prevailing body of opinion. Remember, people were once tortured because they said that the earth revolves around the sun. The quest for conciliation in medicine has led to concepts of integrated medicine. I reject this term somewhat, because it serves to foster the notion of a dichotomy of medical thought and opinion. The dichotomy of opinion in medicine is probably one day going to be characterized as equally as pernicious as any form of discrimination.

The new millennium will bring pluralistic medicine. I have selected this term because I believe it encompasses the idea that only what works and what is most sensible should be applied. Pluralistic medicine implies that a healthcare giver will take the trouble to become enlightened in modern medicine and be willing to select from behavioral medicine and traditional or ancient medical systems that may afford relief to humankind. The body needs some help to heal itself and the idea of attacking a disease without consideration for the entire body is an example of misguided modern science. We are at oneness with our universe—the concept of Gaia.

Gaia may elicit a snigger from the hide-bound medical practitioner, but the theory of being in balance with nature is the fundamental basis of medicine, as practiced from the time of Hippocrates. The idea of global health is found in ancient medical disciplines, such as Ayurveda and traditional Chinese medicine. If one could balance the mind and the gut and restore balance within the gut, functional gastrointestinal disease might be eradicated. Table 1.4 depicts a possible future for medicine that moves from a conventional to a pluralistic approach in which global initiatives are taken.

Table 1.4: Pluralistic medicine and the future.

Pluralistic medicine involves a selection of therapies from all types of medical disciplines and involves more global perspectives in medicine. The idea involves the use of any medical intervention that is safe, effective, and cost-beneficial. The model moves away from care of the sick alone to the domain of wellness. Medicine can no longer be viewed as developing by automatic progression of existing scientific attitudes or knowledge.

PLURALISTIC MEDICINE	CONVENTIONAL MEDICINE
Global	Typically Western
Natural approaches integrated	Physicianic interventions—drugs or surgery
Nutrition of primary importance	Nutrition of secondary importance
Healing orientated	Disease orientated
Body and mind	Physical focus
Blends of synthetic and natural Treatments	Synthetic, single drugs
Sympathetic to belief	Ignores belief systems
Changing traditions	Fixed traditions

CHAPTER SUMMARY

The concepts of functional digestive disease are important to grasp for the new movement of self-diagnosing and self-treating healthcare consumers. Alternative medicine wars with conventional medicine and vice versa. The "winning" of this kind of silly war will result at best in a Pyrrhic victory. Functional gut disorders are among the most common reasons for people to seek medication. New concepts in holistic healthcare recognize the unity of body function. This approach to medicine is somewhat contrary to the idea of "medical specialties" where physicians may direct their attention to a single body system.

Viewing the gastrointestinal tract with its own mind and consideration of its inextricable linkage in the bodymind may be an approach with significant merit, or at least promise, to impact common gut disturbances. Advances in medicine have been viewed as a chronological sequence of automatic progress of current scientific thought and opinion. This model should be challenged.

CHAPTER TWO

WHAT THE GASTROENTEROLOGIST DOES ALL DAY: AN OVERVIEW

HIGH NOON IN ROME

In this book, I am placing specific emphasis on disorders that are not due to readily identifiable diseases or abnormalities of the structure of the guts (see Table 1.1). I propose to walk through the digestive system from mouth to anus and concentrate on discussions about functional problems. I believe that disorders of the guts, not due to organic disease (such as inflammation and cancer), are prime targets for alternative or complementary medical interventions.

In 1990, a group of expert physicians met in Rome, Italy, to discuss and define the many functional disorders of the gastrointestinal tract. (Members of this group must have experienced more than a hiccup or belch from the spicy Italian pasta!) There were several working teams comprised mainly of gastroenterologists, who drew up a general definition of functional gastrointestinal disorders. In brief, this definition (Table 1.1) implied that functional disorders of the alimentary tract occurred with many symptoms that were chronic (long lasting) or recurrent and were not explained by structural disease in the gastrointestinal tract.

The defined disorders were split into their occurrences by anatomic regions, those affecting the esophagus, stomach and/or duodenum (gastroduodenum), biliary tract (gall bladder and bile ducts), bowel (small and large intestines), or the anus and/or rectum (anorectum). However, this ground breaking meeting of the minds did not cover all of the common conditions of the alimentary tract that may bother an individual on a frequent basis. They especially seem to have forgotten the mouth, except for "rumination" where food is regurgitated back into the mouth. They defined the entities that I have referred to as functional gastrointestinal disorders, irritable guts, and sad guts. I would add lip biting, teeth grinding, and other oral tics to this band of disorders, as I sit here and scratch my head in wonder as to why they were left out!

WHAT THE GASTROENTEROLOGIST DOES ALL DAY

The daily routine of the practicing gastroenterologist was examined by Dr. T. Switz in 1976 and published in the prestigious journal Gastroenterology under the title "What the Gastroenterologist Does All Day." Dr. Switz's study drew attention to the fact that functional bowel disease was the most common diagnosis made by a gastroenterologist in routine practice. The same thing is true today, but one could question whether or not these patients would be better handled at earlier levels of medical care such as primary care practice.

I believe that the general medical practitioner may be able to offer a more rounded management approach to a heterogeneous (varied) disorder such as functional gastrointestinal upset. Functional gut disorders are often deeply rooted in psychosocial issues and imbalance of the guts. I do not wish to deny my fellow gastroenterologists their "bread and butter," but several studies of clinical outcomes in patients with functional digestive diseases have not shown overwhelming success, even when managed by the specialist. It is true that no convincing studies have been reported in the scientific literature that show that alternative medicine fares better than conventional medicine in the treatment of functional gastrointestinal disorders. The many studies, however, that show failures of conventional medicine in functional diseases makes holistic healthcare seem an attractive option.

A LABEL BY EXCLUSION

The folly of the diagnosis of functional bowel disease by a process of exclusion is described in a very eloquent and insightful manner by Dr. Joseph P. Glaser, M.D., and Dr. George Engel, M.D., in their lead, review article in *Clinics in Gastroenterology* (Vol. 6, No. 3, September 1977), titled "Psychodynamics, Psychopathology, and Gastrointestinal Symptomatology." These doctors state: "The traditional principle, 'rule out the organic before considering the psychosocial,' is scientifically unsound, economically extravagant, and often damaging to the patient as well."

Modern medicine, driven by fear of litigation in many circumstances, cannot do enough to cover its own tail. It is easy to be critical of the doctor who plays it safe by doing a comprehensive set of medical tests to exclude the organic disease processes. There are a number of issues raised in these circumstances. The doctor with the attention to detail is not necessarily the doctor who is driven by avarice to make money. However, managed care and the "cost containment" mentality react against a physician's inclination to intensive medical testing, even when it is focused and planned. Now it is possible to understand one reason why irritable bowel syndrome (IBS) is a common disorder among medical practitioners themselves!

HOW THE BEARER OF FUNCTIONAL GUT DISORDERS IS SO OFTEN MISTREATED

The individual with functional gastrointestinal disorder is ubiquitous in our society. Many suffer in silence, many shop for self-cures, and some shop until they drop at the many available medical treatment facilities. The prevalence or incidence (occurrence) of functional gastrointestinal disease defies accurate definition. It is estimated that up to 25 million Americans may have significant, recurrent problems with functional abdominal complaints. Estimates of its occurrence among patients who attend doctors' offices imply that IBS is the most common diagnosis among all gastrointestinal complaints. It occupies more than 10 percent of all practice time for a primary care practitioner and more than 40 percent of the practice time of a gastroenterologist.

A person with IBS who has been exposed to a gastroenterology practice will invariably have been subjected to the "negative" endoscopic examination, often of both the upper and lower digestive tract, with or without the expensive exposure to contrast type of x-rays, such as the barium meal or barium enema. Negative endoscopy means that the test reveals no diagnosis of organic disease, but it often provides a negative experience. I can speak from personal experience. When I went through these tests for my own health or research projects, it was not fun!

One may ask why a person with IBS, which apparently affects the lower gastrointestinal tract, would be so consistently subjected to an examination of both the upper and the lower digestive tract. The answer rests in the knowledge that the pain of IBS is felt in the upper abdomen in 33 percent of all cases. Some studies show that in more than one half of cases, the individual with IBS has other upper abdominal symptoms, with or without lower abdominal complaints. Those findings underscore the notion of universal, permeating irritability of the entire alimentary canal.

The gastrointestinal tract is relatively inaccessible, and testing often involves invasive testing such as the insertion of a lighted tube into the bowel or upper digestive tract (endoscopy). This practice of endoscopy is sometimes unpleasant, but it is usually safe. However, sometimes an iatrogenic (healthcare induced) problem can occur during endoscopy of the guts, as a result of a problem with anesthesia or, occasionally, perforation of the lower bowel.

The use of flexible sigmoidoscopy is very safe and it is one of the most important and effective means of making an early diagnosis of colon cancer. Everyone should know this, but brave gastroenterologists have had to fight with stubborn politicians and many insurance companies who do not want to pay for this important preventive, public health measure against colon cancer. In the test of flexible sigmoidoscopy, the inspection of the bowel is usually limited to the lower 60 cm of the colon. Sometimes the problem facing the healthcare giver is how far to go with testing or, sometimes, how often it should be done. It is recognized that the early stages of some diseases show little abnormality during early testing and there may be a need to confirm that serious disease has not evolved. This phenomenon of evolution of disease is seen sometimes in cases of the development of peptic ulcer, cancer, and inflammatory bowel disease.

THE SHRINE OF THE SYNTHETIC DRUG

As members of the baby-boomer generation at medical school in the 1960s, my colleagues and I were taught to worship at the shrine of the synthetic drug and respond to the promise of high technology. The fact is that over the past thirty years, many common diseases such as arthritis, cancer, and chronic inflammatory conditions remain resistant to conventional medical therapy. Nowhere is this failing of conventional medicine more apparent than in the treatment of functional disorders of the alimentary tract.

The drug-induced disappearance of heartburn that is coincidental with the inhibition of the reflux of acid from the stomach into the esophagus is often highly effective. This quick fix may give the individual with heartburn a newfound freedom to continue to engage in activity that normally makes reflux of acid into the esophagus worse. Relief of heartburn can reinforce overeating, dietary indiscretion, smoking, or drinking. This is an example of how the quick fix hampers recovery in the long term. If nobody experienced a hangover, I believe that there would be many more people with alcohol problems.

I am not antagonistic to the availability of safe and effective remedies such as OTC drugs, but they should be purveyed with much advice about their correct use. Not only are OTC drugs sold without enough educational material to permit their correct use by consumers, their sales are pushed sometimes by advertising that is misleading. I am often intrigued when young males admit, with anxiety, that they suffer from heartburn, which on further questioning only seems to occur after they consume a couple of six-packs of beer. Perhaps it is too obvious, but this kind of beverage induced heartburn responds very well to H_2-receptor antagonists! There is a big danger that an individual may rush to take the H_2-receptor antagonist without reducing his beer intake from twelve cans to three cans a day. I do not wish to change the dialogue to a sermon on lifestyle, but the art of self-watching has a lot to do with health maintenance.

Our global pharmacy has graduated to the availability of quick fixes as OTC (drugs), that have become available without the need for a prescription. Examples of these quick fixes (symptom relief) in the treatment of digestive disorders are Mylanta, Maalox, Rolaids, Tums, Zantac, Tagamet, Pepcid, ExLax, Beano, Lactaid, etc. Marketing research of OTC and prescription drugs seems to indicate that it is symptom relief that drives the sales of medications. Incidentally, evidence suggests that quick fixes drive the prescriptions of drugs by doctors. However, after a while the quick fix just won't satisfy the individual with a recurrent problem. The patient's inevitable disenchantment will drive him or her to look for alternative options that may help go to the root of the problem.

When I talk about natural therapies for functional gastrointestinal disease, I may not be armed with the double-blind, controlled, clinical trial to satisfy the scientists. I am armed, however, with an example of the failure of quick drug fixes for gastrointestinal complaints. Highly effective, safe, and efficacious acid-blocking drugs used to treat dyspepsia, peptic ulcer, and gastroesophageal reflux disease (GERD) have occupied coveted space in the *Guinness Book of World Records* as the best-selling drugs of all time—but more than half of the total use of these drugs has been for nonapproved indications, for which they may not be effective.

In many cases of ill health, especially functional bowel disease, the solution rests in a complex intervention that is often multifactorial and strongly related to the correction of adverse lifestyle and restoration of the balance of life. It is of great interest to note that the correction of adverse lifestyle is often the key to sustained relief of many common disorders.

ALL OF OUR HIGH TECHNOLOGY MAY NOT TRANSMIT RELIEF

One big problem area in the management of functional gastrointestinal disorders of the guts is the diagnosis and management of esophageal chest pain. Contractions in the gullet (esophagus) can cause chest pain that is indistinguishable from pain emanating from the heart (angina). The esophagus with functional problems can cause chest pain that is indistinguishable from a heart attack. Specialized gastroenterology clinics have facilities do special tests, such as pressure studies (manometry) or monitoring studies (pH testing), on the esophagus to define chest pain of esophageal origin. However, many patients with chest pain may undergo coronary artery angiography or other expensive and invasive tests of heart function. This occurs because of the important need to exclude heart disease as the source of the pain.

My colleagues and I have shown in one study that some patients with chest pain who undergo coronary arteriography (x-rays of the vessels supplying the heart) and have normal coronary arteries are reassured by cardiologists and rarely "followed up on." Many of these patients have esophageal problems or other causes of noncardiac chest pain. Despite this reassurance, they sometimes engage in the revolving-door phenomenon by repeatedly attending medical outpatient clinics or even emergency services without the prescription of correct interventions or the application of effective therapy. Studies show that patients who have chest pain due to functional disorders of the esophagus and have undergone specialist testing in gastroenterology facilities (in centers of excellence) may also enter the revolving-door phenomenon. Are the physicians at fault? The answer is an emphatic "no!" The condition of esophageal spasm (functional esophageal disease) is very difficult to treat by any conventional intervention. These situations and circumstances are examples where high technology unravels the medical problem or diagnosis but often makes little contribution to selecting a cure for the disorder, (which is difficult to cure).

CONVENTIONAL MEDICINE HEAVEN

For the bold, lateral thinker in medicine there is no place yet in "conventional medicine heaven." There are individuals who claim to have suffered brutal oppression in their attempt to change conventional medical thinking. Interested parties are referred to a book entitled *Dirty Medicine: Science, Big Business and the Assault on Natural*

Health Care by Martin J. Walker (Slingshot Publications, BM Box 8314, London WCIN 3XX, England, UK). This revealing book has been the focus of lawsuits, grief, ruined careers, and even fisticuffs in public. *Dirty Medicine* is a frightening account of big business (pharmaceutical corporations) making war on physicians who question their profits, the efficacy of their drugs, and their approaches to medicine.

I am a wholehearted supporter of the appropriate use of drug therapy in gastrointestinal disease and, like every other gastroenterologist, I have prescribed bushels of antiacid drugs. However, there is a large proportion of patients encountered in practice who have functional gastrointestinal disease that is not effectively managed by drugs. I am not critical of the pioneering research and importance to modern medicine of multinational pharmaceutical giants. However, it is a fact of life that there just aren't the same incentives to pursue the use of nonproprietary, natural therapies or to engage in alternative treatment research.

WHY YOU MIGHT CONSIDER ALTERNATIVE OPTIONS

Alternative and complementary medical practices are holistic and rely on systems of treatment. These systems involve getting to know patients, introducing patients to belief systems or reinforcing patients' own beliefs, and applying specific interventions based on combinations of physical, psychological, botanical, or herbal interventions.

I have referred often to blending the conventional with the alternative in medicine but disciplines of medicine that are labeled as alternative in Western society are already blends of multiple disciplines. There are many examples of old medical disciplines that are treatment systems. Ayurvedic medicine uses herbs and botanicals, but their use does not occur in isolation of belief systems, behavioral therapy, and the consideration of the spiritual dimensions of Ayurveda. The same can be said about traditional Chinese medicine, homeopathy, and even chiropractic or osteopathic medicine.

Pluralistic medicine involves a blurring of the boundaries between conventional and alternative medical options. Alternative medicine can complement or sometimes replace conventional medicine, and vice versa. Furthermore, alternative and conventional medicine may be synergistic (better when applied together). I believe that we shall consider in more detail the blurring medical boundaries in the present millennium.

Herbal preparations are often used as natural remedies and are derived from a variety of sources including whole plants or specific segments of a plant such as the root, stem, flowers, leaves, or seeds. There are no strict definitions of herbal agents versus botanical agents, that are tenable in the contemporary practices of alternative or complementary medicine. Many botanicals are referred to as herbs and vice versa. There have been increasing attempts in Western society to standardize herbal products so that they can be given in formats that produce a reasonably consistent biological effect. Herbal products are not essential nutrients, and they do not have recommended dietary allowances (RDA). Therefore, dosages of herbs are often a "best guess" unless a standardized herbal extract is used. Even standardization of an herbal extract does not always permit accurate dosing information to be given because dose response studies have not been performed in many cases.

It is important to realize that some herbs are quite safe in small doses but quite toxic when given in larger doses. Although herbs are of natural origin, it does not necessarily mean that they are safe. Practitioners of herbal medicine have been criticized for recommending generally that all herbal products used in treatment are safe. However, many practitioners of herbal medicine behave responsibly in their attitude to the safety issues that surround the use of herbal agents. In general terms, herbal medicine is to be avoided in pregnancy and childhood because there is still relatively little information about its safety in these circumstances. The abortifacient (abortion inducing) or teratogenic (growth deforming) or carcinogenic (cancer causing) potential of some herbals and botanicals should not be underestimated.

Much of the alleged benefit of herbal compounds is based on anecdotal reports of success, often transmitted over long periods of time. In fact, some commonly used herbs in medical systems such as Inca medicines, Ayurvedic medicine, and traditional Chinese medicine are used as a result of information that has been passed down verbally from generation to generation. Perhaps the best-documented materia medica in history is that of traditional Chinese medicine. In contemporary writings about herbal medicine, the scientific support for a statement of a potential health benefit is often not clear.

THE USE OF DIETARY SUPPLEMENTS AND THE PRACTICE OF PURGING

Sometimes the gastrointestinal tract is the focus of many alternative therapies, including purgation, detoxification, and the construction of outlandish theories to explain the causation of a variety of diseases. Sometimes the phenomena described in theories of alternative medicine are real occurrences, but these occurrences may sometimes form the basis of illogical ideas or practices. An example of this is the increasing preoccupation with the leaky gut syndrome, a condition that we shall explore in detail later in this book. The "leaky gut" is an important disease entity but it is not the cause of all human ills!

Nowadays, the gastrointestinal tract is the principal pathway for the delivery of a vast array of nutrients, botanicals, herbals, and remedies of natural origin. These agents are described under the umbrella term of *dietary supplements*. Dietary supplements are used to promote wellness, and by law they cannot be used to prevent or treat any disease. These supplements have variable degrees of benefit and occasional toxicity. Some of the more important supplements used in the promotion of gastrointestinal wellness are discussed in later chapters of this book. There is relatively new legislation that controls the sale of dietary supplements in the United States (the Dietary Supplement and Health Education Act of 1994). Conventional medicine is not entirely conversant with this new, liberal legislation that permits the widespread availability of herbs, botanicals, and nutrients in dietary supplement format.

As mentioned earlier, a favorite health pastime for centuries has been to purge the bowel. The idea that one can purge one's way to health possesses a measure of truth, as does the act of liver or colon detoxification, with attempts to introduce friendly bacteria into the gastrointestinal tract (probiotic medicine). Purgation, detoxification, and probiotic therapy summarizes about 90 percent of all current "natural," alternative medical interventions for gastrointestinal disorders. The acts of purgation, probiotic treatments (use of friendly bacteria, e.g., Lactobacilli), and attempts to combat the leaky gut syndrome are gaining great popularity. Despite this popularity among patients, conventional medicine keeps turning its back on these practices. Furthermore, patients are adopting these treatments increasingly without telling their doctors.

It may seem strange that a protagonist of alternative and complementary therapies is prepared to be somewhat critical of these aforementioned alternative interventions. I am not blindly critical. I am raising the point that we have done little to explore the benefits, or lack thereof, of these remedies of natural origin for the management of gastrointestinal disorders. We fail to examine these options in spite of the knowledge that there are a number of failures of conventional medicine in the management of gastrointestinal disease and there are reports (too often anecdotal) of the success of some alternative therapies that deserve more scrutiny. Furthermore, the gastrointestinal disorders that are labeled functional represent an ideal target for natural, gentle, cost-effective, safe options that may replace the synthetic drug or surgical approach.

TOWARD A MORE POSITIVE DIAGNOSIS

No patient or physician relishes the idea of fruitless testing. The mindset that supports the diagnosis by exclusion of disease is slowly changing as symptom-based, diagnostic methodology helps the physician and patient come closer to a positive diagnosis of functional bowel disease (especially IBS). Symptom-based diagnosis relies on the occurrence of a certain set of symptoms in association or a pattern that results in a high likelihood of a diagnosis. This approach helps but does not always dispense with the need to engage in some medical testing to exclude organic disease. Later in this book, we shall examine some aspects of nonconventional testing in gastroenterology.

There are many examples of symptom-based questionnaires or diagnostic instruments that can be used to reach a likelihood of diagnosis of functional bowel disease (or "globus guticus") without frequent recourse to invasive testing. Examples of these diagnostic instruments include the Manning Criteria, a questionnaire contain-ing fifteen bowel-related symptoms for the diagnosis of IBS and the so-called Rome Criteria, which was put together at the famous con-sensus meeting that covered twenty-one types of functional gastroin-testinal disorders—recently revised a decade later!

IS MANAGED CARE WAKING UP?

In 1996, researchers at several major universities, including the University of Michigan, attempted to do economic studies on man-aged-care costs by disease states to define which disorders would be ideal for alternative medicine interventions. It is no coincidence that placebo (sugar pill, dummy treatments) responding diseases and those in which psychosocial issues played a causative role were high-lighted as good options for alternative healing. At the top of this list stands IBS and other functional disorders of the guts.

Functional problems cost the healthcare system dearly and account for a great deal of unnecessary medical testing. I reiterate that conventional medicine is winning in many areas but predictably failing in others. If my reasoning is sound, then even managed-care organizations could see the potential of complementary therapies for functional gastrointestinal disorders, when effective, alternative therapies can often save medical dollars and ameliorate a great deal of suffering from digestive complaints.

MEDICINE AT THE CROSSROADS

The idea of a crossroads between conventional medical practice and the multiple disciplines of alternative medicine has become closer to a spaghetti junction on a freeway or motorway. At this complex inter-section of medical disciplines are several physicians and healers armed with the ability to engage in interference, compromise, vested interest, economic incentives, and altruistic thoughts. There are many healers out there with a cloned mentality, be it alternative or conventional, but there are also those who are would-be integrators of medicine. These integrators are embraced by a small but growing group of pluralistic thinkers.

I position myself with the pluralistic group, where a modern-day healer or physician can be obsessed with what works rather than be hung up on the source or origin of the treatment or healing intervention. The physician of the new millennium is being forced to think in lateral terms, largely because healthcare recipients are fed up with medical parochialism and politics that reject alternative therapies out of hand. Even the most intransigent physician cannot ignore the pestering of the patient who wishes to assert his or her newfound quest for alternative therapies. The rapid stroke of the pen with the "instant drug-name-recall" and resulting prescription is no longer satisfying the average recipient of health care!

CHAPTER SUMMARY

The range and complexity of functional disorders of the gastrointestinal system is daunting. Alternative medicine may offer a safe, cost-effective alternative to conventional medicine in the management of several functional digestive complaints. The movement toward remedies of natural origin is gaining momentum, and these issues require critical appraisal.

CHAPTER THREE

THE MOUTH:
NO-MAN'S-LAND

NO-MAN'S-LAND

The guts begin at the mouth and end at the anus. For many physicians, the mouth and its problems fall into no-man's-land. Many physicians believe that the dentist owns the healthcare of the mouth, but a physician who specializes in diseases of the ear, nose, and throat (ENT) would argue the contrary. The communication gap between the dentist and the ENT physician would put the Grand Canyon to shame. In contrast to these gaps in communication between healthcare givers, the various regions of the gastrointestinal tract communicate with each other constantly, using their phone lines (nervous systems) and "molecules of emotion" (nervous system transmitter chemicals and hormones).

Although the mouth plays a pivotal role as an organ of communication, it rarely gets discussed among healthcare givers in different medical disciplines. Dentists do not often speak to physicians, and vice versa. Primary care physicians or specialist gastroenterologists do not often speak to ENT doctors. Frequently, a patient who complains to a physician about a common disorder affecting the mouth is told to report to his or her dentist. This can create problems because many of the common complaints about the mouth, including dry mouth or bad breath, are related to general disease states or disorders of the body, not just occurrences within the mouth itself. The frustrated dentist may complete the loop by referring the patient back to the physician, after they have exhausted the options in their chosen domain. Patients with mouth problems are often in a revolving door from which they cannot emerge.

Functional disorders of the mouth include halitosis (bad breath), excessive salivation (sialorrhoea), dry mouth (xerostomia), nonspecific mouth ulcers (apthous ulcers), abnormal appearances and feelings of the tongue, and disorders of taste (cacogeusia). Cacogeusia (a bad taste in the mouth) is often associated with halitosis (bad breath).

Halitosis can be due to major medical illnesses such as kidney failure or liver failure, but it is most often quite benign in its origin. Some physicians could perhaps think of only less than a handful of causes of bad breath, but this is one of the most common symptoms to affect humankind.

DENTISTS AND DOCTORS PASSING THE BUCK

It is unfortunate that doctors and dentists rarely work as a team. In fact, the medical literature points to a lack of communication between physicians and dentists. Not only does a doctor fail to share his medical records with a dentist and vice versa, they hardly ever speak to each other in joint consultation concerning a patient. Whenever there is a lack of communication or collaboration in medicine, there are problems in the management of disorders or diseases. Medical authors point to the shortcomings that exist in the management of disorders of the mouth. Not only is there a lack of communication between dentists and doctors, there is an unfortunate and serious lack of communication sometimes between doctors in different specialties who may treat the same region of the body.

The mouth is a classic example of "forgotten territory" for the gastroenterologist. In recent times, the gastroenterologist has made attempts to inspect the upper reaches of the alimentary tract, especially during endoscopy of the upper guts, but this practice is not consistent. The endoscope that is used by the gastroenterologist is not designed to examine the mouth in detail. Many doctors may perceive that symptoms affecting the mouth or throat are not part of their responsibility. Physicians are taught to inspect the mouth as part of a routine physical examination, but medical studies imply that many practicing physicians have little knowledge about disease of the mouth, gums, or teeth. Add to this situation the fact that many mouth symptoms may be functional in nature and one sees the complexity of this problem.

Some of the most frustrated patients that I have seen in a gastroenterology clinic are those who have been passed from primary care physician to dentist to otolaryngologist (ENT doctor) to gastroenterologist, in a variable order or combination of referrals. This merry-go-round may even involve psychiatrists. The simple fact is that healthcare sometimes confuses the ownership of the mouth as an anatomic region for disease management. Our men in Rome who met to discuss functional diseases of the gut neglected the mouth. Surprisingly, the dermatologist (skin doctor) may have more to offer than anyone else in the treatment of diseases of the mouth, because the mouth (and, incidentally, the anus) are essentially extensions of the skin. No wonder there is confusion!

It is a fact of life that health care professionals just do not like to deal with disorders that they know relatively little about. The unfortunate reality is that we still know little about the causes of many disorders of the mouth and even less about disorders of the oral cavity that are not related to the presence of overt disease or structural abnormality. In this chapter we shall examine some of the most common disorders that affect humankind. Disorders of the mouth are often left to the patient to deal with by themselves. Many a thriving business has been built on gimmicks or alternatives to suppress common and unpleasant symptoms that emanate from the mouth.

BAD BREATH

From candy store to grocery store to pharmacy, there are thousands of products and processes that are aimed at dealing with halitosis. Many people just will not accept that halitosis is sometimes a normal occurrence. The simple fact is that people who have transient halitosis often eat food that smells, and despite the vast consumption of breath mints and fancy mouth sprays, it is very difficult to disguise the odor of spicy food.

Whether or not a person has a tolerance for halitosis is often related to culture. In Western communities, it is not desirable to walk around with the odor of food on one's breath, but in other societies, especially in Eastern Asia and on the Indian subcontinent, it is often quite acceptable to have a lingering buccal odor following a meal. Some societies take this to the extreme. In certain regions of mainland China, it is considered good manners to belch after a meal, and this is interpreted often as a show of appreciation for the chef! This after-meal (postprandial) situation in China is quite interesting. Following a meal in China, many people will spend a great deal of time ceremoniously picking their teeth. This action is likely to reduce one of the most common causes of halitosis, which is the trapping of food particles between the teeth, that often leads to plaque formation. There are many people in Western communities who reach for the breath mint but they will not use the toothpick to pick their teeth!

Unfortunately, like a spouse who has been cheated on, the person with halitosis may be often the last to know that they have bad breath. A person with bad breath can adjust to their own mouth odor. This is particularly the case with people who smoke cigarettes, regularly drink alcohol, or subsist on spicy food. Before we enter any discussion about the multiple causes of bad breath, it should be recognized that the most common cause of halitosis is poor hygiene of the mouth. Dirty mouths are like dirty feet—they often smell!

WHAT IS BAD BREATH, REALLY?

There are a large number of people who think they have bad breath when they do not. Bad breath that is not present or real can be called functional halitosis. These unfortunate individuals complain bitterly of halitosis that is undetectable by others. This can become a serious obsession that can result in rituals of mouth cleaning. This disorder can be part of a serious psychoneurosis (mind problem) that requires the aid of a psychiatrist. Like Lady Macbeth, who ritually tried to rid herself of her conscience, neurotic individuals with fictitious bad breath may brutalize their mouth with antiseptics, scrubbing brushes, and even violent attempts to achieve "cleanliness." The commercial world has recognized this by producing electric tongue cleaners. When desperation prevails, the salesman will fill the need!

The effective management of halitosis involves a bit of sleuthing for the cause. Serious, persistent problems are best handled by an expert because it's important to exclude significant diseases of the upper digestive tract or respiratory passages. I'll reiterate that the most common cause of persistent halitosis is less-than-optimal oral hygiene. Food can get trapped between teeth, and in combination with normal bacteria in the mouth, fermentation of the food can cause an odor. Pockets or crevices occur between the teeth and gums, especially in the presence of periodontal disease.

Many people, both doctors and patients, believe that bad breath is a common indicator of poor digestive function and more specifically "lazy bowels" or constipation. I believe that poor digestive function can contribute occasionally to halitosis, but this link is inconsistent.

The link between bad guts and bad breath has not been investigated extensively. In the 1940s, a number of clinical studies were performed to examine the relationship between constipation and halitosis. In human experiments, constipation was induced by taking drugs known to cause constipation and the subjects were assessed for halitosis. Surprisingly, constipation induced in this manner did not reliably cause bad breath. Furthermore, experiments that were undertaken to purge the bowels of people with halitosis did not result in any consistent or measurable improvement in their bad breath.

WHERE BAD BREATH COMES FROM

Poor oral hygiene and/or the common occurrence of gum, or gingival, disease (gingivitis, which is often classed under the term *periodontal disease*) are the main causes of bad breath. Air flows freely through the mouth, nasal passages, throat area, and respiratory passages of the lungs. Diseases that involve inflammation or tissue damage at any site along the passage of air into the body can cause a foul odor.

Inflammation and disorders of the gums and teeth that result in gingivitis and gum pockets are classic examples of periodontal disease. When periodontal disease becomes established, the gums drift away from their junction with the teeth. Mixed infections occur around the lower areas of the teeth at their junction with the gums and this disorder is often associated with the presence of dental plaque. (Plaque is a cheesy concretion that becomes deposited between and around the teeth—left alone it sets like liquid concrete!) Pockets form around gums and bacteria, food fragments and plaque can collect in these pockets or grooves. Sometimes the gums can swell and bleed. Enlargement of the gums (called hypertrophy but it is strictly hyperplasia) may be quite pronounced and surgical correction is required sometimes by a periodontist (a dental surgeon who specializes in these problems). However, it is often possible to avoid the dental surgeon's scalpel by practicing periodontal hygiene. The mainstay of management of periodontal disease involves plaque removal by brushing, flossing, and the scaling techniques used by a dental hygienist.

Teeth are perched in alveolar bones and anchored by ligaments. A tooth has an enamel coating over soft tissue called dentin. Damage to enamel causes cavities. Many factors play a role in preventing tooth decay. Saliva is very important in maintaining healthy teeth and gums. It is alkaline and buffers excess acid, serving the purpose of irrigation in the mouth, fighting infections and maintaining the proper degree of mineral content of teeth.

One of the most destructive influences on teeth is the presence of acidity in the mouth. The pH of the mouth falls (acidity) as a result of the action of bacteria on food particles that are retained along the dental margin. This explains why drinks of low pH (soda) are damaging. Excessive sugar is bad for teeth—bacteria love sugar. Bacteria and food particles work together to cause plaque, which can collect as soon as four to six hours after brushing the teeth. If left, plaque attracts minerals and bacteria to form tartar, a form of hard material that sticks to the teeth. The buildup of plaque and tartar is related to the types of plaque-forming bacteria present in the mouth, rates of flow of saliva, and factors in the diet.

The throat area (pharynx) is a shared route to both the lungs and the upper gastrointestinal tract. In this region, upper gastrointestinal air is exposed to exhaled breath. Any strong-smelling food that has been eaten recently can be readily detected on the breath. Spices, garlic, fish, and alcohol are common causes of breath odor following meals. If food hangs around in the stomach or upper gastrointestinal tract, it can ferment or putrefy. Food that hangs around in the guts attracts unwanted guests in the form of harmful bacteria and microorganisms. This circumstance can result from blockages in the digestive tract, which are often the result of disease or structural problems.

As well as the common occurrence of odors from pungent foods, other gases or volatile compounds can be present in the breath. Volatile fatty acids can emanate from the guts in states of disease. Liver failure or kidney failure can give rise to chemicals that are part of body waste. These include ammonia-based compounds that can result in halitosis. The "fishy" breath of the chronic drunk often signifies the likely occurrence of liver damage.

Odors in the breath can come from sites distant from the respiratory or digestive passages. A number of aromatic substances when applied to the body can be detected in the breath. Experiments performed sixty years ago showed that when garlic was rubbed on the soles of the feet, its odor appeared in the breath.

KEYS TO ORAL HYGIENE

Inflammation around the teeth involving the gums should be taken seriously if teeth are to be retained throughout life. Periodontal disease should never be neglected—it is best managed by professional advice and compliance with home care programs that are designed to treat and prevent this disorder. Recent research points very clearly to the presence of certain bacterial infections of the gums (e.g., Klebsiella species) and cardiovascular disease. Keeping teeth healthy may be related to saving life as well as to saving teeth.

Perhaps the most important tools for good dental hygiene are a decent toothbrush and good toothpaste. It is worth investing in a decent toothbrush and it does not need to be either electric or expensive. The brush should be of medium texture unless occasional hard scaling by a firm brush is desired. Soft toothbrushes are ineffective, in my opinion, and recommendation for their use by people with sensitive teeth is a deception. Sensitive teeth are sensitive to soft, medium, and hard toothbrushes. In addition to brushing, flossing the teeth is an effective way of cutting through and removing plaque. Floss without a wax coating is more effective for removing plaque and food particles.

There are many designs and shapes of toothbrushes but many are just gimmicks and have little in the way of advantages. The ideal toothbrush has bristles of different length with protrusions that permit the bristles to get into crevices around teeth. Different handle shapes of or curved handles of toothbrushes are sales gimmicks. It is not what you have but how you use it!

Perhaps more important than the shape of the toothbrush is the technique of brushing. The brush should be arched over the teeth. The brushing angle should be varied so that one is not merely brushing the same areas continuously while missing other areas. Difficult-to-reach areas of the mouth during brushing are alongside the molars, and many people forget to brush the back of their teeth, as well as the front.

Good tooth-brushing practices should be combined with the use of the right toothpaste. Plain old bicarbonate of soda is one of the best things to brush with, and it is a completely acceptable alternative to toothpaste. The alkaline (high pH) of baking soda promotes the presence of friendly inhabitants in the mouth. Toothpastes that contain baking soda (sodium bicarbonate) and peroxide have become popular. The best formulation of baking soda and peroxide is Peroxicare (Arm and Hammer), although it is not the best packaged or best tasting of these popular toothpastes.

When gingival inflammation and gum recession is present, the use of water piks to clean out crevices between gums and teeth can be very important. A number of devices exist for this purpose, and the objective is to clean out the "trenches," small pockets and channels that form between the teeth and gums. If these areas are left unchecked, there will be a loosening of the attachment of the gums to the teeth and the creation of gum recession.

A water pik can be used to irrigate the crevices. Antiseptics can be added to the irrigating fluid in the water pik. Perhaps the most commonly used antiseptic to irrigate with is a diluted solution of chlorhexidine gluconate. However, this antiseptic can be used only for a week or two in the presence of significant periodontitis, and it presents three problems. First, chlorhexidine gluconate does not taste good. Second, it can stain the teeth when used repeatedly. Third, it can kill friendly bacteria if used for too long and create an environment for the overgrowth of damaging bacteria. This antiseptic has to be used with distilled water because minerals and contaminants in tap water can interfere with its antiseptic properties.

Other additives for irrigation of the gum margins include diluted hydrogen peroxide and a good mouthwash such as Listerine. I do not believe in the continuous use of antiseptic mouthwashes, but they are useful when used intermittently. It should be noted that the setting used on the water pik should be low. A forceful stream from a water pik can loosen the gums, especially if overused. The whole process of irrigation should be performed with care in a gentle manner.

BREATH FRESHENERS

Freshening the breath is big business. Adjacent to the cash register in any general store, a whole host of products are purveyed to assure fresh breath. One has a choice of flavored candies, chewing gum, sprays, tablets, lozenges, mouth rinses, and drinks. The problem is that most of them are quite ineffective, or, at best, they will substitute a strong pleasant odor for a bad odor for a matter of a few minutes. Sometimes an attempt to disguise bad breath with a volatile oil or flavor used in gum can result in a combined odor that is worse than the original odor. Some foods, such as garlic or strong onions, defy any attempt to disguise their smell. One can enjoy the health-giving benefits of garlic, but patience is required for the smell to go away.

INTERNAL DEODORIZATION

We all want to be assured that we smell good. In states of health the body can disguise its own natural odors, but it always needs a bit of help. According to the advertising, help comes in the form of the perfume, deodorant, and cosmetics industries. But the superficial odor from these products will not disguise the smell of sad guts.

This knowledge has prompted people to think of the concept of internal deodorization, and many natural techniques have been applied. I believe that odors from the guts are often due to an imbalance of the inhabitants of the guts, where friendly bacteria are ousted or substituted by unwanted guests. Probiotic therapy (treatment using friendly bacteria) has a lot to offer in counteracting unpleasant gut odors, and it can effectively be combined with certain essential oils from plants (e.g., peppermint and fennel oil). These essential oils have antimicrobial properties and may not disturb the gut flora (bacteria) to the same degree as antibiotics, thereby promoting healthy digestion.

STRANGE TASTES

Halitosis and a bad taste in the mouth may go hand in hand. Often the management of one is similar to the management of the other. A bad taste in the mouth can sometimes be due to sepsis such as a gumboil (root abscess) or a throat infection. Certain types of taste give clues to their cause. Metallic tastes in the mouth can be due to metal used in tooth fillings. Dental amalgams have to be carefully chosen because they may dissolve due to galvanism, the interaction of metals in fillings with saliva and tissues. Some amalgams contain heavy metals that may be absorbed into the body and are an alleged cause of serious illnesses that may be overlooked. The occurrence of galvanism and the dangers of mercury and other fillings in the teeth are discussed later in this chapter.

Salty or bloody tastes may signify the presence of gingivitis. It may come from bleeding gums, excessive tooth brushing, or from trauma induced by lip biting or sucking or chewing areas of the inner lip or cheek. There is a strong mind-mouth interaction. A dry mouth (xerostomia) has many causes ranging from waking in the morning to autoimmune diseases. Substitute lubricants for saliva afford only temporary relief and a search for the cause of the xerostomia is necessary.

With advancing age, areas of the tongue or mouth may atrophy (shrink). Loss of cerebral function such as found in mature individuals with dementia due to Alzheimer's disease or cerebrovascular disease (hardening of the arteries) can cause loss of taste or a bad taste.

Individuals with depression often describe bad tastes in their mouth, but this is sometimes due to medication—in particular, the drying effect that antidepressant medication may have on the mouth. Several antidepressant drugs inhibit saliva production by the salivary glands, expecially tricyclic antidepressant drugs.

Medication is a common and often overlooked cause of a bad taste in the mouth. Several drugs are potent causes of disordered taste. Lithium salts that are used to treat bipolar disorders (manic-depressive disease) invariably disturb taste sensations. Other common causes of disordered taste include the drugs griseofulvin, used for fungal infections, and penicillamine, used for rheumatoid arthritis therapy. The exact mechanism by which these drugs cause abnormalities of taste is not known; but in some cases it is due to abnormal metabolism of zinc, which is induced by the drug. Supplementation with zinc sometimes improves the problem of drug-induced bad tastes in the mouth and there is experience that zinc supplementation may work in circumstances where the cause of the bad taste is not obvious or known.

It appears to many patients that side effects like a bad taste in the mouth from drugs can be abolished with new drug developments. Every couple of months a report or two emerges about a drug that can affect taste. Among the most commonly used new drugs in the treatment of cardiovascular disease and hypertension are ACE inhibitors (angiotensin converting enzyme inhibitors). The ACE inhibitors have been improved in their treatment effects by the discovery of drugs that have more selective effects in antagonizing the angiotensin receptors. One such example of an improved ACE inhibitor is the drug Losartan. This drug seems to cause dysgeusia (a funny taste in the mouth) or complete loss of taste. Moreover, ACE inhibitors are frequent causes of a tickling cough, intestinal colic, and occasional dysphagia, which is not always identified as being due to the use of these drugs.

There are many examples of drugs that cause a bad taste or loss of taste. Those readers who are searching for knowledge in this area are referred to an excellent source of information in a scientific paper by Dr. R. I. Henkin, M.D., entitled "Drug Induced Taste and Smell Disorders," published in *Drug Safety*, 1994 (Vol. II, p. 318–77).

SWOLLEN, BLEEDING GUMS

Swollen and bleeding gums are red flag signs in most circumstances. This condition is never functional in origin. While it is often due to gingivitis, it can be the first sign of serious blood diseases such as leukemia. In children, bleeding and swollen gums are a common presentation of acute leukemia and other malignant diseases of the blood. Some drugs cause enlargement of the gums that can be very disfiguring. Drugs that are used to treat epilepsy, such as phenytoin, produce gum enlargement (hyperplasia) to such a degree that gums can encroach on the teeth. Swollen and bleeding gums should prompt an individual to seek medical consultation.

WATERY MOUTH

Excessive flow of saliva is uncommon, but the dribbling of saliva during sleep is very common. Babies drool because the flow of saliva is many times greater in infancy than it is in later life. Stress may produce drooling especially during sleep, and some people with severe stress can experience excessive salivation with a sense of choking while asleep. Relaxation techniques effectively reverse this problem.

Excessive salivation can occur in individuals with severe disorders of the brain such as Alzheimer's disease, cerebrovascular dementia (hardening of the arteries), and Parkinson's disease. Perhaps the most common cause of a rush of saliva is the occurrence of "waterbrash" that is associated with GERD or sometimes peptic ulcer. In this situation, gastric contents can reflux into the lower esophagus, stimulating salivary flow by a reflex (not a *reflux*) mechanism. It is not the stomach contents that come into the mouth in this situation. In this situation, stimulation of a nervous reflex occurs that delivers a signal for the salivary glands to secrete excessive amounts of saliva. The remedy for waterbrash caused by this mechanism is to effectively treat the GERD.

Excessive salivation of a functional nature is most often stress-related, and the benefits of stress-reduction techniques are often quite apparent. Later in the book we examine the mind-gut connection in more detail and learn techniques to limit stress, improve the sense of well-being, and combat destructive moods such as depression.

Useful remedies of natural origin for functional hypersalivation include St. John's Wort and minor doses of Ma Huang. Several herbs have atropinic effects (interfere with autonomic nerves that drive the salivary glands), but in doses required to suppress excessive salivation, they have side effects. Ma Huang, or ephedra, is a popular component of dangerous weight-loss dietary supplements. It is an herb that has been associated with illness, injury, and death. For this reason, it is best used only under medical supervision.

Conventional medical approaches to the symptomatic relief of excessive salivation include psychiatric therapy, antihistamine drugs, anticholinergic drugs (e.g., propantheline), antidepressant drugs (especially tricyclic drugs), and even phenothiazine drugs (e.g., chlorpromazine). These approaches often fail and the side effects of these drugs are often worse than the problem of hypersalivation.

DRY MOUTH

Numerous diseases and aging may cause a dry mouth, but the most common is excessive mouth breathing, usually associated with stress. Individuals who snore may wake with a very dry mouth. Among the most common causes of snoring are laxity of the soft palate or nasal obstruction. Snoring goes along with obesity, and the number one simple solution to many cases of common snoring is weight loss. Clinics have sprung up that specialize in the management of sleep disorders, and the diagnosis of abnormal sleep patterns is a very important issue in modern medicine. Some disorders of sleep, such as sleep apnea (stopping breathing), are life threatening. The relationship between weight gain and snoring has been underestimated. Serious conditions that cause a dry mouth (xerostomia) include dehydration, diabetes, renal failure, and the sicca syndrome (Sjögren's syndrome). The sicca syndrome has an autoimmune basis, and it is sometimes associated with rheumatoid arthritis.

The simplest therapy for functional xerostomia (dry mouth) is frequent fluid intake. Glycerol of thymol is useful but it cannot be swallowed. A 1 percent or 2 percent concentration of methylcellulose (false saliva) is quite safe and soothing. By far the most important aspect of the therapy of sleep-induced dry mouth is the promotion of healthy sleep. If sleep aids are required, I prefer the use of valerian root and/or kava but not sleeping pills (drugs).

BURNING TONGUE

A burning sensation in the tongue most often affects mature females and, in my opinion, is often related to menopause and probably has a hormonal basis. This hypothesis will surprise many physicians. If obvious abnormalities of the tongue are present, then they may be due to vitamin deficiency, usually of the classic water soluble–type of vitamins. These vitamins include the entire B complex and folic acid. Classic textbooks of medicine draw attention to the smooth red tongue of iron-deficiency anemia, but this is seldom seen in modern times. Furthermore, some studies suggest that this abnormality of the tongue is no more common in the presence of iron-deficiency or iron deficiency anemia (low red-blood-cell mass) than it is in the general population. One characteristic symptom of pernicious anemia, due to vitamin B12 deficiency, is a sore tongue. Pernicious anemia requires treatment by a physician.

The most obvious cause of irritation of the tongue is sometimes overlooked, namely sharp teeth and poor-fitting dentures. The tongue is sometimes a good indicator of general health, and some traditional medical systems have relied heavily on the appearance of the tongue as a diagnostic indicator of various diseases. I believe that diagnoses based on the appearance of the tongue alone are probably wishful thinking in many cases.

Common abnormalities of the tongue are furring, fissuring (cracks), and the so-called geographic tongue, with its lumps and bumps like rough terrain. Most often these problems are not a sign of ill health. Furring of the tongue with cheesy plaques can be seen in yeast infections, especially with *Candida albicans*. Several drugs, such as nystatin, are effective for yeast affecting the mouth. Diluted peppermint oil usually removes this problem, but it can cause an uncomfortable burn if overused and should only be administered intermittently, for no longer than two weeks. The tongue should not be scrubbed or abraded.

Antibiotic therapy can sometimes precipitate abnormalities of the tongue that may respond to the chewing of fennel seeds. Although I cannot explain the mechanism of action, some cases of hairy tongue or nonspecific glossitis (inflammation of the tongue) respond quite well to *Lactobacilli* (a friendly type of bacteria) taken in capsules (but not retained in the mouth). We will discuss the role of friendly and unfriendly bacteria in the functions of the gut in a later chapter of this book.

MOUTH ULCERS

Troublesome small ulcers of the mouth affect millions of people. About one in ten people may have them on a recurrent basis. Almost everyone will say at one time or another that they have had a sore spot in the mouth. This sore spot is often due to the common type of non-specific ulcer called the apthous ulcer. Most often these small ulcers are quite benign and of unknown cause. They are therefore part of medicine's gray area. However, mouth ulcers can be a marker of underlying disease elsewhere in the guts.

The typical apthous ulcer has a white center and a red ring or halo. Because of this concentric appearance, they look sometimes like a miniature target. Apthous ulcers occur more often in women than men, with a female-to-male preponderance of 2:1. They can occur as a result of a triggering event such as irritation of the mouth by a sharp tooth or the edge of a tooth brace or denture plate. There is some indication that apthous ulcers may run in families, but the most troublesome form of this disorder is when it occurs in young females in a cyclical manner, often coinciding with menstruation. Apthous ulcers can add to the discomfort of menstrual tension.

Many cases of apthous ulceration that are severe enough for an individual to seek medical care are those that occur in a cyclical manner with menstruation, suggesting that they have a hormonal basis. These types of ulcers may respond to soy isoflavones, which modulate the action of the body's own hormone, estrogen. Approximately 50 to 80 mg of mixed soy isoflavones (genistein and daidzein) in a dietary supplement is often effective.

Infrequently, apthous ulcers are a sign of serious inflammation or disease elsewhere in the guts. Apthous ulcers in the mouth can signal the occurrence of Crohn's disease, ulcerative colitis, or celiac disease (gluten enteropathy). Celiac disease is due to an immune reaction to gluten that is found in wheat flour and wheat products in the diet. It is of interest that apthous ulcers can occur in the large bowel, and they are often a sign of early inflammatory bowel diseases, especially Crohn's disease.

Apthous ulcers are self-limiting in most cases, but when recurrent, painful, and troublesome, they can be treated locally by the topical application of steroids in pellets that can be placed against the ulcer to dissolve. A more natural approach is to apply clove or a little calendula (available in ointment). However, calendula should be used sparingly because it is not generally taken internally. In females with apthous ulcers, soy isoflavones often do the trick, but, if preferred, black cohosh can be used in an appropriate dose (about 30 mg/day).

Many treatments for apthous ulceration have been used with variable benefit. Some cases respond to multivitamin supplements, and in many cases emotional factors precipitate their occurrence. I wonder if an undetected infectious agent (bacteria or virus) is present in some cases. Remember the medical profession treated peptic ulcers for years on the basis that they were caused by excessive acid, only to find out that they are most often due to a bug (*Helicobacter pylori*). There are viruses that cause ulceration in the mouth, most notably Herpes simplex and Coxackie viruses, but the lesions caused by these viruses are distinguishable from apthous ulceration, and the clinical course of the disorder they cause is very different than that of apthous ulcers.

In summary, in serious cases of mouth ulcers a search for a significant underlying disease is justified; but in most cases, natural approaches with phytoestrogens (soy isoflavones), stress management, and local soothing therapies are effective.

COLD SORES

Cold sores are an example of an organic disease due to a viral infection with herpes simplex type II virus. I include cold sores in this book because they are chronic, recurrent, and become manifest often at times of stress. They can occur with a number of triggering events that are related to lifestyle.

The herpes simplex type II virus causes a chronic infection where the virus most often lives in the nerves supplying areas of the lips and cheeks. Primary infection (initial acquisition) of the virus most often occurs in infancy when an infected mother transfers the virus in saliva to the infant by kissing and close contact. The virus occupies a site in nerves. At times when immunity wanes or stimuli trigger viral growth, the cold sore (herpetic lesion) appears commonly on the lips. The first sign of an eruption of a cold sore is often a painful burning feeling followed by the occurrence of blistering and subsequent scabbing.

Cold sores may be precipitated by a variety of stimuli. They occur very commonly with excessive exposure to the sun, with menstruation, during times of stress, and during a common cold or respiratory infection. Cold sores appear when one is run down which usually means temporary waning of immunity. The herpes virus is quite an opportunist, and in cases of serious deficiency in immunity, such as is found in the acquired immunodeficiency syndrome (AIDS), cold sores can become rampant. Cold sores are a troublesome, painful, cosmetic scourge for millions of people.

The word herpes conjures up great concern for many people who think immediately of genital herpes, which to all intents and purposes represents cold sores of the genitals. Cold sores are painful enough on the lips or cheeks let alone on the penis, vulva, or in the vagina. The virus that commonly causes genital herpes is herpes simplex type I, not the type II, which most often affects the mouth and lips. Unfortunately, type I and type II viruses are somewhat interchangeable in location, and this knowledge has to serve as a major disincentive to unprotected oral sex.

Herpes infection of the mouth or lips and genital herpes infection are strikingly common and should not cause panic. Unfortunately, herpes is for life, but it can be controlled. It is difficult to eradicate but cases of spontaneous disappearance are reported by naturopathic physicians with the use of natural therapies. A cure for herpes is not yet available. A diet that provides extra amounts of the amino acid lysine and lysine supplements are useful. A number of natural agents to stimulate immune function are reported as successful. These include echinacea, zinc, vitamin C, and the herb *Andrographis paniculata*. Antiviral drug therapy may reduce frequent recurrences of cold sores (e.g., acyclovir) when given by mouth or applied topically.

ALTERNATIVE DENTISTRY

Alternative dental care has to do with recognizing the importance of dental health for the overall health of the body. A splinter group of lateral-thinking dentists has established the American Academy of Biological Dentistry. These dental surgeons believe and cite evidence that dental disease can cause or aggravate many chronic degenerative disease, including arthritis, cardiovascular disease, and several diseases that are caused by poor immune function. Their proposals are often well-founded. Conventional dentistry has agreed with this tack to some degree, but its opinions are not expressed as strongly as they are by alternative dentists.

The practice of alternative dentistry (sometimes termed biological dentistry) supports the use and substitution of nontoxic materials for tooth restoration and greatly extends its interests to the role of dental hygiene in general health or disease prevention. The emphasis on general health seems to be much more prevalent in biological dentistry than in conventional dentistry. One of the key issues raised by alternative dentists is the far-reaching, negative health effects of amalgams containing silver, mercury, and other potentially toxic metals.

DANGEROUS DENTAL AMALGAMS

Evidence points to an association between mercury-containing dental amalgams and a variety of diseases (Table 3.1). Amalgams used in modern dental practice are now apparently quite safe, but millions of people still have older types of fillings in their teeth that contain certain toxic heavy metals. Mercury is a highly toxic metal even in small doses, and it strikes me as common sense not to have it in the mouth. It is proposed that mercury can leach into the body from fillings in teeth and cause many problems (see Table 3.1). This heavy metal is a potent toxin to the nervous system and it shares the property of other heavy metals in its ability to depress immune function. For many people, it is an expensive decision to rid the mouth of amalgam. Many people with ill health that has not been explained or effectively treated by conventional or alternative medicine have had their mouth cleared of amalgam, with apparent measurable and sometimes striking reports of health benefits.

Other metals in dental amalgam may cause problems. These metals include copper, tin, zinc, and silver. The metal in tooth fillings can interact with saliva to produce electric currents, a phenomenon mentioned earlier that is called electrogalvanism. With a lot of metal in the mouth, electric currents are generated in many directions. Electrons that spin can produce magnetic fields. It is known that electromagnetic fields can have powerful effects on body function. The criss-crossing of currents in the mouth caused by metal fillings has been reported to cause serious problems within the mouth such as tooth erosion. In addition, this has been implicated as a cause of neurological (nervous system) complaints, according to some dentists. It sounds farfetched, but I can assure you that electromagnetism has significant biological effects, some good and some bad!

It would be wrong to give the impression that the dental profession has a consensus opinion that mercury/silver amalgams are dangerous. This issue has become one of the most controversial debates

Table 3.1: Diseases and symptoms that can be linked to the presence of mercury amalgam fillings.

Tendency to allergies	Chronic inflammatory disorders
* Chronic debility	* Neuroticism
* Depression	* Metallic taste in mouth
Abdominal upset (vague)	Disturbed immunity
* Mixed neurological complaints	Coronary artery disease
Chronic fatigue syndrome	

* Denotes circumstances where a very plausible causal relationship exists, in the author's opinion. Note the association of mercury tooth fillings with neurotic behavior. This is used as a spurious reason to indicate by some that the associations of disease with amalgam fillings are all neurotic and amalgams are safe.

in modern dentistry. Some societies and advocates of conventional dental practice have labeled the removal of serviceable mercury amalgams from patients' teeth unethical. Furthermore, the American Dental Association and State agencies that license dentists have applied sanctions and penalties against some dentists who dared to recommend removal of tooth fillings with metal amalgams on grounds other than "failure of the fillings."

The general public should be aware that there are alternatives to metal amalgams and safe, compatible, and effective materials are available for tooth restoration and prosthetic replacements. One of the best alternatives to mercury amalgams is the composite amalgam that contains metals of low toxicity. While dentists in most Western countries no longer use obsolete amalgams containing heavy metals, they are often used in third world countries. The high price of dentistry in Western communities has motivated many people to seek dental treatment in less well-developed countries. These bargain-basement shoppers must be aware of what they are buying!

DISEASES AND ORAL HEALTH

Thirty years ago, Professor Samuel C. Miller, D.D.S., of the New York School of Dentistry proposed a relationship between poor dental hygiene and many different diseases. His work was ignored for a decade until these relationships were further examined. In particular, there seems to be a close link between a variety of cardiovascular diseases and dental health.

Several studies reported in the medical literature indicate the possibility of bacterial translocation (migration and travel) to the bloodstream. Bacteria that are found in the mouth can collect in atheromatous plaques (cholesterol deposits) that are found in arteries throughout the body. Organisms that have been identified as having this translocation potential include *Helicobacter pylori* (associated with gastritis and peptic ulcer) and *Chlamydia pneumoniae* (a common cause of lung infection).

In animal experiments performed at the University of Minnesota, dental researchers showed that bacteria from dental plaque were able to escape into the bloodstream and produce small blood clots. In these experiments, large amounts of certain bacteria (*Streptococcus sanguis* and *Porphyromonas gingivalis*—common oral inhibitants) caused irregular heart beats and early signs of a heart attack. It appears that these common bacteria that are present in the mouth have clotting factors on their surface that cause blood to coagulate (especially *Streptococcus sanguis*).

Scientific studies at the University of Toronto, Canada, have shown the presence of immune markers from oral bacteria in cholesterol-containing plaques (atherosclerosis)—suggesting but not proving a relationship between oral bacteria and atherosclerosis. These findings are supported by population studies from the National Institutes of Health and the State University of New York that links the presence of gum disease with the occurrence of cardiovascular disease, coronary heart disease, and stroke.

The associations of poor dental hygiene and heart disease have been extended to lung disease and peptic ulcer disease. Overall, it seems that dental health is a much more important determinant of general health than medicine has previously recognized.

NOVEL APPROACHES TO DENTAL HEALTH

Dental health has more to do with general health than most individuals think and vice versa. Dental health is not possible without adequate nutrition, measures for oral hygiene, and dental care. Toothbrushing and the use of dental floss can be supplemented by the use of chewing sticks such as a meswak (*Salvadora persica*), a popular practice in the Middle East. Several other natural, dental products exist that can improve dental hygiene, including herbal toothpastes and mouth rinses.

The herb bloodroot (*Sanguinaria canadensis*) contains substances that prevent bacterial formation of plaque, but it is toxic and therefore cannot be swallowed or used by pregnant women. Tea tree oil and calendula have been used for their antimicrobial effects in the mouth but, again, toxicity is a problem. One effective anti-bacterial agent is goldenseal (*Hydrasis canadensis*), which is often used in herbal preparations for dental use. Goldenseal contains berberine, which has been shown to have antibiotic properties in laboratory studies. In addition to the direct application of herbs, physicians with an interest in natural therapies may often use herbals, botanicals, or nutritionals that stimulate immune function (e.g., vitamins A, C, and E, and echinacea, andrographis paniculata).

NATURAL ENZYMATIC DIGEST AND BIOCLEANSING

Prevention of oral disease must concentrate on a variety of issues affecting oral health, including: oral hygiene, the nature of plaque-forming bacteria, retained food residue in the mouth, salivary flow, general immunity, and nutritional or dietary habits. The sequence in which some foods are eaten and the interval between their consumption have been shown to be important. For instance, if cheese is eaten shortly after a sugary item, the acid formed from the sugar is neutralized by the cheese.

Oral hygiene involves meticulous attention to the gums, teeth, and mouth, and it is expensive, time consuming, and often poorly undertaken. In order to simplify the approach, my colleague Nikolaus Smeh and I developed a rapid and effective way of cleaning the mouth with an enzymatic digest toothpaste that is based on natural ingredients. This novel toothpaste has a base of soluble fiber that holds water and is quite sticky. Added to this base are enzymes (papain, from papaya). When this natural enzyme in a matrix of sticky fiber is rubbed on the teeth, plaque and debris around the teeth are loosened and partially dissolved. In order to enhance the mouth cleanup and control of bacteria, several natural agents are added that have powerful antioxidant actions. These natural additives include green tea extract and vitamin C.

The use of vitamin C for dental health has been undervalued. In one study, vitamin C supplementation of the diet (500 mg/day) in young boys resulted in a cleaner mouth, regardless of how well or how poorly these boys brushed their teeth. It appears that vitamin is quite important in the prevention of gingivitis.

ARE ROOT CANALS A ROOT OF EVIL?

Root canals are used to preserve teeth and to achieve cosmetic success. Their benefit is too often overshadowed by the problems they create. I recall a patient who was regarded as a "difficult diagnostic problem." This individual presented to his doctor with recurrent fevers of unknown origin. For weeks, this patient woke up at night drenched in sweat, suffering severe malaise, and ultimately landed in the hospital to have almost every blood test, x-ray, scan, and test known to medicine. The case was presented at a medical meeting to a large audience of physicians. The secret was hiding in the patient's mouth. It was an infected root canal. I suspect one or two doctors looked in the patient's mouth, but the infection passed unrecognized, while the hospital bill ran up to more than $40,000.

I am not proposing that everyone now rush to have their expensive root canals ripped out. We should be motivated, however, to prevent the need for root canals and prosthetic teeth by preventive dentistry. Sounds good, but multiple prostheses are regarded as a cosmetic blessing that is here to stay, at least for those who can afford the dental work.

Some distinguished dentists have made claims that ripping out root canals can sometimes reverse some types of heart disease and renal (kidney) failure. We need a lot more research in this area. However, a badly created root canal is a ticking time bomb that can be the seat of chronic infection and act as a generator of problems that can affect general health.

THE TEETH AND ACUPUNCTURE MERIDIANS

It is believed by some alternative/complementary physicians that each tooth in the mouth has a close relationship with an acupuncture meridian or site in the body. The concept that a diseased tooth at a specific site can cause disorders in the organ of the body that is represented in an acupuncture meridian is an interesting thought. For example, the meridians of the gonads and kidneys are claimed to be related to the front teeth. I believe in the general art of acupuncture, but more evidence for the use of focused acupuncture in the mouth is required.

TEMPOROMANDIBULAR JOINT (TMJ) PROBLEMS

Put your teeth out of alignment and you put your jaw and the lower part of your face out of alignment. The burden of stress that occurs as a consequence of misalignment of the teeth and jaw is felt usually in the temporomandibular joint (TMJ). This joint is located on either side of the head immediately in front of the ears. It functions every time the mouth opens.

Loss of alignment of the jaw can result from tooth problems induced by disease or sometimes dentists. Very often the poor alignment of the jaw is just an imperfection of human development. Unfortunately, problems of the TMJ can be very painful, and they may also cause other more general symptoms. Some physicians are convinced that TMJ problems can cause insomnia, depression, poor memory or concentration, headaches and even backache. I accept these relationships as possible, but direct evidence that TMJ problems have such far-reaching health consequences is in dispute. The treatment of TMJ disorders focuses on methods to realign the jaw. There are a growing number of "jaw chiropracters." Perhaps dentists should be required to learn the Alexander technique of the mouth. The Alexander technique is an alternative medicine discipline that concentrates on correcting poor posture of the body, especially the spine.

One important aspect of therapy in conventional medicine to treat TMJ problems is surgery of the mouth, jaw, or TMJ itself. My tip is to avoid that if you can. Some complementary medical techniques are available that offer real benefit for TMJ problems. These include mouth balancing with the wearing of braces, homeopathic remedies, cold laser therapy, and perhaps acupuncture (general acupuncture theory). For more complete information on alternative approaches to dental care, the reader is referred to the American Academy of Biological Dentistry, P.O. Box 856, Carmel Valley, California, 93924, USA.

CHAPTER SUMMARY

The mouth should not remain no-man's-land in medicine. Striking evidence exists that poor dental health may cause chronic disease. Remedies of natural origin provide exciting alternatives for dealing with common disorders of the mouth.

CHAPTER FOUR

SWALLOWING
AND PUSHING INTO
THE STOMACH

THE ESOPHAGUS OR
SWALLOWING TUBE

Moving attention from the mouth into the gullet (throat and esophagus), we reveal a number of functional problems including globus hystericus (a lump in the throat), difficulty in swallowing (dysphagia), painful swallowing (odynophagia), regurgitation or vomiting, rumination (merycism), and chest pain that may be due to spasm (muscular contraction or "colic") of the esophagus. The connection of the mouth to the esophagus constitutes the throat, or pharynx. This area of the digestive tract is now receiving much more attention from gastroenterologists, who tended formerly to leave this domain to the ENT doctor.

The gullet or esophagus joins the stomach, and this is an important junction called the gastroesophageal junction. This junction works normally like a kind of flapper valve. This means it works to let food into the stomach and then acts to keep it there.

HOW TO SWALLOW

The act of swallowing is one of the supreme events of the body. The mind and body function during swallowing to protect the respiratory passages. This coordinated action is achieved by both conscious (vol-

57

untary) control and acts that do not surface to the conscious level (involuntary actions). During swallowing, speech and breathing become second place.

Swallowing starts by the approximation of the tongue to the soft palate. It is followed by an opening of the back of the throat in a manner that protects the upper airways. This phase of swallowing is sometimes referred to as the oropharyngeal (mouth-throat) phase of swallowing. The events involved in transfer of food from the mouth to the upper gullet (esophagus) occur in less than one second. So well orchestrated is this event that minor deviations from the order of events due to any cause can result in alarming discomfort.

The esophagus is responsible solely for the passage (transit) of food from the throat to the stomach. The esophagus has active submucosal glands in its lower portions that secrete alkaline fluid similar to saliva. The function of these glands has been generally ignored. It is a unique portion of the guts. The esophagus has two guarded portals that serve the dual purpose of entrance and exit. The upper guarded portal is the contracted muscular area called the upper esophageal sphincter (high-pressure zone), whereas the lower portal is the valvelike mechanism termed the lower esophageal sphincter (a kind of flapper valve that is assisted by the "pinchcock" mechanism of the diaphragm—the muscle between the guts and chest).

The term *sphincter* merely means that there is a measurable high-pressure zone in the digestive tube. There are several sphincters in the gastrointestinal tract, including the upper esophageal sphincter that is kept closed by nerve action at the back of the throat. The lower esophageal sphincter is kept closed by nervous and hormonal actions at the junction of the stomach and esophagus. Other sphincters of the gut include: the sphincter of Oddi, where the bile duct tips into the upper intestine, and the ileocecal valve that separates the small bowel from the large bowel. The terminus of the gut tube, the anal sphincter, exists at the anal margin, which separates the lower bowel from the world. The anus has two sphincters. The external sphincter is under voluntary control and the internal sphincter is not. The gut has a number of other anatomic sphincters that have collected eponyms derived from surgeons and anatomists of old.

Sphincters play a role in the overall motor function (movements) of the gastrointestinal tract. The guts function to push food, fluids, and gas from the mouth to the anus. The gastrointestinal tract in health moves its contents in a beautifully coordinated manner from mouth to anus (aboral, away from the mouth). I belabor the point of ideal movement in one direction in the healthy gut because of its pivotal importance.

Sphincters in the gastrointestinal tract have complex neural (nervous) controls and in many cases hormonal and chemical controls. Sphincters are quite responsive to the "molecules of emotion" (Pert's concept). The controls function to let the zones of the sphincter move digestive contents in one direction, away from the mouth. Disordered (troubled) sphincters are poor gatekeepers and they let contents of the guts move backward. In health, the overall direction from mouth to anus is assured. In general, backward flow through sphincters causes problems. This backward flow of contents across sphincteric zones is termed reflux. The classic example of reflux causing problems is a circumstance that affects the lower esophageal sphincter at the junction of the lower esophagus and stomach. Poor function of the lower esophageal sphincter results in GERD, where acidic stomach contents move backward, into the lower gullet.

DIFFICULTY IN SWALLOWING (DYSPHAGIA)

Disorders of the mouth (oro) and throat (pharynx) that cause oropharyngeal dysphagia were discussed in chapter 2. We need to focus some attention on the later phases or completion of the swallowing process, which is largely the function of the main body of the esophagus. If we imagine the esophagus to be a simple tube, then we can think about the organic causes of the obstruction to the flow of contents. Any factor in the channel of the esophageal tube, in the wall of the tube, or pressing on the wall of the tube will cause blockages and result in dysphagia. To provide some examples, an obstruction of the esophagus can be due to something stuck in the inside tube of the gullet, such as an impacted bolus of food or foreign body (commonly coins in children). Some disorders affecting the wall (e.g., cancer or inflammation) and things that compress the esophagus from the outside (e.g., a tumor in the chest) can cause difficulty in swallowing.

These disorders are serious and they present themselves with a sensation of food or fluid getting stuck or hung up in the chest.

The symptom of difficulty in swallowing must always be taken very seriously and should precipitate a visit to a health care practitioner. In anyone over the age of forty years, a new onset of difficulty in swallowing must be suspected to be cancer unless proved otherwise. In the case of obstruction from an anatomical abnormality, the difficulty in swallowing is usually greater for solid food than for liquids.

In this book we are focusing our attention on functional disorders. In clinical practice, the occurrence of functional dysphagia is more common than hitherto supposed, and it is often difficult to manage. Functional dysphagia is sometimes due to poor chewing, eating during periods of stress, or spastic contractions in the esophagus that are stimulated by stress. Relaxation techniques and mind body interventions that are described later in this book are first-line options for functional disorders of the esophagus. Drugs and surgery are not ideal first-line options.

NORMAL REFLUX FROM THE STOMACH TO THE ESOPHAGUS

Studies of the complex factors that control the pressure in the lower esophageal sphincter (LES) have been a pastime of many academic gastroenterologists, including myself. It is known that at least three types of mini–nervous systems control the LES in concert with hormonal influences that can increase or lower pressure in the LES. Anything that lowers pressure in the LES will tend to facilitate backward flow of stomach contents into the gullet. There are many agents (including stress, posture, food, and drugs) that can lower the pressure in the LES and provoke reflux. Welcome to the world of GERD, the most common esophageal problem, causing recurrent symptoms in at least one quarter of the population; even excluding the almost universal phenomenon of reflux in pregnancy. Ask a mother about heartburn in pregnancy and she will cringe.

Synchronous with a swallow, the LES relaxes and contractions in the gullet (peristalsis) gently push food and fluid down the esophagus into the stomach, with the assistance of gravity. The stomach expands to accommodate the food by a process of relaxation of its upper portions (fundus of the stomach). This process is called receptive relaxation. Following a meal, food initially lies around in the stomach, which then secretes acids and churns the food to make a semisolid mass of liquefied contents. This semisolid material is delivered (emptied) in a controlled manner through the outlet of the stomach into the upper small intestine or duodenum.

In the early period following a meal, it is not uncommon for small amounts of gastric contents to reflux into the esophagus, but this normally occurs silently and does not produce any symptoms. Although minor reflux occurs, the healthy lower esophagus can rapidly clear the refluxed material back through the LES into the stomach.

The ability of the healthy esophagus to rapidly clear its contents is a key issue. Failure to clear refluxed, acidic, gastric contents from the esophagus can cause a burn of the lining of the lower gullet. When the residence time of the contents of the esophagus is prolonged, problems arise. The burn of acid causes esophagitis (*esophag* = esophagus, *itis* = inflammation).

BURNING, BELCHING, ACID REGURGITATION

Just as it is known that acid secreted by the stomach can burn the lining of the lower esophagus, it is recognized that the most common symptom produced by reflux is a burning sensation experienced behind the breastbone. This symptom is called heartburn. Heartburn is typically experienced after meals when reflux occurs most commonly. After a meal the stomach is occupied by material that can be refluxed. At other times, heartburn occurs when circumstances favor the reflux of acid from the stomach to the esophagus. Such circumstances occur when an individual is lying down or sleeping, or following the ingestion of foods that commonly irritate the esophagus. Examples of direct dietary irritants to the lower esophagus are tomato juice and orange juice. Exercise can provoke acid backwash from the stomach and give rise to exercise-induced heartburn (an alarming symptom that can be confused with angina or pain from the heart). Reflux is common following overeating, which causes overdistension of the stomach. Overdistension of the stomach increases the pressure below the diaphragm which tends to cause backwash of stomach contents. This circumstance is very likely to occur with the ingestion of fatty (or "heavy") foods following excessive alcohol ingestion, or smoking. These factors reduce the pressure in the LES and inhibit its gatekeeper functions.

SYMPTOMS OF GERD

Symptoms of GERD can be mild, moderate, or severe. The degree of damage occurring in the lower esophagus as a consequence of reflux can also be mild, moderate, or severe. Mild symptoms of GERD with transient heartburn can vary with cycles of severe symptoms where the burning pain can be intense or prolonged and associated with acid regurgitation in the mouth, and even dysphagia.

Dysphagia is a sensation of food being stuck in the gullet, and it can occur as a result of inflammation, with poor clearance function in the lower esophagus. It seems reasonable to presume that mild symptoms are associated with mild inflammation in the lower gullet. However, this is not always the case. Sometimes severe and intractable symptoms of heartburn are associated with negligible signs of inflammation in the lower esophagus and vice versa. This lack of a relationship between the severity of acid-related inflammation and the severity of symptoms is well recognized.

Severe inflammation of the lower esophagus (esophagitis) can result in erosions (breaks in the lining) and ulcerations (craters in the lining). The lining cells of the esophagus can change into cell types that are premalignant (forerunners of cancer), known as Barrett's epithelium. This inflammation can partially heal or progress to narrowing of the esophagus (stricture) where a permanent anatomic deformity can occur. In severe cases, the so-called "peptic stricture" of the esophagus occurs. This can result in a permanent narrowing of the esophagus that causes severe dysphagia (difficulty in swallowing) and it may require stretching during endoscopy or even surgery in certain cases to correct the problem. Surgery for reflux in the esophagus has to be carefully considered by the patient and surgeon because it does not have an unblemished record of success.

A LUMP IN THE THROAT: THE GLOBUS SENSATION

The condition globus hystericus is experienced almost universally when one gets a severe fright or shock. It is a classic sensation of a lump in the throat. Some experts have argued that this alone does not constitute globus and that true globus involves an inhibition of or interference with the act of swallowing. I do not subscribe to this opinion, but it should be recognized that globus has a number of manifestations. Rather than a sensation of difficulty in clearing the throat during swallowing, some individuals complain of a sensation that they want to "bring something up from the throat."

The back of the throat is kept closed by constant excitation of the muscles of the pharynx (cricopharyngeal muscles). Swallowing occurs by inhibition of this continuous excitation of the muscles. In the condition of globus, the normal ability to inhibit these muscles is affected and the coordinated contraction of other muscles is disturbed. The result is that the sensation of globus occurs almost constantly. It can be entirely unrelated to the act of swallowing. Stress is often at the root of the globus symptom.

The problem patient with the globus sensation (a sensation of something continuously or intermittently stuck in the throat) is often not taken seriously by the healthcare giver. In more than one half of all cases, the globus sensation occurs secondarily to reflux disease, retrograde flow of stomach contents into the lower esophagus, termed GERD or esophagitis. We shall learn more about the typical and atypical manifestation of GERD later. The individual with a globus sensation caused by GERD may not have frank manifestations of GERD, such as acid regurgitation or heartburn.

The term *globus* is sometimes qualified by the term *hystericus*, implying the presence of neurosis. *Globus hystericus* is a useful term to point to the importance of emotional factors in its causation. However, globus is seldom due to hysteria but it is often associated with feelings of depression and unexpressed or repressed grief about a distressing life event. This psychological reaction contributes to gastrointestinal disease as part of the phenomenon of the conversion reaction.

GERD OFTEN MASQUERADES AS GLOBUS

When globus is present, it is sometimes useful to treat this disorder as though the individual has GERD. This treatment involves the avoidance of esophageal irritants, intermittent administration of antiacids, sleeping propped in bed, and the occasional use of courses of drugs that effectively reduce gastric acid secretion. Sometimes individuals with globus have a choking sensation when lying flat. This is due to acid moving back up the gullet from the stomach. Such people can have a burning sensation in their throat or a sour or bitter taste in their mouth. Infrequently, an alarming coughing spell can occur as acid tickles the throat or vocal cords. This situation can be dangerous because on occasion a reflux of stomach contents can enter the windpipe and respiratory passages, causing major lung problems. It takes only a small amount of gastric acid in the respiratory passage to provoke violent coughing, airway constriction (asthma), and severe lung damage.

Occasionally, the reflux of small amounts of acid on an intermittent basis can trigger asthmatic attacks, especially at night, and this situation is a perilous situation in infants. People with chronic bronchitis or emphysema can have their condition triggered or made worse by reflux in the esophagus. The occurrence of GERD and its effective management in the patient with chronic or acute lung disease may be overlooked.

The acid contents of the stomach do not need to travel all the way up to the back of the throat to cause globus sensations or even lung problems. These disorders can be produced by a reflex mechanism induced by the reflux mechanism. Thus globus and pulmonary (lung) disorders may be a consequence of the "reflex effect of the reflux effect."

About one half of the cases of globus are functional in nature, meaning that they are not caused by GERD or other diseases. In this circumstance, stress is usually at the root of the problem. The use of stress-relief techniques with occasional reliance on natural techniques for relaxation, such as hydrotherapy, meditation, aromatherapy and the use of dietary supplements such as kava or valerian root, are all useful interventions. These interventions can be used in a variable combination with good effect, and they are discussed in the chapter on remedies of natural origin for gut problems.

SCHATZKI: THE DOCTOR KNOWN FOR HIS RING

In 1964, Dr. R. Schatzki described his theory of the evolution of the globus sensation in the *New England Journal of Medicine*. In brief, Schatzki proposed that an anxious individual can develop an awareness of the act of swallowing, and a reduction of salivary flow occurs with anxiety. This sets up a vicious cycle of events where swallowing results in discomfort or irritation and spasm of the muscles of the back of the throat. This results in the globus sensation. Whatever the cause of globus, Schatzki's observations appear plausible and reinforce the role of the mind in causing globus and the use of natural relaxation techniques to deal with this problem.

Dr. Schatzki is better known for his description of a membranous ring in the lower esophagus that sometimes causes food to stick in the gullet. It is treated best by stretching the gullet, a maneuver reserved for the gastroenterologist or surgeon.

ASSESSING SWALLOWING

Measuring pressures in the muscles of the back of the throat or definition of the lack of coordination of muscle action by manometry (a pressure-measuring technique) can help in diagnosis. However, manometry is uncomfortable, and it may not alter management unless a severe organic disease is diagnosed. Examples of these severe diseases are muscular dystrophy or primary or secondary neurological disorders (nervous system diseases) that affect swallowing.

There are more comfortable ways of assessing swallowing using small doses of radioisotopes and the taking of scans. In a technique, a small amount of liquid containing a radioisotope is swallowed while sitting in front of a gamma camera. Also, one can use x-rays after swallowing a radio-opaque (x-ray detectable) marker to watch the act of swallowing. X-rays can be taken in sequence to make a video. This is called cine-video-fluoroscopy and it can be used to diagnose and plan treatment for swallowing disorders that are caused by abnormalities of the mouth, throat, or upper esophagus. These diagnostic techniques are limited to special diagnostic and treatment centers only.

THE SWALLOWING CLINIC

Specialized clinics have become established in several major medical centers to specifically deal with swallowing problems, arising out of the need for a multidisciplinary medical approach. In these clinics, swallowing problems are investigated and discussed among teams of specialists.

The team is often led by a gastroenterologist but is composed of speech therapists; psychologists; ENT specialists, and gastrointestinal assistants. The speech therapist is often called upon to treat the oropharyngeal swallowing problem, and these experts have advanced knowledge of the complex workings of the muscles of the mouth and throat that control the early phases of swallowing. These therapists can teach exercises to help swallowing.

LOOKING AT THE LES

A variety of normal events may provoke the reflux of gastric contents into the esophagus but adverse lifestyle and stress are major causes of reflux. Stress and poor lifestyle habits also play a role in making preexisting reflux worse. The pressure in the LES acts like a one-way valve system that favors passage of food and fluid into the stomach. This valvelike mechanism can be affected by many factors that alter the control of pressure in the LES including the nerve connections, hormonal influences, and even simple physical events like pressure on the abdomen (tight clothes) or exercise.

The pressure in the LES is altered by the type of food eaten. Fat will tend to lower the pressure in the normal LES, whereas carbohydrate in the diet has little effect. In contrast, protein intake in the diet may increase the LES pressure. These simple facts have an important bearing on the type of food that rests well in the stomach. The other simple fact is that overeating will tend to cause rising pressure in the stomach that will promote the backwash of gastric contents. Adding these observations together, it is prudent for the person with reflux to eat low-fat, proteinaceous meals (preferably vegetable protein) in modest amounts with the avoidance of caffeine-containing beverages, fizzy drinks, alcohol, and agents that are direct irritants on the esophagus, such as orange, cranberry, or tomato juice. One other frequent pleasure best avoided is chocolate. Chocolate contains compounds called methylxanthines that can act like drugs to lower the LES pressure and promote reflux. The veteran refluxer will not thank anyone for after-dinner chocolates.

Several drugs or agents found in the diet can have a pharmacological action (druglike effect) on the LES. This circumstance is easily overlooked. It is well recognized that smoking causes a reduction in pressure in the LES and provokes reflux. Alcohol relaxes the LES, but certain types of alcoholic beverages have the added effect of irritating the gullet in some people. Notable culprits are red wine and some of the more pleasant liqueurs such as Drambuie and Crème de Menthe. Crème de Menthe is a particular problem because it contains peppermint, which relaxes smooth muscle and lowers the LES pressure. Furthermore, the liqueur is a direct irritant, and the alcohol content itself lowers the LES pressure. I have yet to find a person with heartburn who can tolerate Crème de Menthe!

Many drugs or natural agents that tranquilize or relax the body can also cause the same effects on the upper gastrointestinal tract. The occurrence of heartburn and constipation in the depressed individual who is placed on tricyclic antidepressants can cause concern for patients and occasional bewilderment for the psychiatrist. Many drugs used to treat depression have an effect that interferes with certain types of nerves called cholinergic nerves. Predictably this is called an anticholinergic effect. Cholinergic nerves supply many organs in the body, including the heart and digestive tract. Inhibition of these cholinergic nerves that supply the gut causes reductions in pressure of the LES, thereby promoting reflux, and they can delay the emptying of the stomach. Delaying the emptying of the stomach causes food and fluid to hang around longer in the stomach, and the stomach contents remain available longer for reflux. Antidepressant drugs with anticholinergic effects can also inhibit bowel movements and cause constipation, as well as more generalized side effects like a dry mouth, rapid heart rate, and blurred vision. The gastrointestinal side effects of antidepressants (especially tricyclic drugs) are a common reason for people to stop taking their medication.

MANAGEMENT OF GERD

The management of GERD involves accurate diagnosis, assessment of the severity of the disorder, and appropriate medical therapy. The main goals of treatment include prompt relief of symptoms, the healing of esophagitis, and steps to change the clinical cause of the disorder over time. In particular, the avoidance of complications of GERD, such as narrowing of the esophagus and the development of changes in the lining cells of the esophagus, which predispose to cancer, must be avoided.

We have reviewed some of the principal factors that cause GERD, but many complex mechanisms operate (Table 4.1).

Table 4.1: Factors involved in the pathogenesis causation of gastroesophageal reflux disease (GERD).

Antireflux barrier	Decreases pressure in lower esophageal sphincter (LES) Intraabdominal segment of esophagus Angle of entry of esophagus Mucosal rosette Transient LES relaxation Gradient between stomach and esophagus Hiatal hernia?
Gastric factors	Gastric secretion Gastric emptying delay Duodenogastric reflux (pepsin, bile) Volume of ingested meals
Motor disorders	Delayed clearance of acid, pepsin, or bile Weak peristatic contraction
General defense	Factors that determine antireflux barrier Mucus Squamous, mucosal integrity Saliva Regenerative ability of squamous mucosa

CAUSES OF GERD

GERD occurs as a result of prolonged contact of refluxed gastric or duodenal contents (or both) with the lining of the distal esophagus. The causation of GERD can be considered a disruption of the delicate balance between aggressive factors (e.g., acid reflux) and mucosal (lining) defense mechanisms in the lower esophagus (Table 4.1). Acid contact in the lower esophagus is a key determinant of esophagitis that is related to the frequency, duration, and volume of fluid that is refluxed from the stomach. Changes in the gastroesophageal antireflux mechanisms in GERD are commonly associated with reduced pressure in the LES. Recently, inappropriate transient relaxation of the lower esophageal sphincter has been identified as a major cause of repeated reflux, but the neurohormonal and other physiological variables that contribute to this relaxation of the sphincter are poorly defined. Abnormal movements in the upper gastrointestinal tract may result in prolonged contact of refluxed material due to reduced clearance of this material as a consequence of impaired peristalsis or contractions (clearance mechanism) in the lower esophagus. In addition, delayed gastric emptying may result in a large volume of fluid available for reflux, especially following meals.

Much attention has been focused on acid as an aggressive factor in GERD,but the presence of bile and proteolytic (protein splitting) enzymes that originate in the duodenum plays a role. Indeed, suppression of acid secretion with histamine (H_2) receptor antagonists has become the mainstay of medial management of GERD, but not all cases respond to this therapy. This has led to the use of more powerful types of acid-inhibiting drugs called proton pump inhibitors, of which the drug omeprazole is a classic example.

MEDICAL TREATMENT OF GERD

The range of severity of GERD has led to a proposed staged lifestyle and drug treatment plan for this disorder. Gravitational infleunces have been stressed frequently as important in the management of patients with GERD; controlled clinical observations have indicated that elevation of the head of the bed together with administration of an acid-lowering drug (H_2-receptor antagonist) is significantly more beneficial than the administration of an H_2-receptor antagonist alone.

General patient advice that helps to decrease in the pressure gradient between the stomach and the esophagus is often highly effective. For example, patients should be advised to flex their knees and crouch rather than stoop during exercise; tight-fitting garments should be avoided; and exercise-induced reflux, which may occur during aerobic exercise or sexual intercourse, may be dealt with by prior administration of an antacid or correction of posture. The role of obesity in the causation of GERD remains poorly defined, but many patients may report accelerated weight gain in the period prior to symptomatic presentation. Weight reduction is advisable for obese patients and may result in a lower pressure gradient between the stomach and the esophagus.

Several agents, including orange juice, tomato juice, and certain alcoholic beverages, exacerbate reflux symptoms by a direct irritant action. Effective management of a patient with GERD requires an understanding of the factors that influence LES pressure. These neurohormonal controls (and molecules of emotion or drugs or substances of abuse) are summarized in Table 4.2).

Table 4.2: Agents that influence the pressure of the lower esophageal sphincter (LES).

INCREASE PRESSURE	DECREASE PRESSURE
Gastrin (pentagastrin)	Secretin
Motilin	Glucagon
Prostaglandin (F2)	Prostaglandin E1, E2, A2, I2
•Substance P	Vasoactive intestinal peptide
Cholinergic agents	Anticholinergic agents
Vasopressin	Gastric inhibitory peptides
Anticholinesterase agents	Progesterone
Histamine (H1)	Histamine (H2)
Metoclopramide	Dopamine
Domperidone	Fat
Antacids	Chocolate
Protein meals	Alcohol
Indomethacin	Theophylline
	Caffeine
	Smoking
	Calcium-blocking drugs
	Meperidine

REAPPRAISAL OF GERD THERAPY

Given the introduction of omeprazole and other similar drugs into clinical practice, it is time to reappraise the use of H_2-receptor antagonists in the treatment of GERD. It appears appropriate to stage antisecretory intervention in the treatment of GERD in a manner similar to that in which the overall therapy of GERD is staged. The key to selecting an appropriate antisecretory medication is now dependent on an assessment of the severity of disease, which will determine therapeutic intervention. For the treatment of mild to moderate reflux esophagitis, H_2-receptor antagonists appear to be safe and efficacious, and they achieve acceptable levels of symptomatic relief and, probably, healing. Overall, it seems reasonable to prescribe an H_2-receptor antagonist for patients without severe esophagitis if antacids or other interventions have failed.

Early-stage treatment for GERD may involve the administration of antacid preparations or alginates. It is interesting that despite the widespread use of antacids in the management of GERD, clinical evidence of any major benefit derived from their administration is lacking. Except in mild cases, antacids can be considered only an adjunct to the symptomatic relief of heartburn. To date, H_2-receptor antagonists have become the mainstay of treatment for significant GERD.

Omeprazole seems to be ideally suited for the treatment of patients with severe esophagitis or for those who have recalcitrant symptoms, in whom investigations have excluded other disorders (e.g., esophageal infections or cancer). Whether omeprazole therapy is beneficial in the management of complications of esophagitis (e.g., peptic stricture, Barrett's epithelium) remains to be further clarified. However, omeprazole may heal Barrett's esophagus. It appears that omeprazole and other substituted benzimidazole drugs (types of proton pump inhibiting drugs) are being used more freely in the treatment of all acid-related disease in the upper gastrointestinal tract. However, the use of such potent acid reducing drugs so frequently could be questioned. Are physicians using a sledgehammer to crack a nut?

Our understanding of factors that may predict which patients may respond to various therapeutic interventions remains inadequate. It appears clear that the degree of esophagitis is an important determinant of the outcome of therapy, with severe forms being more resistant to treatment. There is a suggestion that patients who fail to have diminution in the frequency or duration of acid reflux, as a result of antisecretory medication are those who may not respond adequately to H_2-receptor antagonists.

Although it is difficult to predict who will respond to medical treatment, it is equally difficult to predict which patients may have recurrence of symptoms. However, clinical research has indicated that patients with low pressure in the LES and those with severe forms of esophagitis may relapse more frequently. It is interesting that we may have been somewhat misled in our belief that low-dose H_2-receptor-antagonist therapy may prevent relapse. Furthermore, successful healing of erosive esophagitis (severe esophageal inflammation) with some objective improvement in the pressure in the LES is not consistently associated with a reduction in relapse of GERD. Further investigations are required to define patients who may tend to relapse so that adequate therapy can be instituted in such circumstances.

In the absence of predictors of recurrence, how do we manage GERD that has a tendency to recur when medical treatment has stopped? Because we are uncertain about how long medical treatment should be continued to induce remission, and because the natural history of the condition GERD is variable, it appears reasonable to institute a short course of maximum treatment (approximately two months) and to use pulsed therapy when relapse occurs.

If medical treatment rarely produces long-term cure of the symptoms of reflux, what is the place of surgery? There is no general agreement about the indications for antireflux surgery—even in the presence of peptic stricture of the esophagus. Though a hiatus hernia predisposes to reflux, it does not make it inevitable. Only when such a hernia is large and is causing mechanical problems is it an indication for surgery. Attempts to assess the severity of GERD by using such criteria as endoscopic findings, pH studies, and other tests have shown that these do not correlate well with the outcome of surgery. The combination of the lack of accepted predictors of successful outcome and the knowledge of the potential adverse effects of surgery accounts for the difficulty in deciding about surgical intervention and its timing.

The surgeon's aim in treating reflux disease is to correct any substantial hiatus defect, to restore the intraabdominal esophagus, to potentiate the efficacy of the LES, and, if possible, to improve the efficacy of the crural sling and the mucosal flap valve. These goals have to be achieved without impairing esophageal emptying. Most techniques use some form of fundic (upper stomach) wrap around the esophagus, either partial or complete; the most widely used is Nissen fundoplication. This technique of fundoplication has been said to control reflux symptoms in over 75 percent of cases, but in large series of patients other adverse effects have resulted in less than half of those treated being completely free of symptoms. Sometimes the surgery required is major, and reoperation for unsatisfactory results has been associated with great risk.

Perhaps the general lack of confidence among surgeons in the commonly performed surgical antireflux procedures (Nissen, Hil, and Belsey) was shown a few years ago by the enthusiasm with which the Angelchik antireflux prosthesis was adopted. The role of this device is contentious; it has been abandoned.

Optimizing the results of fundoplication seems to be a job for the highly skilled, experienced, and specialized surgeon. This should not preclude the development of simple and technically reproducible operations based on sound physiological principles. Endoscopic methods for preventing reflux are appealing but require much development. Doctors will undoubtedly use more omeprazole, and this may reduce the number of antireflux operations in a similar manner to the reduction of peptic ulcer operations that occurred as a result of the introduction of cimetidine tagamet, twenty years ago.

The outcome of drug and surgical therapy for reflux is inconsistent and may prompt some to examine alternative approaches, despite their equally inconsistent outcome.

NATURAL THERAPIES FOR GERD

Natural approaches to the management of mild degrees of GERD are to be commended. A balanced diet and the avoidance of offending foods is important. The management of significant GERD cannot be undertaken with predictable success by alternative medical strategies. Lifestyle adjustments are important in the management of GERD but several herbal agents and belladonna extracts are outdated for clinical use. Botanical alternative therapies such as licorice and probiotic therapy with friendly bacteria lead to unpredictable outcomes. In general, alternative medicine affords little that is specifically helpful for GERD—at least at present.

LARYNGITIS DUE TO REFLUX

A lot of people suffer from an intermittent, often mild forms of inflammation of the larynx (laryngitis), which is often ascribed to a temporary infection. Laryngitis, however, is clearly associated with GERD, but the mechanism of damage to the larynx is not clear. The link between laryngeal disorders and GERD was first described at the turn of the twentieth century by Dr. L. Coffin, but this brilliant observation lay essentially dormant in medical thinking until the 1960s.

The common symptoms associated with inflammation of the voice box (larynx) are a husky voice (hoarseness), squeaky voice (vocal fatigue), chronic cough or throat clearing, and even a globus sensation. Of course, all of these symptoms are very well explained in terms of chronic smoking, but smoking worsens GERD and strongly predisposes a person to throat cancer.

Reflux laryngitis is one example of several conditions linked to GERD. Others include: stenosis (narrowing) of the glottis, contact ulcers from acid, spasm of laryngeal muscles, laryngeal nodules, and possibly laryngeal cancer. Recent data suggest that careful control of reflux is required in the condition of reflux laryngitis, and this circumstance seems to be a clear indication for the use of potent acid-blocking drugs (high doses of H_2-receptor antagonists or the use of proton pump inhibitors, such as omeprazole).

DEPRESSION: THE ULTIMATE CAUSE OF SAD GUTS

Depression itself causes stress, which can provoke reflux and a general slowing down of the guts. Depression teaches us about the power of the mind-gut interaction. In this disorder, the function of the guts reflects the mood. In fact, one very common presentation of depression to a doctor is the occurrence of abnormal digestive symptoms.

It is unfortunate that the most commonly used therapies for depression may actually aggravate the effects of depression, per se, on the guts. No wonder some patients reject certain antidepressant medication and some prefer their state of mild depression instead of the side effects of tricyclic antidepressant drugs. This may be one of many reasons for the galloping popularity of natural treatments such as St. John's Wort (referred to popularly as nature's blues buster).

The reaction of the guts to medication can make the treatment worse than the disease. It is not just antidepressants that cause gut side effects. Minor tranquilizers such as benzodiazepine drugs (e.g., Valium and Librium) and sleeping tablets can cause reductions in LES pressure and promote reflux. Sleeping tablets are usually taken at night, when most people will be lying down. This is just the time when reflux is worse! Many studies, including those of my colleagues and I, have shown the relationship between acid damage to the esophagus and reflux in the supine position.

A pernicious cause of gastrointestinal problems are some drugs that are used in the treatment of cardiovascular disease. Many drugs that are used to lower blood pressure in people with hypertension can cause unpleasant gut symptoms. A group of drugs that are called calcium-channel-blocking drugs are used often in the treatment of coronary heart disease and hypertension. These drugs work by blocking calcium entry into cells and cause smooth muscle relaxation. Blocking calcium entry into cells can relax cardiac (heart) muscle and smooth muscle in blood vessels, which is the desired effect in the treatment of cardiovascular disease. However, these calcium-channel-blocking drugs are potent relaxants of smooth muscle in the upper gastrointestinal tract and they are effective at abolishing the high-pressure zone of the LES, that guards the junction of the stomach and esophagus. Incidentally, certain plant essential oils (e.g., peppermint and fennel) contain anetholes and menthol that are natural calcium-channel-blocking agents.

Classic examples of calcium-blocking-drugs are nifedipine and diltiazem. When these drugs are given to control cardiac chest pain (angina), they can cause reflux that itself can cause heartburn or occasional chest pain. There are some patients with coronary artery disease that have increased chest pain with the use of calcium-channel-blocking drugs. This pain is relieved sometimes by stopping the drug, especially when the added pain is caused by reflux (GERD), that is induced by the calcium-channel-blocking drug. It is notable that calcium channel blocking drugs have found a role in the treatment of esophageal spasm. This condition is a serious functional disorder where the esophagus goes into a spastic phase of contraction causing pain and dysphagia. My colleagues and I showed in the late 1970s that the calcium blocker nifedipine was useful in the treatment of esophageal spasm. Dilute pepermint oil may have a similar effect.

OBESITY, HIATUS, HERNIA, AND GERD

It has been suspected for years that obese people tend to have more problems with GERD, but these relationships were clarified only recently by Dr.'s Wilson, Wenzhou and Hirschowitz (*American Journal of Gastroenterology*, 94, 10:2840–2844, 1999). These physicians have shown that obesity is an independent risk factor for hiatal hernia and esophagitis. This association seems to occur more often in whites than African Americans.

It has surprised many patients and physicians that gastroenterologists have not become more vested in the management of obesity. The control of body weight is very important in GERD and other aspects of general health.

THE HEART OR THE GUT?

The heart and the lower esophagus lie together in the lower chest. Pain from both of these organs is often experienced in the same place behind the breastbone. Therefore, pain from the heart is often confused with pain from the esophagus and vice versa. More important, up to one half of all mature people with coronary heart disease and angina may have GERD, and perhaps as many as 10 percent of mature people with GERD may have coronary artery disease. The characteristics of pain from the heart usually differ from those of pain arising from GERD, but on occasion the gullet can go into spasm and produce a pain that is indistinguishable from angina.

The heart carries a special charisma in medicine as *the* vital organ in the body, but other organs are equally vital for life. However, the perception of the vitality and indispensability of the heart occupies the minds of both physicians and patients. This is reflected in medical approaches to the diagnosis of chest pain, where it is always seen as a priority to confirm or exclude the heart as a source of chest pain. I am not minimizing the significance of heart disease, but I am proposing that preoccupations can sometimes lead to expensive testing and treatment failures.

The average person with chest pain usually thinks about the heart as the primary source of the pain. However, there are many structures within the chest that can cause pain sometimes similar to cardiac pain. Most notable is the occurrence of spasm in the esophagus (esophageal colic). As previously mentioned, in the lower chest the esophagus touches the back of the heart and therefore, problems in heart or esophagus emanate from the same anatomic location. A source of pain that is quite common and often overlooked is the chest wall, which consists of a complicated series of joints, muscles, and ligaments. Pain and tenderness around the breastbone is sometimes called Tietze's syndrome or costochondritis.

Other less common causes of pain in the chest that do not originate from the heart include diseases of the lungs and abdominal conditions that are felt in the chest. There is a curious type of nonspecific chest pain that is described in heavy smokers. Of course, smoking is associated with diseases of the lungs, heart, and esophagus, but chest pain is sometimes experienced by smokers without evidence of disease in these organs. Surprisingly, it does not always respond to smoking cessation.

ESOPHAGEAL SPASM OR IRRITABLE ESOPHAGUS SYNDROME

There are a complex group of disorders of movement of the gullet that are termed esophageal motor disorders. A normal wave of contraction occurs in the esophagus to push food toward the stomach. This wave of contraction is propagated down the esophagus in a coordinated manner, and the esophagus facilitates the transfer of the bolus (lump) of food or fluid to the stomach by an apposition (moving together) of the walls of the esophageal tube. In simple terms, the walls have a sort of pinching mechanism to push the bolus down the esophagus. Gravity helps to facilitate the clearance of food or fluid down the esophagus, but a healthy gullet will empty efficiently even if a person is lying flat. Many an ancient Roman laid flat and symptom free during feasts and binges!

The peristaltic activity of the esophagus can become weak, feeble, or absent, but on occasion it can be forceful and squeezing, with contractions that produce a kind of colic. A sustained contraction in any part of the tubular portions of the guts can cause protracted colic. Colic generally gives rise to a severe pain that is often short-lived, lasting a few seconds to a couple of minutes. This sustained contraction or colic with severe chest pain gives rise to the disorder called esophageal spasm, which is a condition that is very often stress-related.

In cases of esophageal spasm, the esophagus may be more sensitive to all types of stimuli. The size, consistency and temperature of a swallowed bolus of food or fluid can alter the movements in the gullet and the speed of transit through the esophageal tube. Most people recognize the discomfort of swallowing large chunks of solid matter that have not been chewed or mixed with saliva. Good chomping (mastication) produces a lubricated bolus that can slide through the esophagus with ease. Larger-sized lumps of food produce measurable increases in the strength of contraction in the body of the esophagus. In esophageal spasm, any food can cause abnormal motor responses.

Hot fluids can irritate the esophagus, but ice-cold beverages can bounce around in the esophagus for a while (seconds to minutes), and they are effective at provoking spasm in the esophagus in susceptible individuals. The mechanism of this effect of cold beverages causing esophageal spasm is not known, but it is probably due to the direct effects of cold on the function of the muscle of the gullet. Such an effect can be reproduced in the laboratory by cooling strips of muscle that have been isolated from the esophagus of animals.

Some gastroenterologists have questioned the role of stress in the causation of esophageal spasm. However, there is no doubt that people with symptoms due to esophageal spasm have a worsening of their problems of chest pain and difficulty in swallowing during periods of emotional stress. My colleagues and I have measured pressure changes in the esophagus in normal individuals and patients with esophageal spasm. A definite relationship exists between high-pressure contractions in the esophagus and stress of different types (e.g. emotional upset and excitement), such as occurs during sexual intercourse. Some inconsistency of response to stress in the esophagus is observed but overall stress of all types "whips up" contractions in the responsive gullet.

STRESS AND SPASM IN THE GULLET

Contemporary observations of the ability of stress to alter the movements of the esophagus in healthy people confirm observations that were made over half a century ago by Dr. S. Wolf and Dr. T. P. Almy. These doctors reported studies in 1949 where they showed that the induction of stress caused increases in the number and force of measured contractions in the gullet. These contractions result sometimes in obstruction of the esophagus. Using x-ray techniques it can be shown that the passage of a radio-opaque medium (e.g., barium) through the esophagus can be delayed in states of stress.

There is a group of uncommon disorders of movement of the esophagus that may evolve in a proportion of patients who present with symptoms of esophageal spasm. These conditions are diagnosed by special pressure testing of the esophagus (with manometry), and they require carefully selected therapy with drugs or sometimes surgery by an expert. The prevalent type of these uncommon motor disorders is called achalasia, which is characterized by the failure of coordinated opening of the gullet sphincter (LES) and the absence of significant, propagated contractions or the presence of spasms in the body of the esophagus (vigorous achalasia).

Achalasia is an example of an uncommon but well-defined motor disorder of the gullet. This condition is due to disorders in the nerves supplying the lower esophagus. Achalasia is often progressive, and it commonly gives rise to difficulty in swallowing, which more often affects the swallowing of fluids than solids. In standard medical teaching, it is emphasized that obstruction in the esophagus from cancer or inflammation, causing narrowing (stricture), usually affects the swallowing of solids more than liquids. It is not thought that achalasia and its variants are caused by stress per se, but stress definitely makes the condition worse when it is established. In these motor disorders of the esophagus, degeneration of nervous tissue supplying the esophagus occurs, and stress facilitates the cause of unpleasant symptoms such as dysphagia and intermittent chest pain.

FUNCTIONAL VOMITING

In order for a person to throw up, the body has to cause an initial relaxation of the stomach. The stomach is then compressed within the abdomen by becoming squashed between the front wall of the abdomen and the diaphragm. The LES relaxes and the gastric contents are expelled with varying force through the esophagus into the mouth and nasal passages. The act of vomiting is often, but not always, preceded by nausea, hypersalivation, and retching. Dry heaves occur when most of the gastric contents have been expelled or in the initial phases of vomiting.

Some people can train themselves to vomit on demand, and others can easily promote vomiting by tickling the back of the throat with their fingers. Some babies seem to delight in this practice for no apparent reason. This trained vomiting is seen in eating disorders such as bulimia (characterized by overeating and vomiting).

Functional causes of vomiting are less frequent than organic causes. Almost any disease or adverse reaction experienced by the body can be associated with vomiting. The unpleasant act of vomiting is best approached during its occurrence by passivity. Attempts to restrain the act of vomiting can be dangerous. One important example of a need to go with the flow of vomiting is following excessive food or fluid intake, especially excessive alcohol intake. A state of intoxication with alcohol can often give rise to nausea and welcome vomiting. This act is the body's defense against excessive intake of alcohol, which in high doses is an effective poison. Unfortunately, vomiting that occurs when the senses are dulled (e.g., by alcohol intoxication) can result in respiratory obstruction and a risk of death due to inhaled vomit.

More serious damage to the esophagus with total rupture (splitting the full thickness of the wall of the esophagus) can be seen in the circumstance of violent vomiting, with or without a preceding binge. This condition is referred to commonly as von Boerhaave's syndrome, after the Lord High Admiral of the Dutch Navy who may have suffered this fatal event.

THE CHINESE RESTAURANT SYNDROME

Many people will experience a sweaty feeling after a Chinese meal. This is because Chinese food often contains monosodium glutamate (MSG). MSG is used as a preservative and flavor enhancer in Chinese and other foods, and it is capable of causing a rather complex array of symptoms. People who are very sensitive to MSG can experience tingling sensations, sweating, abdominal discomfort, rapid heartbeat and even severe short-lived chest pain with fainting. Diarrhea and abdominal pain are prominent features of more severe types of this disorder, which is sometimes called Kwok's Quease or MSG toxicity. Many restaurants now advertise MSG-free food because of the common and unpleasant side effects of MSG. A person with functional abdominal pain should search for MSG in his or her food and cut it out.

INTEGRATED ACTIVITIES IN THE GUT

The motor functions of the esophagus secure an orderly transit of food and fluid to the stomach. However, abnormal movements in the esophagus often go hand in hand with abnormal movements of other areas of the guts. We have learned that the body of the esophagus and junction of the esophagus with the stomach react to distant events in the guts. For example, the initiation of swallowing provokes events lower down in the esophagus.

It is recognized that people with reflux symptoms may have a delay in the rate at which their stomach empties. This leaves food around in the stomach for a long time following meals and promotes reflux of stomach contents into the esophagus. There are other examples of the complexities of the interrelationships between various parts of the gut, which in some circumstances is related to the fact that there are nerves, hormones, and other molecules of emotion that have effects on multiple parts of the gastrointestinal tract. There is a subset of patients with IBS that has coexisting symptoms of GERD and a subset that has dyspepsia or symptoms of functional stomach disorders in association with bowel complaints. As we move into the stomach in the next chapter, the importance of considering the guts as an integrated series of regions with connections and inter-actions will become more apparent.

CHAPTER SUMMARY

GERD is very common and it is effectively treated in the short term by potent acid-reducing drugs. Lifestyle factors are important in potentially changing the clinical course of reflux disease, which, if left untreated, can cause permanent damage to the esophagus and a pre-disposition to esophageal cancer. The esophagus is very responsive in the body-mind link, and holistic medicine has a great deal to offer, even though specific herbal or botanical agents have not been identi-fied as reliable therapy for esophageal disorders.

CHAPTER FIVE

THE
EMOTIONAL
STOMACH

THE STOMACH RECEIVES THE FOOD

Anatomically the stomach is connected to the upper portions of the small bowel called the duodenum. Therefore, many disorders in this area are referred to as gastroduodenal because of the intimate relationship between the distal (terminal) portions of the stomach (gastro) and the upper small intestine (duodenum). Everyone is aware at some time of bloating in the upper abdomen, belching, and the presence of pain around the area of the solar plexus (upper abdomen or epigastrium). Pain that is indistinguishable from the type of pain experienced by a person with an ulcer of the stomach or duodenum can be functional in origin. This functional problem has been called non-ulcer dyspepsia—that is, upper abdominal complaints in the absence of an ulcer that are similar to ulcer symptoms.

Nonulcer dyspepsia is another example of a functional upset of the guts that is a diagnosis that is most often made by the exclusion of ulcer or other disease. People with persistent nonulcer dyspepsia who seek a medical consultation will inevitably receive several tests on their upper guts. Often, these tests may not reveal structural problems or disease. The medical investigations used in the diagnosis of dyspepsia often include at least an x-ray (barium meal), and probably an endoscopy (gastroscopy). Endoscopy involves the passage of a lighted tube through the mouth into the upper reaches of the gut.

This tube (the endoscope) permits a doctor to visualize the lining of the upper digestive tract. In many circumstances dyspepsia patients receive a test on their gall bladder, such as ultrasound. Pain from the gall bladder is sometimes indistinguishable from pain originating in the stomach or duodenum (See chapter 13).

There is a type of upper abdominal discomfort that has been called dyspepsia due to dysmotility (disordered movement of the stomach or duodenum). This sounds complicated but it is quite simple. Motility in the guts means movement of the guts. If movement in the stomach or the intestines is abnormal, then food or fluid is not pushed along the tubular digestive tract in an efficient manner. In the case of abnormal movement of the stomach (gastric dysmotility), then food or fluid hangs up in the stomach. A delay in the emptying of the stomach often produces bloating and pain in the upper abdomen. This simple relation between failure of the stomach to empty and the presence of symptoms of pain or bloating in the upper abdomen is easy to understand. However, when one tries to measure the rate at which the stomach empties and relate it to the presence of symptoms, there is not always a viable relationship between abnormal movement and the symptoms of hang up of food or fluid in the stomach.

This unclear situation, together with other mismatches in the relationships between symptoms and tests of gut function, has caused some doctors to deny the importance of abnormal stomach movement (dysmotility), as a well-defined cause of dyspepsia. However, the general consensus is that when the stomach does not empty properly, then an individual will tend to have symptoms of dyspepsia. This situation can be relieved often by lifestyle adjustments or the use of medication or natural interventions that facilitate the emptying of the stomach.

OBSERVATIONS OF AN EMOTIONAL STOMACH

The healthy stomach is a kind of bag that receives food, mixes it with acid to initiate the process of digestion, and then empties its contents in a controlled way in the upper reaches of the small intestine (duodenum). Anger and strong emotion affect the blood flow, movements, and secretions of the stomach. Resting the mind rests the stomach. This is evidenced by the changes in the activity of the stomach that can be induced by relaxation, hypnosis, and acupuncture. There is a long and colorful history surrounding the studies of relation between the brain and the stomach. Some of the most important observations on the functions of the stomach were made more than one hundred fifty years ago by an American physician, Dr. William Beaumont. I go back this far in medicine not because of historical sentimentality, but more to show how the medical profession cannot always learn their own lessons.

Dr. Beaumont studied the exposed stomach of Alexis St. Martin, a fur trapper from Canada. St. Martin was wounded in the abdomen and chest by a musket in June of 1822. Dr. Beaumont treated St. Martin's wound when he was in the service of the American army. The surgery left St. Martin's stomach permanently exposed and visible on the abdominal wall so it could easily be studied. Over a period of many years, Dr. Beaumont was able to experiment on Mr. St. Martin and study the movements and secretions of his stomach by direct observations under a variety of circumstances.

So protracted and complete were Dr. Beaumont's studies on St. Martin's stomach that these studies formed the basis of an entire book entitled *Experiments and Observations on the Gastric Juice and the Physiology of Digestion*, printed by F. P. Allen in Plattsburgh, Pennsylvania, in 1833 (reproduced by Oxford Historical Books, Abingdon, Oxon, England, UK, 1989). This book would have been perhaps better titled "Looking through a Hole in Alexis St. Martin's Stomach."

Dr. Beaumont made some very important observations about the human stomach. In 1833, he was able to make fifty-one significant conclusions about the workings of the stomach, which he was modest enough to describe as "inferences." These conclusions are the focus of continuing modern-day research. He noted the importance of the differences in the way the human stomach handles solid and liquid food, and his obsession with gastric juice (stomach acid and some enzymes) permitted an understanding of its pivotal role in health. The lesson about the importance of gastric acid for health has been somewhat forgotten in the modern era of popping pills that eliminate acid from the stomach. These pills include the most frequently taken drugs in Western society (e.g., Zantac, Tagamet, Pepcid, Axid, Losec, Prilosec, etc.).

Despite Beaumont's descriptions of the stomach during periods of anger and rage experienced by St. Martin, these observations did not figure prominently in Beaumont's list of fifty-one inferences. However, in the prelude to the reporting of the experiments, Beaumont makes some powerful statements that summarize a great deal about the effects of emotion on the stomach.

BEAUMONT: OF SATISFACTION AND SATIETY

Beaumont recognized the negative health consequences of the "theory of excess." In simple terms, if you eat too much, you may be likely to drink too much, smoke too much, lie around too long, work too much, play too much, etc. Beaumont's work is so replete with messages for modern medicine in its dealings with indigestion and dyspepsia that I highly recommend that the modern, high-tech-oriented physician take a moment to glance at Beaumont's writings.

Dr. Beaumont stated in 1833:

> In the present state of civilized society, with the provocation of the culinary art, and the incentives of high seasoned food, brandy and wines, the temptations to excess in the indulgence of the table are rather too strong to be resisted by poor human nature. It is not less the duty, however, of the watchmen on the walls to warn the city of its danger, however in may regard the premonition. Let them at least clear their own skirts from the stain of unfaithfulness, whatever may be the result.
>
> There is no subject of dietetic economy about which people err so much, as that which relates to *quantity*. The medical profession, too, have been accessory to this error, in giving directions to dyspeptics to eat until a sense of satiety is felt. Now, this feeling, so essential to be rightly understood, never supervenes until the invalid has eaten too much, if he have an appetite, which seldom fails him. Those, even, who are not otherwise predisposed to the complaint, frequently induce a diseased state of the digestive organs by too free indulgence of the appetite. Of this fact the medical pro-

fession are, generally, not sufficiently aware. Those who lead sedentary lives, and whose circumstances will permit of what is called free
living, are peculiarly obnoxious to these complaints. But by paying
particular attention to their sensations during the ingestion of their
meals, these complaints may be avoided. There appears to be a
sense of perfect intelligence conveyed from the stomach to the
encephalic centre, which, in health, invariable dictates what quantity of ailment (responding to the sense of hunger, and its due satisfaction,) is naturally required for the purposes of life; and which, if
noticed, and properly attended to, would prove the most salutary
monitor of health, and effectual preventive of, and restorative from,
disease. It is not the sense of *satiety*, for this is beyond the point of
healthful indulgence, and is nature's earliest indication of an *abuse*
and *overburden* of her powers to replenish the system. It occurs
immediately previous to this, and may be known by the pleasurable
sensation of *perfect satisfaction, ease and quiescence of body and
mind.* It is when the stomach says *enough*, and is distinguished from
satiety by the difference of the sensations—the former feeling
enough—the latter, *too much.* The first is produced by the timely
reception into the stomach of proper aliment, in exact proportion to
the requirements of nature, for the perfect digestion of which, a definite quantity of gastric juice is furnished by the proper gastric appa-
ratus. But to effect this most agreeable of all sensations and conditions—the real Elysian satisfaction of the *reasonable* Epicure—timely attention must be paid to the preliminary processes, such as thor-
ough mastication, and moderate or slow deglutition. These are indis-
pensable to the due and natural supply of the stomach, at the stated
periods of alimentation; for if food be swallowed too fast, and pass
into the stomach imperfectly masticated, too much is received in a
short time, and in too imperfect a state of preparation, to be dis-
posed of by the gastric juice.

Beaumont also noted: "I consider myself but a humble inquirer
after truth—a simple experimenter. And if I have been led to conclusion
opposite to the opinions of many who have been considered the great
luminaries of physiology, and, in some instances, from all the professors
of this science, I hope the claim of sincerity will be conceded to me,
when I say that such difference of opinion has been forced upon me by
the convictions of experiment, and the fair deductions of reasoning."

Notice the timidity with which Dr. Beaumont was informing his
colleagues about the errors of their ways and understanding. In the
nineteenth century and earlier, the questioning of prevailing medical

bodies of opinion by anyone was at least equally as hazardous as it may be as we enter this millennium.

Beaumont related that many prevailing thoughts of the early nineteenth century about the functioning of the stomach were screwed up. He pointed to the direct evidence of a strong relationship between the guts and the mind. He was pointing a way to recognize the obvious impact of adverse lifestyle habits on gut function, but he was notable in his lack of attempts to look for a quick fix. I believe that Beaumont was proposing alternatives in the management of digestive disturbances by pointing out the links between excesses in life and the powerful effects that these choices had on the functioning of the human stomach. Indeed, Beaumont was talking about issues that we are beginning to readdress with our newfound knowledge of neurohormonal controls.

The next great contributions to our understanding about the function of the human stomach came from the work of Walter Cannon, M.D. in the early part of the twentieth century, but it was three physicians, doctors Ivey, Grossman, and Bachrach, who were the last great crusaders, prior to the explosion in pharmaceutical research and its domination of medicine after the Second World War. These doctors focused their attention on the causation of peptic ulcer in the classic book entitled *Peptic Ulcer* (York, Pennsylvania: The Blakiston Company, Maple Press Co., 1950).

Dr. A. C. Ivey and his colleagues elected to discuss dyspepsia and indigestion by indicating that it was foreign to the purpose of their book to give a complete account of these disorders. I find this strange because fifty years ago one could not be entirely sure whether or not one was treating dyspepsia in the presence or absence of an ulcer! The symptoms of these disorders (peptic-ulcer-induced dyspepsia or dyspepsia without an ulcer) are indistinguishable by a consideration of symptoms alone. Furthermore, I believe that much of the indigestion treated these days is somewhere between an ulcer and dyspepsia, if one roughly defines dyspepsia as a functional disorder; meaning abdominal pain in the absence of readily identifiable disease or overt structural or tissue problems in the stomach or duodenum.

Doctors Ivey, Grossman, and Bachrach referred to dyspepsia in 1950 as a group of symptoms that would suggest to a physician that the stomach or duodenum (upper part of the small intestine) is not functioning properly. We shall see later in this book how our ideas have not advanced much from this position over the past fifty years. These three wise men talked about four types of dyspepsia, modern researchers talk about at least five types and our medical experts who met in Rome in 1990 to define functional diseases of the guts talked about even more types!

There is a type of dyspepsia where the symptoms of digestive upset in the upper abdomen are cause by some reflex mechanism elsewhere. Hence, an upset of the kidneys, gallbladder, colon, or other organs in more distant locations can cause dyspepsia. Of course, dyspepsia can be due to any major illness or upset. For example, when one experiences flu or pneumonia, nausea and upper abdominal discomfort can prevail without evidence of structural disorders in the stomach or duodenum. Even a bang on the head often makes people feel sick to their stomach!

WHAT CAUSES THE DIFFERENT TYPES OF DYSPEPSIA?

Our three wise men (Ivey, Grossman, and Bachrach) indicated that prior to 1930, between one in five and one in ten cases of dyspepsia were due to ulcer and the rest were due to reflex (not reflux) causes or general disease or functional causes. In fact, about one in four causes of dyspepsia in those days was said to be due to functional causes, meaning the absence of overt disease to account for the dyspepsia. The exact occurrence of functional dyspepsia in the 1990s is difficult to define, but depending on the source of information, it is present in anything from one in four to three in four cases of all causes of dyspepsia. I believe that the realistic situation is that about three quarters of all cases of dyspepsia are due to functional causes. Again, we recognize that cases of functional disease of the guts are more common than organic disorders.

Classic medical teaching would have us believe that there are at least two types of functional dyspepsia. I reiterate that our men in Rome, who looked for definitions and criteria, discussed many more types of functional dyspepsia, but how constructive their definitions have been remains contentious. Dr. Ivey and his colleagues recognized dietary habit dyspepsia and psychoneurotic dyspepsia. What were they really talking about?

First, dietary habit dyspepsia provokes a reaction of déjà vu to the observations of Dr. Beaumont more than one hundred years earlier. It surprises me that Dr. Ivey and his colleagues thought that this type of dyspepsia was due in part to "unhygienic habits." Even the most anti-septic person gets dyspepsia! It is no surprise that bad eating habits were highlighted as a cause of dyspepsia by the three wise men. The variability in the tolerance of certain individuals for overeating or dietary indiscretion is important to consider. A powerful but simple message emerges. Adverse lifestyle, in many cases due to poor diet, causes illness both in the short and long term. Now, we enter the realm of holistic care. This information may be enough to stop some sufferers of dyspepsia from reading one more word in this book!

The discussions of psychoneurotic dyspepsia in the medical liter-ature have been amusing, intriguing, often very valuable, and some-times worthless. We are not strangers to the power of the mind over the stomach and duodenum. Dr. Ivey and his colleagues introduced and referred to terms like *gastric neurosis, dyspepsia of chronic nerv-ous exhaustion, nervous indigestion, chronic non-ulcerative dyspepsia, functional dyspepsia*, and, believe it or not, *dyspepsia of the constitu-tionally inadequate*.

DYSPEPSIA OF THE CONSTITUTIONALLY INADEQUATE

In this label, we can use see how classifying disease can result in bar-riers to appropriate therapy. The acceptance of the notion of consti-tutional inadequacy is so judgmental that a healthcare giver who sub-scribes to this kind of idea could become quite nihilistic. Believe it or not, there is still a little bit of the old guard in medicine that recog-nizes the notion of constitutional inadequacy, especially when dealing with psychiatric illness. If the constitution is wrong, does that mean that no intervention can work? To the nihilistic physician or patient, the answer is yes! This is nonsensical thinking.

There is an important concept in medicine involving the idea of the seed and the soil. The seed, for the sake of the present discussion, is the agent or factor that causes the disease, for example, a virus or a toxin. The soil is the body or organ of the body, that is the site of the disease where the seed germinates. A farmer knows that a seed will not grow in bad or ill-prepared ground. Prepare the stomach by insulting it with toxins and any seed will grow, if you throw enough seeds you will get some to grow . . . the concept goes on! I discuss this analogy of seed and soil because it returns us to natural concepts and the idea of nature's balance in the promotion of health.

We act like kamakazi farmers every time we pop an irritant pill or drink alcohol excessively. Anyone who gobbles a few aspirins or nonsteroidal anti-inflammatory drugs (NSAIDs like ibuprofen, naproxen, suldinac, etc.) will damage their stomach. Gobbling too many of these seeds will result in the growth of an ulcer. We are able to characterize the adverse effects of aspirin and NSAID as a major public health concern. These drugs have frequent, serious, and sometimes life-threatening effects on the stomach and duodenum (and lower bowel, liver, and kidneys!).

ENVIRONMENTAL STRESS AND DYSPEPSIA

There have been several population studies to show that stress can cause grumbling guts. A number of studies of the effect of stress on dyspepsia of all causes have been performed among members of military forces. Cumulatively, these studies show a definite relationship between the stress of being a combat soldier and both organic and functional gastrointestinal upset, including such conditions as IBS, nonulcer dyspepsia, and peptic ulcer disease.

During times of crisis, hospital admission rates for peptic ulcer complications and symptoms increase. Several scientific studies have shown such trends during stressful events such as the air raids and bombings of the Second World War and the stock market collapse in Hong Kong in 1987. Dr. H. Tidy, an English physician, published some interesting results on the medical effects of stress in the population in 1945, in an article *British Medical Journal* entitled "The Incidence of Peptic Ulcer at St. Thomas's Hospital" (*British Medical Journal*, Vol. I, 319, 1945). Dr. Tidy's work memorializes the impact of stress on gut disease. He recognized the mind-body interaction to be complex in his statement: "psychoneurotic stimuli may pull the trigger [referring to peptic ulcer complications], but some other hand has previously loaded the gun."

LOADING THE GUN

If you do not treat your pet dog well, it is likely to bite you. The same applies to your own stomach. Our diet is loaded with the wrong things, and we may even eat too much of the right thing. The balance of health rests with lifestyle choices, and we are all tired of being told that Western diets are disease provoking. Perhaps this mind-set is stopping some people from improving their nutrition.

The habits of the twentieth century, including smoking and a greater consumption of alcohol, drugs, and caffeine, have played a major role in the causation of dyspepsia. Our pal *Helicobactor pylori* is at the root of a lot of dyspeptic symptoms but this bacterium (microorganism) is quite opportunistic. Insult the gastroduodenum or debilitate the body and *Helicobacter pylori* will take hold. Many factors tax the resistance of the lining of the guts to maintain its health and integrity.

HELICOBACTER PYLORI

The bacterium *Helicobacter pylori* is clearly recognized as playing a major causative role in chronic gastritis, peptic ulcer (stomach and duodenum), and the development of gastric cancer. Dr. Barry Marshall and his colleague Dr. J. Robin Warren from Australia discovered the association of HP with dyspepsia in the early 1980s and since then, scientists have toiled to explain the mechanisms of the damaging effect of *Helicobacter pylori*.

In general, *H. pylori* does not act like a virulent infectious agent— it sits beneath the mucus layer of the stomach mainly where it goes about its business of creating havoc with the lining of the upper digestive tract. How does it create this havoc?

H. pylori causes immune responses, which result in inflammatory processes to rid the body of the organism. A number of antibodies to *H. pylori* are readily detected and measured. The most interesting observations, however, of the damaging effects of *H. pylori* relate to its ability to generate free radicals (or reactive oxygen species). Free radicals are discussed increasingly in conventional and alternative medicine as a primary cause of many acute and chronic diseases.

Many books describe the importance of free radicals as generators of disease. An understanding of free radicals involves a look at the role of oxygen in body tissues. Oxygen is necessary to sustain life but it can change its state and combine with body tissues causing oxidation. This is the general example of the free radical chain of oxidation, a circumstance that causes unwanted effects on tissues called oxidative damage.

The body has well-developed mechanisms to deal with small amounts of unstable oxygen molecules that cause oxidation and a number of chemicals in our diet can help prevent this unwanted oxidation. These chemicals are called antioxidants or free radical scavengers. Antioxidants are compounds that can break the unwanted chain of reactions involving free radicals (unstable oxygen species) and body tissues. A number of natural substances are powerful antioxidants. Examples include vitamin C, A, and E and a whole range of phytochemicals—substances found in plants, such as soy isoflavones, catechins in green tea, and curcumin from turmeric.

Returning to *H. pylori*, it can be shown in the laboratory that adding *H. pylori* to stomach lining cells results in the generation of free radicals or reactive oxygen species. This damage can be reversed by the addition of antioxidants such as superoxide dismutase, catalase and vitamin C. The degree of damage seen in the lining of the stomach bears a close relationship to the presence of inflammatory white cells that are attracted by chemicals secreted by *H. pylori*. It is known that these white cells are potent generators of free radicals. The chemistry of *H. pylori* that involves the generation of free radicals is quite complex but, overall, the most important issue is that the damage from *H. pylori* may be minimized by antioxidant use—a useful step that can provide added benefit to the conventional use of antibiotics combined with antisecretory drugs to eradicate *H. pylori*.

Predictably, levels of antioxidants such as vitamin C are found to be depleted in the stomach secretions of patients with gastritis. Vitamin C in secretions from stomachs infected with *H. pylori* is present mainly in a reduced or biologically inactive form. These findings have garnered great interest recently, but it is worth noting that similar observations were made almost thirty years ago by Dr. T. V. Taylor in Manchester, England—where individuals with complicated peptic ulcer disease were found to have low leucocyte levels of vitamin C in their blood.

An important issue in the treatment of *H. pylori* infections is that eradication of the organism, which is associated with indirect evidence of less free radical generation, results in a rise of vitamin C levels in gastric juice. The "antioxidant issues" in *H. pylori* infection are not clear cut because studies show that other antioxidant vitamins, notably vitamins A and E are found in normal amounts in the stomach infected by *H. pylori* and they do not appear to play a role in the protection of the stomach lining free from radical damage.

This whole area of nutritional research in *H. pylori* infection requires greater scrutiny. It provides some very interesting options for the application of remedies of natural origin and it helps explain indirectly another mechanism whereby why antioxidants are chemopreventive against cancer. To illuminate this issue, we know that *H. pylori* is associated with a risk of gastric cancer, and this risk may be due to free radical damage induced by *H. pylori*. The anticancer benefits of green tea, soy isoflavones and herbs like turmeric may be well explained by the actions of the antioxidants they contain—epi-gallo-catechin gallate (in green tea), the isoflavones daidzein and genistein (in soy), and curcumin (in turmeric).

Longstanding *H. pylori* infection seems to be associated with precancerous changes in the lining cells of the stomach (metaplasia). Given scientific evidence to date, antioxidants should be considered a must in the treatment of *H. pylori* associated, acid-related disease of the gut. The benefits of antioxidant therapy are well recognized in alternative medicine, and they seem highly portable to conventional management of *H. pylori*.

DOCTORS CANNOT AGREE ABOUT DYSPEPSIA

Dyspepsia is usually manifest by upper abdominal pain with or without the presence of other dyspeptic symptoms such as belching, heartburn, bloating, nausea and vomiting, and so on. If one says one has a queasy stomach, then this is a form of dyspepsia. The problems of definitions of dyspepsia have become increasingly apparent. To quote a cute title of one informative paper by Dr. David Peura, M.D., a distinguished gastroenterologist, we can have "dys" or "dat" type of dyspepsia.

My colleagues and I performed a study called "Probing Perceptions of Dyspepsia," which was presented at the World Congress of Gastroenterology in 1994. I felt that defining this disorder was very important if a doctor or healthcare professional were to give advice about therapy. In other words, there should be some general agreement about what constitutes categories of different types of dyspepsia, if people are to get useful advice or treatment that matches their complaints.

In this attempt to probe the knowledge of healthcare givers about dyspepsia, a questionnaire was administrated to a group of doctors, pharmacists, medical students, and nurses in a major university hospital in New York. The results were quite startling. Only 10 percent of the group felt that a patient with dyspepsia should see a doctor! The respondents were given a widely accepted definition of dyspepsia, as published repeatedly in the peer-reviewed medical literature, but only 13 percent accepted the definition. In summary, only 16 percent even believed that dyspepsia could be adequately defined. This study is not novel nor is its message new. If healthcare givers cannot agree upon a definition of dyspepsia, what chance is there that consistent or standardized treatment advice will be given to the millions of people who suffer with this problem?

CONFUSION ABOUT TREATMENT

The study just discussed implied that much confusion prevailed about dyspepsia among doctors and healthcare givers. Therefore, it prompted my colleagues and I to look at attitudes and knowledge toward common medications that are used to treat dyspepsia. In particular, we focused on the use of OTC medications that are used to self-medicate for dyspepsia. In 1994, these drugs had just started to move from prescription status to OTC status. This second study performed in 1994 provided evidence of even more revealing inadequacies about knowledge in the general use of OTC medications.

In this study of understanding of and attitudes toward OTC drugs for dyspepsia, among healthcare givers in a university hospital, opinion was divided and knowledge was highly variable. First, 76 percent of the respondents did not think that drugs that were powerful at reducing gastric acid secretion should even be available as OTC medications. A very interesting contradiction, because we should recall that only 10 percent of this group expressed the idea that a patient with dyspepsia should see a doctor! The drugs under scrutiny in the study were Pepcid, Zantac, Tagamet, and Axid, together with other antacids in many branded formats (e.g., Maalox, Tums, Rolaids, Mylanta, etc.). Obviously, the results of these studies were context specific, but they exemplify divided opinions in medicine.

If healthcare givers cannot agree on the availability of drugs or their use for dyspepsia (which they cannot always define), then the would-be self-medicator who is faced with OTC treatment options, but no medical training, has a problem in selecting appropriate treatment. This situation is a mess because effective OTC drugs can be effective only if used correctly for the right problem. Putting this situation in different terms, a new dilemma is faced by healthcare recipients. If they do not have the knowledge to use OTC medications (or alternative therapies) appropriately, then they will not derive the required health benefit with any consistency. This dilemma faces the treatment of many disorders for which powerful OTC medications are now available. We must ask ourselves whether or not the condition we are trying to treat is readily amenable to self-diagnosis, before we even select the treatment option or consider its potential safety or efficacy.

"HOW DO OTC DRUGS AFFECT DISEASES?"

I was asked to answer this question by the editor of the medical journal *Drugs* in 1993. The question was posed to me prior to the switch of some gastric-acid-reducing (antacid) drugs (Zantac, Pepcid, Tagamet, and Axid) from prescription-only status to OTC availability. For me, this raised more questions than answers. Questions about the effects of any major health initiative often take many years to answer, and in my opinion, most of them in this case have remained unanswered for almost a decade now.

Although there are many very difficult questions to answer about OTC acid-reducing drugs, they are worthy of much thought. Concerns about the widespread availability of OTC drugs that were once available only by prescription from a licensed medical practitioner involve a complex combination of political, medical, social, business, and ethical issues. Maybe it is safer for physicians not to discuss these issues?

Despite the importance of the increasing trend of switching prescription drugs to OTC drugs in healthcare, the general public has been somewhat protected from these decisions. They are told very little about the potential benefits or adverse outcomes of this increasing practice of switching prescription drugs to OTC status. This switch of drugs could be good, but there are many areas where it is potentially bad. I shall expand on this reasoning, which is a revealing process.

Research on acid-reducing drugs (like Pepcid, Zantac, Tagamet, and Axid, examples of H_2-receptor antagonists) to move them to OTC status was performed to support sales that could have been threatened by expiration of patents on these drugs at that time. Patent expiration, and other things, motivated pharmaceutical companies to review and develop extensive research and development programs to evaluate the safety and efficacy of H_2-receptor antagonists for the self-treatment of self-diagnosed dyspepsia. The results of many of the OTC studies with H_2-receptor antagonists performed by pharmaceutical companies were not disclosed in the medical literature, because each company was looking for a competitive edge as it rushed to be first into the OTC market. In general terms, it is known that first to market with a new drug category usually wins the commercial race. Furthermore, it may be a shock for some readers to know that many studies of OTC antacid drugs did not reveal convincing benefit for their use as OTC treatments for dyspepsia! However, the pharmaceutical industry learned rapidly to construct clinical trial protocols that could satisfy a focused measure of efficacy.

REGULATIONS ARE WORLDWIDE

The FDA and other regulatory authorities around the world have instituted special OTC divisions of staff that evaluate prescription-to-OTC switches. The approval of an OTC product requires comprehensive support to assure safety and efficacy of the candidate drug. There is a need to demonstrate that a suitable target population exists with a medical disorder that is amenable to self-diagnosis and self-treatment. It is known that self-diagnosis is a real problem. We know this for certain in the realm of dyspepsia.

Stringent criteria are proposed for a submission to government agencies for the approval of the nonprescription use of drugs. These criteria were attainable for H_2-receptor antagonists, at least in terms of safety and limited efficacy. Such criteria focus on issues such as direct toxicity or drug interaction potential, together with a broad-based knowledge and experience with the drug in prescription form. The importance of a well-defined surveillance program to detect drug-related problems has been recognized, but how good is the surveillance? Alternative medicine also needs to focus on this issue because no postmarketing surveillance exists in the dietary supplement industry to monitor adverse effects of herbals, botanicals, or nutrients (nutriceuticals).

THE PHARMACIST'S ROLE

To counteract the potential problems of a precipitous transition from prescription to general availability of an H_2-antagonist, these drugs could have been placed into a transition class for a period of time. This transition status exists currently for several drugs in a number of countries, but not in the United States. It would mean that the drug could be used only as recommended by a pharmacist or other healthcare professional with advanced training in therapeutics. Incidentally, I would support the placement of several remedies of natural origin (dietary supplements) in a transition class because their unsupervised use could be dangerous (e.g., ephedra or Ma huang).

Some professional organizations in the United States have petitioned the FDA to establish a class of compounds that would be available without a physician's prescription, but only with the advice of a pharmacist. This is an appealing option that is consistent with a long-overdue call by pharmacists to have an increased engagement in therapeutic decisions.

Pharmacists have been "spurred" on by falling incomes as dispensing charges are reduced by cost-containment initiatives. In the middle of all of this, pharmacists are showing a great thirst for knowledge about alternative therapies in the form of dietary supplements. The American Pharmaceutical Association (APA) has recognized the importance of continuing medical education (CME) for pharmacists on natural remedies and herbals. Nowadays one will find a pharmacist less willing to refer a client to a health food store, and he or she is playing an increasing role in promoting remedies of natural origin.

WHY DOCTORS PRESCRIBE DRUGS

The hierarchy of importance of the components of a physician-based decision to use any drug usually involves consideration of safety, efficacy, and cost. This order of importance of the properties of a drug may be changed when the consumer is making a decision for self-treatment. The consumer in the OTC domain may tend to be an individual who wants convenience and quick relief from an illness that he or she may not perceive as severe. Of course, this reality signals some dangers.

An important component of OTC drug use (or dietary supplement use) by a self-medicator may be the belief that the OTC drug or supplement will be safe and effective for the particular disorder. Symptom relief drives the prescription use of H_2-receptor antagonists, since it has been estimated that more than 60 percent of the revenue derived by manufacturers from the sale of prescription H_2-receptor antagonists may have emanated from the use of these drugs for nonapproved indications. I suspect a lot of the OTC use of these drugs is also for the wrong reason! The same problem faces the use of dietary supplements.

THE POWERFUL INDUCEMENT TO TAKE DRUGS

The pharmaceutical industry has promoted the use of OTC drugs by obtaining the endorsement of pharmacists or healthcare professionals. However, the greatest influence to use of H_2-receptor antagonists has come from the consumer purchase decision, which has been influenced by widespread media promotion. This latter tactic has become quite widespread in recent years, with inducements for patients to take an increasing role in the interpretation of their own symptoms and in their own treatment decisions.

The increasing practice of advertising prescription drugs is wrong in my opinion. The pressure induced by a patient or physician to receive or recommend a prescription drug does not need to be compounded by television commercials. Enormous pressure can be placed on a doctor to have a low threshold for drug prescription. The average patient wants what they ask for, sometimes even if they do not need it. If they do not get the prescription they want or think they need, they will shop around for another doctor. Doctors must keep patients—no patients, no practice, no pay! More drug demands from patients mean more prescriptions and escalating costs of healthcare.

GUT DISEASE: A MIXED BAG OF TRICKS

Another confounding factor is that there is considerable geographical variation in the prevalence and severity of dyspepsia or acid-related disease (peptic ulcers) within countries, let alone between different countries. This variability in ulcer disease is readily apparent when we look at placebo (sugar pill) healing rates in duodenal ulcer patients. In the pre-Helicobacter era, placebo healing rates in clinical trials of duodenal ulcer healing in London, England were around 20 percent, whereas those in Lausanne, Switzerland, were of the order of about 60 percent. Thus, an ulcer in Switzerland does not behave like an ulcer in England—this story is not so simple, but it makes a point about the variable nature of different diseases. Duodenal ulcer does not breed true, and dyspepsia must be regarded as the ultimate mongrel!

WHAT ARE OTC DRUGS USED FOR?

Despite the great deal of effort expended to review or define the safety and efficacy of H_2-receptor antagonists for OTC use, few studies so far have attempted to define the target population that may use these drugs. In addition, the indication for which the drugs may be used (i.e., dyspepsia or other acid-related symptoms) may be particularly difficult to define because of a lack of consensus on the definition of dyspepsia and a continuing lack of knowledge about the causation of dyspepsia or the generation of acid-related symptoms. For example, there is much we do not know about the relationship between *H. pylori* and NSAID and the causation of dyspepsia.

Considerable evidence has accrued that adverse lifestyle behaviors such as smoking or excessive alcohol consumption and perhaps stress, may be important determinations of dyspepsia in the community. The availability of H_2-antagonists as nonprescription drugs may unfortunately lead to less interventions to correct an adverse lifestyle. Adverse lifestyle is very common in patients with gastrointestinal symptoms, and its importance cannot be underestimated in terms of its pivotal role in the causation of most chronic diseases that afflict society. Alcohol is a major cause of dyspepsia. Excessive drinking as a cause of gastrointestinal upset frequently masquerades as a functional digestive disorder. Substance abuse in general can be linked to digestive upset.

The efficacy of H_2-receptor antagonists in the treatment of nonulcer dyspepsia is variable and sometimes disappointing. It appears that individuals who have predominantly GERD-like symptoms could be the group who may respond favorably to OTC H2-receptor antagonists, but this is not entirely clear. Certainly, beverage-induced heartburn seems amenable to successful symptom relief from H_2-receptor antagonists. You will recall that opinions vary on whether discrete types of nonulcer dyspepsia are readily identifiable.

NOT EVERYONE CAN BE TESTED IN DETAIL

The incidence of dyspepsia in the community is so frequent that it is not current practice or even practical to investigate, by medical testing, most individuals with upper gastrointestinal symptoms. Special diagnostic and treatment considerations may be required in certain patients, however, such as the elderly who may present with vague gastrointestinal symptoms. Any gastrointestinal symptoms in the elderly must be taken seriously because of the increased occurrence of gut cancer with age.

Dyspeptic symptoms are among the most common reasons for geriatric patients to consult a physician. It is clear that more attention should be paid to the development of risk indices that help characterize the severity and prognostic implications of certain forms of acid-related disease, so that those groups of individuals who should avoid self-medication can be identified. There have been moves in this direction, but so far we have little evidence of any widespread use of risk indices by the medical profession.

DOCTORS AND DYSPEPSIA

Dyspepsia is very common, and about 1 percent of the population may present to their primary care physician with upper abdominal pain each year. Only a small proportion will receive comprehensive assessment, of which one-third may have nonulcer dyspepsia. Furthermore, only about one-third of patients who actually experience dyspepsia may attend their physician. This leaves a large proportion of the population that may incur considerable cost and suffering. Earlier in this chapter I suggested that various subtypes of nonulcer dyspepsia exist, including reflux type, ulcerlike, dysmotility type, or unspecified dyspepsia, but considerable overlap exists among these dyspepsia subtypes. There is a suggestion that various subtypes of dyspepsia may be more amenable to one form of anti-dyspeptic therapy than another. Many dyspeptic individuals are recurrent intermittent seekers of healthcare.

DYSPEPSIA DUE TO DISORDERED MOVEMENTS OF THE STOMACH

Several studies have shown that H_2-receptor antagonists or antacids may be of limited benefit in the treatment of certain forms of nonulcer dyspepsia. This occurrence has been explained to some degree by the suggestion that abnormal emptying of the stomach (a lazy stomach) or abnormal motility (motor function) is the cause of dyspepsia in many individuals who do not respond to drugs that reduce gastric acidity. There are drugs that can be used to speed up delays in stomach emptying (e.g., metoclopramide and cisapride) and these drugs have shown benefit in relieving dyspepsia in some people. Although approximately one-half of groups of individuals with nonulcer dyspepsia may have delayed gastric emptying, the relationship between disturbed gastric motility and symptoms is often unclear. Thus, it appears quite difficult to select therapy for dyspepsia, at least when using clinical grounds as a means of attempting to match treatments with presumed types of dyspepsia.

The availability of OTC H_2-receptor antagonists could result in the mistreatment of a large group of individuals with dysmotility-like dyspepsia who could benefit from drug therapy that corrects the lazy stomach. Treatment Trials of drugs for dyspepsia are gaining acceptance in uninvestigated patients with dyspepsia. Perhaps the first consideration in any attempt to classify patients with dyspepsia on clinical grounds (those who do not have tests) should be the immediate exclusion of dyspepsia with danger signs. This can be defined as dyspepsia with symptoms or signs of serious organic disease, such as gastrointestinal bleeding, weight loss, or dysphagia. Remember, this is dyspepsia with red flags that signal a high likelihood of serious disease. Red flags may fly but they are not always seen!

DO OTC DRUGS REALLY SAVE HEALTHCARE COSTS?

Despite the substantial social or economic costs of dyspepsia, few attempts have been made to measure the potential social or economic benefits of OTC drug treatments. The assumption that self-medication, with a reduction in physician contact, may have economic benefit needs to be challenged until it is shown to be the case. Follow-up periods in clinical trials with many drugs have been short, and adequate measures of quality of life are not always applied in research studies of acid-related disease. Please note that these arguments apply equally to dietary supplements and alternative medical interventions. Short-term benefits in clinical trials that use only symptom improvements as a principal criterion for benefit are likely to create an illusion of long-term benefit for the drug intervention. However, the placebo response to dyspepsia may be very high. All of this dialogue means that something is just not right with OTC drugs and some nutriceuticals. Enter the realm of holistic care!

THE CONSTANT DANGER FOR SELF-MEDICATORS

Self-medication with H_2-antagonists could result in masking of a number of disorders and delay interventions for conditions where early detection and treatment could result in improved prognosis. The symptoms of cancer of the upper gastrointestinal tract, especially gastric cancer, can be similar to any type of dyspepsia of functional cause. In the United States, about twenty-six thousand new cases of gastric cancer occur per year, and there are approximately fourteen thousand deaths caused by it annually. The risk of masking gastric cancer is real because symptoms of cancer can sometimes temporarily respond to acid-lowering drugs, and a delay in diagnosis could occur and has probably occurred, at least to some degree.

Recent studies have drawn attention to the changing pattern of gastric cancer. A decrease in the occurrence of cancer affecting the gastric antrum (terminal part of the stomach), which may be associated with *H. pylori*, infection has been accompanied by an increase in the incidence of cancer affecting the gastric cardia (upper part of the stomach), which may be more smoking-or alcohol-related. Researchers have studied groups of patients with early gastric cancer who presented over a twenty-year period, and they found that 91 percent of these individuals presented with dyspepsia that was indistinguishable on clinical grounds from peptic ulcer symptoms or nonulcer dyspepsia. Most cases of gastric cancer occur in individuals aged over forty-five years, implying the importance of the adequate investigation of a new onset dyspepsia in later life.

GUT INFECTION IS A RISK WITH NO ACID

Some specific circumstances exist where low gastric acid may be considered undesirable. AIDS is an increasing cause of upper gastrointestinal symptoms in many urban areas worldwide. These symptoms occur most often as a consequence of opportunistic infection of the esophagus, especially with the yeast *Candida albicans*. Individuals who are infected with HIV tend to have reduced gastric acidity, with a tendency to develop enteric infection. Concern may be expressed about the general unsupervised use of OTC H_2-receptor antagonists in this group because of the possible further reduction of the gastric acid, which serves as a barrier to infection of the guts. Acid is known to be a very important body defense, and we may not be doing the right thing for health by encouraging a mass reduction of gastric acid with antacid medications.

THE NSAID SCOURGE

Anyone with miserable joint pain or the pain of an acute injury has enjoyed the temporary benefit provided by non-steroidal anti-inflammatory drugs (NSAIDs). Practitioners of alternative medicine have attacked rheumatologists (doctors who specialize in diseases of bones and joints) concerning the use of NSAIDs. It is frequently stated that NSAIDs are only a quick-fix approach because they do not alter the clinical course of arthritis in general, and they do not go to the root of the cause of arthritis. Furthermore, NSAIDs may damage joints further in some cases, and they have alarming side effects.

Many practitioners of emergency medicine have spent a lot of time dealing with the alarming side effects of NSAIDs, especially life-threatening bleeding from the gut. Gastroenterologists work in concert with rheumatologists—linked by NSAID use that causes bleeding from the guts. Some people may consider this remark cynical but it has more than a measure of truth.

My colleagues and I spent a good deal of time in the 1980s trying to define the adverse affects of NSAIDs. Population studies show that more than 60 percent of patients with life-threatening bleeding from the upper reaches of the gut have been taking NSAIDs for both the wrong and the right reasons! I want you to understand with clarity that there is a vast range of NSAIDs that are dished out by prescription or freely available to purchase OTC. If there ever was a category of "me too" drugs, NSAIDs are the best example.

Like all drugs, NSAIDs have a generic name and a trade name. Consumers of NSAIDs should read the label on the products. The user of NSAIDs should concentrate on generic names to be certain that they know what they are taking. The most striking literature on NSAIDs damage to the gastrointestinal tract is now somewhat historic. The writing was on the wall that NSAIDs are not safe drugs as early as the start of the 1970s.

THE AMERICAN COLLEGE OF GASTROENTEROLOGY SEEKS "ALTERNATIVES"

After years of evidence that NSAIDs are a major cause of bleeding from the gut, the American College of Gastroenterology (ACG) has produced a consumer education brochure called "Understanding GI [gastrointestinal] Bleeding." The booklet is worthy of close scrutiny. The brochure appears to have been produced in association with support from the pharmaceutical industry. Therefore, it comes as no surprise that the suggested alternative to NSAIDs is another drug.

The patient booklet states that:

Patients who need to use NSAIDs regularly should consult regularly with their physician to be alert for any potential GI effects. Since problems may arise with few, if any, symptoms, ongoing monitoring with your physician is important. If problems do arise, and are recognized early, there are a variety of ways to minimize or reverse any adverse effects, either by using *alternatives* to NSAIDs, or through your physician prescribing medications that can reduce any adverse effects.

The implication is that by using acetaminophen for arthritic pain, one can avoid the gastrointestinal side effects of NSAIDs. However, acetaminophen is a classic quick fix. It can effectively relieve pain but only for an hour or two, and it is a relatively poor anti-inflammatory, which renders it not useful in treating many types of arthritis. Add to this the potential liver damage that can occur when excessive acetaminophen is taken, and one has in acetaminophen a less-than-adequate alternative to NSAIDs. Acetaminophen is valuable as an occasional alternative to NSAIDs for pain control only, and many physicians have recognized its limitations for the treatment of arthritis.

There is a second rub in the preceding statements by the ACG. The physician has another alternative, quote: "or through your physician prescribing medications that can reduce any adverse side effects [referring to NSAIDs]." This refers to the ability to use an ulcer-healing medication, such as an H_2-receptor antagonist or a prostaglandin to prevent or treat an ulcer caused by an NSAIDs. This is the classic example of iatrogenic multiplication or polypharmacy, where medical treatment causes a problem with a drug (an NSAID) and the side effect is treated with another drug! There has to be a better way.

It is accepted that NSAIDs are a major cause of gastrointestinal bleeding, liver problems, and kidney damage. These effects are most apparent in elderly people, who are the ones who use vast quantities of NSAIDs for their painful joints. When one demands an alternative from modern medicine, the usual response is another drug with a claim of less side effects. Many studies show that certain NSAIDs have fewer side effects than others. Overall, these studies have provided little evidence to suggest that ibuprofen is less damaging than ketoprofen or different from naproxen (or any NSAID) in its ability to cause gastrointestinal ulceration. There is not much to choose from in the safety profile between commonly used NSAIDs; they are all potentially dangerous.

In the past decade, we have heard the promise that new NSAIDs, e.g., COX-2 inhibitors, will have fewer side effects, but this promise has not been completely fulfilled. According to early studies, the COX-2 inhibitors may be effective with less gastrointestinal upset. However, early studies do not usually show us the true side-effect profile of any new medicine.

NATURAL ALTERNATIVES TO NSAIDS

Are there really alternatives? The good news is that there are many natural compounds that can be used effectively to promote bone and joint health, and these are available as dietary supplements, not drugs. Recent reports of a randomized, double-blind, controlled trial of glucosamine in the treatment of osteoarthritis of the knee show both symptomatic improvement and objective improvements in the structure of joints. Many thousands of patients have discovered the benefits of shark cartilage, glucosamine, chondroitin, mixtures of these agents, and Ayurvedic herbs such as Boswellia. Boswellia not only suppresses joint inflammation, it does so without causing any significant irritation or ulceration in the gut and can be considered an herbal agent with activity like an NSAIDs—without the side-effect profile. Popular books have focused on these alternatives, e.g. *The Arthritis Cure*, by Brenda Addersley, Barry Fox, and Jason Theodosakis (New York: St. Martin Press, 1997) and The Power of Cartilage, by Stephen Holt and Jean Barilla (New York: Kensington Publishers, 1998). However, the conventional physician remains often quite reticent to try or recommend such alternatives. Despite evidence of the awful side-effect profile of NSAIDs and the efficacy of these natural alternatives, these alternatives remain underutilized in modern medicine.

DOING AWAY WITH NSAIDS

Although we have new kinds of NSAIDs drugs that are selective inhibitors of cyclooxygenase (COX-2) inhibitors (preferential types of NSAIDs are Etodolac, Lodine, Lodine XL, nabumetone, Relafen, celecoxib, Celbrex, rofecoxib, and Vioxx), whether or not these drugs will relieve symptoms without the risk of damage to the gut that is posed by traditional NSAIDs remains to be demonstrated. The COX-2 inhibitors are not innocuous for gastrointestinal structure or function, and it is not common knowledge that the COX-2 inhibitor plays a role in ovulation, bone formation, and endocrine function (especially affecting insulin-secreting islet cells in the pancreas). With increasing use of COX-2 inhibitors, the list of side effects of these drugs is likely to grow.

There are now well-controlled clinical observations that clearly demonstrate that remedies of natural origin can effectively improve the symptoms of arthritis. More than a quick fix for symptom relief, several of these natural agents may go to the root of the problems in arthritis. I cover many of these issues in my book with Jean Barilla, M.S., entitled *The Power of Cartilage*.

So important and neglected are these agents that they are now prominently summarized:

- *Glucosamine:* shown in prospective clinical studies to improve symptoms of arthritis and assist in regeneration of joint cartilage.
- *Chondroitin*: similar actions to glucosamine, with a common anti-inflammatory effect, but poorly absorbed from the gut.
- *Shark cartilage* (researched as cartilade): a holistic mixture of glucosamine-like components (glycoaminoglycans), chondroitin, type II collagen, calcium, phosphorous (2:1 ratio), and antiangiogenic proteins.
- *Hydrolyzed collagen*: type II collagen of bovine, shark, or chicken origin is effective in arthritis (especially inflammatory arthritis or rheumatoid disease) by mechanisms of immune tolerance.
- *Boswellia serrata*: a natural anti-inflammatory with actions similar to NSAIDs, without any gastrointestinal side effects.
- *Methylsulphonemethane (MSM)*: a sulphur containing natural anti-inflammatory with credible evidence of improvements in pain and inflammation in joints.
- *Others*: cetyl myristate, ginger, sea cucumber, green-lipped mussel, with variable evidence of benefit in arthritis.

These remedies of natural origin are safe and quite effective alternatives to NSAIDs. One drawback, however, that is these natural agents, with the exception of Boswellia and perhaps ginger, take time to be effective. Comparisons of the treatment benefits of glucosamine with NSAIDs show equivalent or better symptom control, but in some cases it takes glucosamine up to twelve weeks to be maximally effective. Obviously, the arthritis sufferer needs immediate relief, and the introduction of these agents is best achieved by tapering off existing medications. At the least, natural therapies can drastically reduce the need for NSAIDs.

Solutions for rapid pain relief are at hand with topical capsaicin creams that have facilitated absorption by the use of liposomes (little fat bubbles in the cream). Capsaicin blocks substance *P*, a molecule that is a principle pain transmitter to the brain. When used regularly, it can take three days or so to reach maximum effectiveness (longer without liposomes). Immediate analgesic effect can be achieved in natural pain relief creams by adding the cooling essential plant oils of menthol and camphor. Topical creams and lotions have been developed with variable combinations of capsaicin (to block pain) and menthol and camphor (to provide immediate analgesia) in bases of shark cartilage, bovine cartilage, aloe, MSM, and other natural agents. This natural approach of using capsaicin is approved by the FDA as effective, and these products have received an OTC drug claim on their label.

Finally, I wish to note that studies of the topical application of capsaicin for pain control have resulted in reductions of the need for NSAIDs in some patients by a factor of 80 percent. What are we waiting for, in the face of dangers of NSAID usage and the presence of effective, safe natural options for bone and joint health?

THE AGING GUT

Like the general features of the aging body, such as reduction in agility and movement, the aging gut becomes sluggish in its movements. A discussion of the characteristics of the aging gut is very important for several reasons. First, the elderly are the most avid seekers of remedies for general digestive upset. Second, they are the target of bone and joint disorders and they are most likely to suffer the adverse consequences of NSAIDs usage. And third, they have the highest prevalence of many functional symptoms of deranged gut function, especially reduced appetite, dysphagia, dyspepsia, and constipation.

Antiaging strategies are a key initiative in alternative medicine, and they evoke modest interest these days in conventional medicine. It is staggering when one reviews the magnitude of this interest among medical personnel. For example, the Anti-Aging Society of North America holds an annual meeting that has almost six times more registrants than the meetings of the ACG, even though there are more than six times the number of gastroenterologists than clinicians engaged in the focused practice of antiaging medicine.

The hallmark of the aging gut is changes in normal coordinated gut movements. However, changes in gut absorption and glandular function also occur with aging. Dysphagia affects up to 10 percent of the population greater than 60 years of age, and it is present in almost one-third of all people in retirement or nursing homes. Swallowing mechanisms change with age to include feeble contractions in the main gullet with retention of good contractions in the throat (pharynx), but a narrowing of the upper sphincter of the esophagus. The rate at which the stomach empties tends to decline with age, perhaps resulting in early satiety and anorexia or dyspepsia. More than 10 percent of elderly people can lose weight as a consequence of these changes.

Advancing years bring a tendency to suffer constipation and almost universal changes in strength of movements and coordination of the anus and rectum. There is a decrease in sensation that is experienced in the rectum, and neuromuscular problems affect the squeeze pressures in the lower bowel. In addition, there is delayed transit of stool in the colon. Paradoxically, the tragic and distressing occurrence of incontinence of stool in the elderly most often relates to constipation rather than diarrhea. This circumstance makes natural and gentle ways of facilitating bowel actions an attractive option for the elderly. (See www.antiagingmethods.com for more information).

In general, remedies of natural origin that combine herbals, nutrients, and phytochemicals may have a major role in retarding the aging process, and they can be used to help correct the consequences of aging (symptoms). In contrast, conventional approaches (drugs) deal only with the consequences of aging. Antioxidant therapy, nutrients to support gut function, and modulating the structure and alternatives of the microclimate or ecology of the bowel by probiosis are exciting options for the management of the aging gut. Some of these options are discussed in more detail in later sections of this book.

CHAPTER SUMMARY

The stomach fits snugly into our bodymind concept. Dyspepsia is so common that we can all expect to experience it at some time. The past decade has witnessed a complete turnaround in attitudes toward the treatment of peptic ulcer disease and significant forms of gastritis, given the discovery of the role of *Helicobacter pylori* in these disorders.

With more scrutiny, we see that *H. pylori* seems to exert a great deal of damage by virtue of its ability to generate damaging, free radicals. The quenching of free radicals is one of the most important areas in the application of nutritional and natural medical therapy for certain gut diseases, by the revision of antioxidants as supplements. Clearly, more work is required to see if antioxidants can play an adjunctive role in the area of *H. pylori*–induced upper gastrointestinal disease, bearing in mind that the issue of eradication of *H. pylori* with appropriate, conventional medical therapy is the most important option.

Alternative medicine has provided a major alternative to the serious gastrointestinal problems caused by NSAIDs. While alternative medicine may not star in its approach to the therapy of peptic ulcer disease, it has provided a pathway to avoid NSAIDs—the most common, residual cause of complicated ulcer disease.

CHAPTER SIX

BELCHING,
FARTING, AND BLOATING

THE "TO AND FRO" OF GAS

Gas passes freely into and out of the gut in states of health. The tubular digestive tract contains gas by virtue of its communication with the atmosphere and as a consequence of the production of gas in the gut. Gas is produced in the gut as a result of bacterial fermentation and as a consequence of the interactions between food and digestive juices. It has been argued by some that gas serves no useful purpose in the gut, but I subscribe to the notion that it aids digestion, facilitates the positioning of the guts, and it causes a sensation of relief when it passes freely out of the guts. In many Western societies the acts of belching and passing wind are considered somewhat antisocial. The free expression of gut gas is definitely taboo in many social circles.

Most people can exert a degree of control over the passage of gut gases to the exterior but many cannot. Some individuals can experience examples of loss of control in response to a variety of events or causes. Even those who cannot control the urge to belch or fart can often exert an influence on the process to produce a disguised or silent release of gas. However, no individual can readily exert any control over the smell of the gas that they eliminate from their guts.

The grumbling sound of gas can be a great embarrassment to some individuals. It is believed commonly that all gas is generated within the bowel or stomach from food. We shall learn that a good portion of the gas present in the guts, particularly the stomach, occurs as a consequence of swallowing air (aerophagia). The amount of gas found in the guts varies tremendously from one person to another, depending on an individual's diet and states of emotional and physical health.

Overall, three basic factors control the amount of gas in the guts. These factors are swallowing of air, the composition of the diet, and the bacteria or microorganisms found in the gut. A significant amount of gas enters the gut, usually by swallowing. Gas can enter the colon through the anus and some individuals are quite adept at sucking air into their lower bowel and discharging it in a controlled manner.

The act of farting may fascinate certain segments of the population, and it is a source of endless amusement to many teenagers. There are a number of people who have normal bowel function and gut function who can train themselves to fart or belch at will.

The famous nineteenth century vaudeville star Monsieur Petit-Pas from Paris, noticed that while swimming he could store water in his lower bowel and discharge it at will. He graduated from the sea to the land and found that he could store gas in his rectum and lower bowel with the same skill. So adept was Monsieur Petit-Pas at this act, that he learned to play the trumpet with his anus, and he entertained many an audience with his antics.

I am raising the story of Monsieur Petit-Pas to give the reader some insight into the degree of learned control that some individuals can exert over bowel or gut function. While few people may desire to develop the skill of Monsieur Petit-Pas, they can be reassured that they can have better control over gut function with practice than they may have hitherto supposed. This anecdote is useful to know for those who are troubled by lack of control of the passage of flatus or by incontinence of stool. Alternative medical disciplines that focus on mind-body control (e.g., Yoga, biofeedback training, etc.) can be invaluable to the person with excessive gut gas.

SWALLOWING GAS

Up to a teaspoonful of air (2–3ml) enters the upper portions of the gut with each swallow, and more air seems to enter the stomach while swallowing liquids compared with solids. Many popular carbonated beverages are heavily and loaded with gas (carbon dioxide). Over the past decade, there has been a twofold increase in the sale of carbonated beverages in the United States. We can learn some important points from babies who are bottled-fed. During a bottle feeding, an infant's stomach can expand by a factor of up to five times, due largely to swallowed air. Interestingly, babies' stomachs do not blow up like this when they suck their thumbs or an empty bottle, or when they breastfeed. Therefore, it is no surprise that the breastfed baby is somewhat protected from gassy colic.

The person who suffers frequently from excessive belching is almost always an air swallower with a nervous disposition. The act of air swallowing in these people is so overt that other people can actually observe them swallowing air repeatedly. After swallowing air, they regurgitate the air. The individual who does this may be difficult to convince about the simple cause of their problem. One of the best pieces of advice is to have the individual look in a mirror for a while. They will observe themselves swallowing air. This is a first step in managing aerophagia. The habit of swallowing air can be broken when the person with aerophagia is willing to accept that this is the cause of his or her belching.

FOOD AND FLUID AS SOURCES OF GAS

Food and certain fluids are sources of gas, and they may contribute to excessive belching or flatus. Carbonated beverages (fizzy drinks) when consumed in regular servings can generate as much as one-half of a liter of gas in the stomach. The shape of the stomach is adapted to the presence of a gastric bubble of air (located in the upper part of the stomach, or fundus of the stomach). The rapid drinking of a carbonated beverage is often followed by belching. In many people, this can cause a pleasing and sometimes comfortable sensation. Effervescent drinks are sometimes used as agents to cause temporary relief of gastric distress through belching.

Excessive flatus is often caused by intestinal fermentation, especially in the colon. Various bacteria, molds, or yeasts occupy the colon in states of health. These microorganisms can use a variety of agents in the diet as substrates to form gas. Undigested food provides more available substrate (material) for microorganisms to produce gas. Bacteria within the intestines are versatile in their ability to ferment almost all major classes of nutrients in the diet.

Diets high in fruit and vegetable intake provide a large indigestible residue that is presented to the colon, and it often causes excessive flatus. This situation is common when dietary fiber supplementation occurs in the diet. Fermentation of soluble and insoluble fibers, such as cellulose, are common causes of excessive release of anal gas. Several foods are particularly flatogenic (gas forming), and these include legumes, cabbage, cauliflower, broccoli, and some root vegetables. In addition, a high intake of fruit and vegetables presents a high load of complex or indigestible carbohydrates. For example, soybeans contain oligosaccharides (complex sugars) such as raffinose and stacchyose, which are potent causes of excessive flatus in animals or humans who eat them. These carbohydrates in soy are associated with health, and they play a role in the encouragement of the growth of friendly bacteria in the colon (discussed in chapter 10).

Many food items contain air, but this may not be obvious. Apples and pears may have approximately one-quarter of their entire volume composed of air. Other foods are specially prepared to contain air to improve their appeal. Examples include ice cream, soufflés and light bread. Several fruits or their juices are quite flatogenic. Bananas, prunes, apple or grape juice, apple puree and raisins can often increase hydrogen production in the bowel. In contrast, apricots, apricot nectar, and orange juice may be less flatogenic.

Several controlled clinical experiments have been performed where gas production in response to different diets has been studied. It is known that switching to bean-prominent diets can cause increases in the rate of gas production in the colon to an approximate average of 17 ml per hour. When bean intake is increased to account for up to 30 percent or 60 percent of the total calorie intake, then gas production in the bowel can increase to a range of fourfold to tenfold, respectively. These studies support my proposal of the syndrome of the "Cowboy's Colon."

We also have to be tolerant of some of the normal effects of certain foods. Legumes, such as soybeans, peas and lentils, often cause a bit of gas, especially if they are not consumed on a regular basis. These foods are often good foods for health. Everyone is aware that fruit and vegetables may stimulate bowel function due to their fiber and other unabsorbable carbohydrate content. Vegetables, including beans, contain indigestible fiber and some complex carbohydrates, which can resist digestion by the human gut. Bacteria that are normally present in the large bowel can ferment fiber and carbohydrates, producing gas. Since we know the potential health benefits of fiber and some complex sugars, it may be prudent to accept a certain amount of gas from health-giving vegetables. The passage of flatus from the bowel is often accompanied by the desirable occurrence of a comfortable, soft bowel movement. Science shows us that increasing fruit and vegetable intake in our diet decreases our overall risk of many types of cancer and other chronic diseases.

FRUCTOOLIGOSACCHARIDES (FOS)

Fructooligosaccharides (FOS) are naturally occurring types of complex carbohydrates that tend to support the growth of friendly bacteria. The use of friendly bacteria (probiotics) in the treatment and prevention of gut disorders has become a big issue in alternative medicine, and this is discussed in detail in chapter 10. The use of FOS has increased greatly in recent times, and they are used as flavor enhancers, sweeteners, humectants (moisturelike mouth feel), and flavor enhancers in food manufacturing. There is no doubt that FOS are potentially health giving, and they are used as components of dietary supplements in increasing amounts. Ancient treatment disciplines have revered the value of FOS. For example, soy flour with a high content of FOS (stacchyose and raffinose) is identified as a longevity factor in branches of traditional Japanese medicine.

With the renaissance of interest in FOS must come the acceptance that these carbohydrates often cause loose stool and gas. The friendly (and some unfriendly) bacteria in the bowel use FOS as a source of energy and produce gas. In fact, a consideration of the FOS contents of certain foods is a good guide to their ability to generate gas. In descending order, the following are examples of foods high in

FOS: soybeans (crude), onion family (includes garlic), artichokes, barley, rye, wheat, bananas, and asparagus.

FOUL GAS

Flatus can be tolerated in moderate amounts by many people, but it becomes intolerable when it has an offensive odor. The composition and volume of gases in the gastrointestinal tract varies greatly from one person to the other. In general, foul gas is often produced if methane- or sulphur-containing gases are produced by bacterial fermentation.

Many foods have sulphur-containing compounds that can be changed into chemicals with unpleasant odors such as hydrogen sulphide or volatile mercaptans. Hydrogen sulphide is a common component of stink bombs that are sold in joke shops—it smells like rotten eggs. Excessive intake of eggs and meat provides a large load of sulphur-containing substances. The flatus induced by meat or egg protein can be particularly offensive due to its content of sulphur-containing gases.

Other odoriferous gases contribute to the clinical problem of excessive flatus. These gases include ammonia, skatol, indole, volatile amines, and short-chain fatty acids. The human nose can be extremely sensitive to the detection of these gases in dilutions of only one or two parts per million in environmental air. All gases in the gastrointestinal tract can be absorbed, transported in the blood, and expired through the lungs. Thus, gases produced in the guts can often appear in the breath. Scientific studies suggest that as many as 250 gases or volatile substances can be detected in human breath, and most are produced by bacterial metabolism in the colon.

Excessive flatus and belching are most often benign in origin, but they can be an indicator of malabsorption, inflammation, or cancer in the, gastrointestinal tract. In many diseases, the bacterial flora of the gut and the handling of food by the gut can be changed, resulting in major differences in gas production. When excessive gaseousness is accompanied by abdominal pain, change of bowel habit, or other red-flag symptoms, then medical investigation is required to exclude organic disease. The combination of food, bacteria, and digestive juices in the bowels form the "digesta" which is discussed in greater detail in chapter 8.

COMPLAINTS OF TOO MUCH GAS

Common misconceptions about complaints of excessive gas exist in medicine. Scientific studies have shown that in many subjects who complain of too much gas, the actual amount (volume) of gas present in the guts may be no greater than normal. Such individuals seem to be more aware of the presence of gas in their guts. Doctors Bond, Levitt, and Lasser showed in the 1970s that two-thirds of a group of patients who complained of gaseousness had much more discomfort when gas was introduced into their guts than did individuals without such complaints.

In clinical experiments, these researchers actually pushed (infused) gas into the guts of these subjects and monitored symptoms. In six of eighteen individuals, the infusion of gas caused quite severe pain and discomfort that resulted in a need to discontinue the experimental process. Thus, the amount of gas in the guts may be less important than the ability of an individual's guts to handle the gas. When researchers examined the subjects who could not handle the gas, they found that movements of gut contents were feeble or delayed. In particular, the time taken for gut contents to pass through the guts (transit time) was prolonged. I propose that natural medicines (fibers, herbs and botanicals) that facilitate transit can really help in this circumstance.

RECENT SPANISH STUDIES

Dr. Juan-R Malagelada and his colleagues at the Autonomous University of Barcelona in Spain, have performed very elegant experiments on the dynamics (movements and activity) of intestinal gas and its tolerance in humans. These results were reported in the journal *Gastroenterology* (115:542–550, 1998). The findings of these studies were similar to the earlier observations of doctors Levitt, Bond, and Lasser (*New England Journal of Medicine*, 293:524–526, 1975).

The Spanish investigators infused gas into forty-six healthy sub-jects for three hours and measured symptoms, anal passage of gas, and abdominal girth. Even with relatively high infusion rates of gas, most of the subjects were able to expel the gas. The researchers noted that six of the forty-six healthy subjects retained gas (greater than 400 ml), but only five of these six developed abdominal disten-sion and untoward symptoms.

The importance of these studies is the clear demonstration that most people can deal with excessive gas without any problems. The guts appear to have inbuilt protective mechanisms against the accu-mulation of gas. There are several issues to consider about the caus-es of "excessive gut gas" that are relevant to the planning of treat-ment for this common problem. Knowledge of the generation of the symptoms is one of the most pivotal issues in deciding the manage-ment of gaseous disorders. Discussing this issue in a different man-ner, there are three questions posed about symptoms of excessive gas. These are:

1. Is there gas overload caused by too much gas entry into the gut or by excessive gas generation in the gut?
2. Is there an impaired handling of gases by the gut?
3. Is there just an increased perception by some people of gas in the gut, or is there a lack of tolerance for modest amounts of gas in the gut?

The answer to these questions in many individuals will determine the correct primary treatment approach. For example, if the main problem is a lack of tolerance of the gas itself, then relief is likely to be gained by the application of somewhat difficult measures of dietary restriction to reduce gas production. I believe that many indi-viduals who are bothered by gas may inappropriately exclude health-giving foods, such as fruit and vegetables in their diet in the false hope that they can improve their symptoms.

COMPLAINTS DUE TO GAS

Perhaps everyone at some time in his or her life is bothered by gastrointestinal gas. While excessive gas may be the apparent complaint, close questioning often reveals that it is an inability to pass gas by belching or farting that is the real problem. Earlier in this chapter, the problem of aerophagia was addressed. This condition has been termed the Magenblase syndrome.

The Magenblase syndrome is most often due to ingested gas that causes problems. It is often related to anxiety but it is aggravated by many factors, including: excessive chewing of gum (a common American pastime), mouth breathing (often forced by allergies or nasal blockages), the presence of irritation in the mouth or pharynx, and problems caused by corrective dental appliances such as braces or poorly fitting dentures. The nervous, brace-wearing teenager who chews gum is a sitting duck for aerophagia. It is important to recognize these simple circumstances that lead to air swallowing and belching before the individual reaches for the bottle of antacids, Beano, or other medications that are alleged to have an almost universal control of excessive belching or gas. In chapter 3, we discussed problems of excessive saliva production and swallowing. This disorder may be associated with repetitive air swallowing that, in turn, can cause abdominal complaints. In the most severe form of aerophagia, individuals can swallow and retain a couple of liters of air in their stomach, with resulting gross fluctuations of abdominal girth.

An uncommon and often overlooked cause of excessive gas accumulation in the upper digestive tract is starvation or malnutrition. Studies of holocaust victims and patients with anorexia nervosa show that these individuals may have gross delays in stomach emptying. On rare occasions, this can lead to life-threatening acute gastric dilatation (the stomach blows up like a balloon). However, the gas in this severe situation results probably from a combination of air entry into the stomach and the production of gas within the upper bowels. The latter mechanism has been proposed because some studies have shown a preponderance of carbon dioxide in the stomach gas of these individuals.

I discuss this extreme example of gas lodgment in the stomach because people who engage in prolonged fasting in the cause of "health" may notice a bulging abdomen, which may reinforce their perceived need to fast if weight loss is a goal. Inappropriate weight loss is sought in anorexia nervosa, bulimia, and crash dieting, especially by teenage girls. Thus, dieting that is very strict can actually contribute to a potbelly caused by gas! One overlooked reason why popular high-fat/high-protein diets (e.g., Atkins or Zone Diet) may apparently work is that the exclusion of carbohydrates eliminates fermentable products for the gut bacteria. Therefore, reduction of abdominal girth on these diets is just sham weight-loss. Another major reason is that these diets cause water loss from the body in their early phases of application.

When gas accumulates in the small intestine, gurgling noises (borborygmi) and abdominal cramp can occur. There are certain portions of the bowel where gas accumulation can cause quite distinctive and alarming symptoms. Gas pockets around the bends in the colon, close to the spleen (splenic flexure) in the upper left side of the abdomen can cause pain that is felt in the left lower chest. On occasion, this pain can be quite severe, and it can be confused with pain originating from the heart. This condition has been termed pseudoangina (pseudo = false, angina = from the heart).

TREATMENT AND PREVENTION OF GAS

There are a few situations in medicine where a common complaint, such as excessive gas, leads a physician to scratch his or her head or offer abrupt advice. The individual who presents to a physician with the common complaint of excessive gas often represents a difficult circumstance of management to the healthcare giver. The key to the problem in most cases is the identification of a specific source of the problem, e.g., air swallowing or dietary factors, and its correction. The most common cause of excessive gas production, per se, is diet. Despite this knowledge, studies that have looked at dietary changes and relief of the complaints of excessive gas have not tended to show universally favorable outcomes. A major reason for this poor outcome is the inability of certain individuals to handle amounts gas in their guts of greater than 200 ml. The cumulative difficulties in the management of excess gas makes certain alternative medical options such as yoga, hypnosis, and biofeedback attractive treatment approaches.

"BALANCE" THERAPY FOR GAS

I believe that complaints of excessive gas are a classic but simple example of a lack of balance in a natural process. The treatment should therefore be aimed at restoring the balance. Any attempt at treatment that focuses on the elimination of excessive gas in the guts without an attempt to correct the circumstance of intolerance of the gut to gas will often fail.

The exact reasons why some people can and others cannot tolerate gas in the guts remains unknown. Studies have shown that approximately one in six people may have a diminished ability to tolerate excessive gas, which means that as many as forty million Americans may have variable problems with excessive gas. One sees a reason why billions of dollars' worth of digestive aids are consumed on an annual basis in the United States.

In recent studies of the human tolerance to gut gas, Dr. Malagelada and his colleagues studied apparently healthy and normal individuals. Of course, the definition of normality requires a foolproof way of selecting "normal people," and no such way exists. Dr. Malagelada and his associates tried to select individuals without functional gut problems by using questionnaire techniques and clinical examination. However, these researchers concluded that apparently healthy individuals who cannot tolerate excessive gas may ultimately develop a functional gut problem—a "cute" proposal.

Similar suggestions to explain gas intolerance in some individuals are found in earlier literature. I extend this suggestion by adding that the intolerance of some individuals to gas may be an intermittent phenomenon, which I believe is most likely related to a mind-gut interaction. Therefore, I believe that the therapy of gaseousness should be similar to some of the more effective types of intervention that are used to treat functional gut disorders such as IBS. Functional gut disorders are due to imbalances of nature, and I propose that natural therapies may have a lot more to offer than drug interventions. When one examines the therapy of many functional gut diseases, one is impressed by the failure of conventional medical approaches that reach preferentially for drug therapy.

Accepting that the cause of excessive gas is multifactorial (many causes), then an appropriate approach is to focus on teaching ways of tolerating excessive gas in the guts as well as obvious measures to correct the production of excessive gas or diminish excessive entry of gas into the gut (Table 6.1). The lesson learned from Monsieur Petit-Pas, the vaudeville star now becomes very important. Individuals can learn to tolerate the sensation of excessive gas, and this process is more effective when the gas excess is recognized as the cause of the symptom. In the ensuing chapter on IBS, one will accept the modern evidence that education is a powerful intervention in functional digestive disturbance. Holistic medicine involving diverse disciplines of alternative or pluralistic medicine hold the key, in other words, hypnosis, Yoga, Ayurveda, relaxation therapy, biofeedback, and so on.

TREATMENT PLANS FOR EXCESS GUT GAS

A proposed treatment plan is shown in Table 6.1. A detailed dietary history is very important, with a specific focus on offending dietary items. One common cause of excessive flatus is lactose intolerance and the elimination of nonfermented dairy products is a simple and often effective approach. Diets that are low in dietary fiber will tend to be low in fruit and vegetables, and such diets are not healthy. Although these diets produce less gas, they also tend to delay the transit of the gut contents, including gas, and, in my opinion, should be avoided unless specific circumstances dictate the need for reduced fiber intake.

My advice may seem contrary, but I am suggesting to many people that their opinions about gas in the gut should change. The passage of gas is a healthy body function. Both Hippocrates and the Roman emperor Claudius proclaimed the benefits of the release of gas. Dr. J. H. Pollock, in his excellent book titled *Gaseous Digestive Conditions* (Springfield, IL: Thomas Publishing, 1967), quotes Claudius in the following statement: "All Roman citizens shall be allowed to pass gas whenever necessary."

VALUABLE NATURAL THERAPIES FOR GAS

Table 6.1: Some strategies for excessive gas in the guts.

Note, an accurate diagnosis of the cause of the problem is a prerequisite for any intervention.

Enhancing the tolerance for gut gas	• Acceptance of gas—"Claudius' decree"* • Relaxation techniques • Yoga • Education • Learned maneuvers to pass gas • Control mood
Decreasing gas production or entry	• Avoid excessive single dietary offenders, e.g., beans, milk products • Observe and avoid air swallowing • Fix specific problems, e.g., stress • Avoid excessive animal protein • Avoid drugs that impair gut movements • Use carminatives • Consider a supervised "colon cleansing" • Consider probiotic therapy with added prebiosis • Supervised use of formulas of friendly bacteria can be effective • Selected use of absorbents ,e.g., charcoal, kaolin, pectin

* The Roman Emperor Claudius decreed that citizens were allowed to pass gas in an unencumbered manner.

Table 6.1 summarizes many nonconventional approaches to the management of excessive gas, but the relative importance of these interventions is not apparent. The most obvious initiative is lacking in Table 6.1, namely correction of adverse lifestyle habits. Adverse lifestyle is a primary cause of gut imbalance. In many cases, the move toward a healthy diet, exercise, and the promotion of psychological well-being can cause excessive gas to go, almost as fast as it comes!

In my own experience, I have found that the use of herbs, spices, and botanicals with carminative actions are very valuable (Table 6.2). They represent a pleasant, less expensive, and highly effective alternative to many digestive aids. Of great importance are the essential oils of peppermint, fennel, dill, and caraway. The use of peppermint oil is of particular benefit because of its antifoaming effects, smooth muscle relaxing effects, and deodorizing capabilities. Peppermint oil is best presented in delayed release (enteric-coated) formats because of its pungent taste and occasional irritant effects on the upper digestive tract. For less severe types of complaints, it can be consumed in dilute elixirs or herbal teas. The value of peppermint and other carminatives is reviewed in detail in chapter 7. Herbs and botanicals that can help relieve gas are listed in table 6.2.

ACTIVATED CHARCOAL: DOES IT WORK?

Table 6.2: Carminatives and soothing agents that can be used for excessive gas in the guts.

Peppermint, fennel, caraway, and ginger are highly effective at relieving gas in the author's clinical experience.

AGENT	COMMENT
Allspice	Used in Jamaica for many years. Contains eugenol, which stimulates the enzyme trypsin.
Anise	Essential oil of seed is effective.
Caraway	The oil is used in canamoa tincture.
Catnip	Effective, but only small doses are safe.
Cinnamon	A classic Chinese antiflatulent.
Dill	Mashed dill seeds produce a carminative oil.
Fennel	Essential oil with monoterpenes.
Ginger	A classic antinauseant and carminative.
Marjoram	Active ingredient unknown.
Papaya	Contains enzymes.
Peppermint	Very effective—see chapter 7.
Thyme	Ancient Roman remedy after feasts.

Activated charcoal (burned wood) has been used for three thousand years to treat a variety of diseases ranging from epilepsy to infections (Hippocrates), through to its modern-day use for the treatment of excessive volumes of—and bad smells due to—gut gas.

The main gases in the gut are nitrogen, oxygen, carbon dioxide, hydrogen, methane, and trace gases, especially those containing sulfur. Sulfur-containing gases such as hydrogen sulfide and methanethiol are responsible for much of the bad smell associated with passing gas. While these gases are smelly, they are also quite toxic and can play some role in general feelings of ill health, and a causal role in worsening inflammatory conditions of the bowel, especially ulcerative colitis.

Activated charcoal certainly binds these noxious types of gut gases, but recent studies show that charcoal does not seem to materially effect the liberation of bowel gas. The generation of the gas is a function of the contents of the digesta, the bowel contents. While activated charcoal may afford some limited symptomatic benefit for excessive, smelly gut gas, the key is to effect changes in the microflora (bacteria in the gut) which is an active component of the digesta. The significance of microflora in health and disease is extremely important in medicine and it is discussed in detail in chapter 10.

VISCEROPTOSIS—RED HERRING?

When the abdomen is bloated, the bulging is usually caused by fat, fluid, or flatus. Gaseous bloating can result in gross displacement of the guts. Displacement of the guts within the normal confines of the abdomen (excluding herniae) is termed visceroptosis. These gut displacements have been often erroneously considered to cause serious gut disorders, but the esophagus, stomach, and bowels are usually able to function quite normally regardless of their position.

In medical literature as recently as forty years ago, discussions of visceroptosis were quite common. The question remains whether or not visceroptosis is a true cause of gut symptoms. The answer, probably is only on rare occasions. There is a condition sometimes referred to as Glenard's disease that is believed to be related to poor body posture (the asthenic habitus), characterized by a straightening of the spine, stooping shoulders and variable protrusion of the abdomen. Aging tends to move many people towards this type of posture—especially men.

Certain circumstances tend to promote visceroptosis including multiple childbirths, loss of a large amount of weight, and loss of abdominal wall strength due to age or sedentary lifestyle. There are a group of patients in whom visceroptosis may cause stretching of mesenteric (bowel) attachments. In these individuals, chiropractic interventions and the use of posture therapy (Alexander technique) or exercise can improve nonspecific abdominal complaints. Acupuncture is very beneficial for drooping of the guts, while surgery to correct visceroptosis is most often not a good idea. Conventional medicine doubts the significance of visceroptosis, but in selected cases its correction may be beneficial.

CHAPTER SUMMARY

When the serious or specific causes of excessive gas have been excluded, the most appropriate approach is to attempt to restore balance to the guts. Intolerant guts can be made more tolerant by natural means. This approach has more to offer when applied in a holistic manner than any current drug intervention. The magnitude of the problem of excessive gas in the guts has not received the attention that it deserves from modern medicine. Problems associated with excessive gas in the guts are a prime target for natural therapies.

CHAPTER SEVEN

IRRITABLE
BOWEL SYNDROME

IRRITATING THE GUTS: IBS

Irritability of the intestines is universal. Dr. John F. Fielding, an Irish gastroenterologist, coined the phrase that I have used in this book: "All bowels are irritable and all bowels are irritated." Every time food passes our lips, the guts are stimulated into action, but in health those stimuli produce no adverse sensations or are quite unobtrusive. In addition, the sight or smell of food can whip the guts into action. Stress or anxiety is a well-known stimulus to gut function but its effects are usually transient. Thus, short-lived gut reactions are normal. However, when irritability of the bowels is persistent and organic disease is absent, the condition of IBS can be said to be present. Just as the definition of IBS is often a definition of exclusion, the diagnosis of IBS is often a diagnosis of exclusion (of organic disease).

ENDLESS DEBATES, DEFINITIONS, AND TERMS

Despite the common nature of IBS, modern medicine has failed to fully understand what causes IBS. When a condition is poorly understood in medicine, it creates a monster list of labels and a lack of consensus on definitions. We shall learn that IBS is a mixed bag of tricks.

IBS has been otherwise called the irritable gut syndrome, the irritable colon syndrome, irritability of the intestines, spastic colitis, spastic colon, mucous colitis, unstable colon, functional bowel disease, and so on. Each of these terms has a basis for its use, but the term *irritable gut syndrome* is probably ideal because it recognizes that irritability in IBS is global in the gut in many cases. In different terms, a person with an irritable large bowel is more likely to have irritability elsewhere in the guts, such as in the small bowel, stomach, and esophagus.

The general and widespread nature of irritability in the guts commonly presents a problem in treatment. Symptoms of irritability of the colon frequently dominate the clinical picture, but they are not often the whole problem. Modern medicine has tended to restrict thinking and diagnostic intervention to the colon in the disorder of IBS. These focused thoughts may have been an impediment to its management. The recognition of subtypes of IBS such as pain-predominant types and diarrhea-predominant types, is an example of focused thinking. The situation is exemplified by the heterogeneous types (many different types) and variable locations of motor problems that form the complex disorder of IBS. To simplify matters, I shall use the abbreviation IBS (Irritable Bowel Syndrome) throughout this chapter, but this will refer to the global gut disorder that is known to comprise "irritable gut syndrome."

IBS: ONE OF MANY FUNCTIONAL GUT DISORDERS

There are many working definitions of IBS, but the Rome criteria (1990) give us the best description because they tend to remove the focus of medical thoughts from the colon alone and take the global approach. This Rome definition of functional gut disorders indicates that they comprise "A variable combination of chronic (long lasting) or recurrent gastrointestinal symptoms, attributed to the pharynx esophagus, stomach, biliary tree, small or large intestine, or anorectum (anus and lower bowel) that are not explained by structural or biochemical (body chemistry) abnormalities."

By now, the reader may be lost in concepts and definitions. I started to discuss irritable bowels and I have ended up back in the upper portions of the guts. I am not shadowboxing, I must reiterate the global nature of the movement disorders (motor dysfunction) that are encountered in the guts, before a focus is made on the colon).

DEFINING IBS

IBS can be simply stated to generally conform to a definition that includes the presence of chronic (long lasting, greater than three months) or intermittent (recurrent) abnormalities of bowel habit, with or without lower abdominal pain or discomfort. The pain or discomfort of IBS can be felt anywhere in the abdomen and sometimes in the chest. The most important issue in the definition is that it is *not* explained by any structural (anatomic problems or disease) or metabolic (altered body chemistry) causes. IBS is the most common "type" of functional gut disorder. Therefore, it gets a great deal of attention.

There are other quite distinct functional disorders of the bowel. These include functional abdominal bloating, fullness or distension (a blown-up belly), functional problems with functional diarrhea and disorders of the evacuation of the bowel. The latter condition has been referred to as "dry heaves of the rectum"—attributed to Dr. S. Phillips. The complexity of the abnormalities of the function of the bowels, independent of IBS, now becomes apparent. In my opinion, these disorders are often lumped under the diagnosis of IBS, and failure to characterize this varied group of functional bowel problems could be a handicap to the management of these disorders.

TALKING TO PATIENTS

The complex nature of the symptom pattern of IBS requires the taking of a meticulous patient history. Unfortunately, the pressures of modern medicine leave only small amounts of time for a physician to speak to patients. Furthermore, it has been argued that medical reimbursement provides some disincentives to take extensive patient histories, which may define the global and complex manifestations of IBS.

This situation became acutely apparent to me during an evening book signing and lecture that I gave at a Barnes and Noble bookstore in New York. I was surprised to find that the audience who had come to hear about my book *Miracle Herbs*" contained several medical residents (trainee doctors). During the question-and-answer period, it became obvious that these medical residents had recognized the importance of addressing some of the newfound patient demands for information about botanical and herbal therapies.

The doctors in the audience were raising issues about their understanding of standards of care when I discussed the unwillingness of conventional medicine to embrace or pay for remedies of natural origin, even though they were demanded frequently by patients. One trainee doctor quoted his understanding of standards of care. According to his teachers, he had been told to spend a minimum of fifteen minutes in a follow-up visit, write a minimum of focused notes in the chart, and finish his treatment plan with a drug prescription.

The reaction from the nonphysicians in the audience was quite negative. Of course, the interests of the audience were skewed toward alternative medicine. They had seldom had to face the reality of how medicine may have to be practiced by algorithm (a form of recipe) to satisfy standards of care. When several members of the audience asked, who set the standards of care, the medical resident replied that it was a condition of reimbursement and written guidelines of quality of care. Clearly, the art of medicine is being stripped out of medical practice.

THE NON-IBS FUNCTIONAL DISORDERS

Some individuals are bothered by a sensation of bloating or fullness in their abdomen, which does not appear to be related to abnormal digestion. This situation can occur in the presence of IBS or functional dyspepsia or as an isolated phenomenon. Sometimes, the cause becomes obvious by the taking of a careful dietary history. Individuals who eat significant amounts of nondigestible substances such as excess dietary fiber or excess legumes (e.g., beans, lentils, peas, soybeans) may have their symptoms alleviated by moderation of intake of these foods. However, the distended belly can be present without these causes, and it represents, in my opinion, one of the many manifestations of the lack of the balance between the mind and the guts or the "mind" of the guts. The answer to this kind of problem is a natural way to restore this balance, not the use of current drug therapy.

There are people who have difficulty with bowel evacuation in the absence of IBS. These problems are manifest by infrequent opening of the bowels (less than two times per week), incomplete evacuation of their bowels (or a sensation of incomplete passage of stool), and the passage of pellets of hard stool. There are many people who complain of rabbitlike stools. Rabbit-type droppings in humans are most often a function of fiber roughage deficiency in the diet. It is important to realize that a number of functional disorders of the anorectum affect stool appearance. These are discussed in chapter 8.

Perhaps the most perplexing condition of all is plain bellyache in the absence of IBS or other common causes of pain, such as PMS (premenstrual syndrome) or excessive eating. This condition has been given a label of the destitute with the meaningless term *chronic functional abdominal pain*. Again, I believe this is a problem of mind-body balance, and it is not likely to respond to any popular drug therapy.

As I dig further into the many variants of functional gut disorder and the related conditions that confuse the picture, one may be sympathetic to my opinion that conventional medical approaches may not help solve these common problems. Of course, this opinion depends on a definition of what constitutes conventional therapy. Expressed differently, existing drug therapy will not do the trick in many cases. A much more holistic approach to IBS is required.

IBS: A COMMON AND WIDESPREAD PROBLEM

Descriptions of IBS have been around for a long time, and it is apparent that this disorder knows no social or ethnic boundaries. IBS is more common in females (accounting for 60–75 percent of cases) and its occurrence seems to decline with age. Perhaps the mind and body learns to coordinate more with time or perhaps sensitivities decrease with age. Without engaging sarcasm, it is impossible to detect IBS following a frontal lobotomy! Overall, up to one-quarter of the population of several Western societies experiences IBS, with a range of occurrence of about 10 to 25 percent. Of course, the occurrence of IBS depends on the criteria that are used to make a diagnosis, and many people with the disorder do not seek healthcare.

Population studies of attendances at medical facilities with IBS show that as few as one in five people with IBS will seek medical attention for their symptoms. At the most only about one in two sufferers may seek attention. Where do these people go and what do they do?

THE IBS SUFFERER

Not only do a large proportion of sufferers of IBS not go to a physician, but those that do attend a medical facility complain frequently that they do not often obtain relief from medical therapy. One could write a complex and lengthy book on why people seek healthcare. Bars to medical services include cost, cultural beliefs, psychological factors, social issues, and the construct of medical services themselves. America and many other countries may not have produced generally portable or user-friendly healthcare services.

I believe that the majority of individuals with IBS self-medicate. They often pace the aisles of pharmacies, health food stores, and grocery shops looking for OTC digestive aids. The problem is that IBS is not a condition that is readily self-diagnosed and sufferers cannot easily match over the counter OTC digestive aids with their problem. When they do, they realize often that many such aids do not work. It is not uncommon for self-diagnosis to result in a wrong match of an OTC digestive remedy. You might be surprised by the number of people taking upper digestive aids (e.g., H_2-receptor antagonists) for lower digestive problems. Ask a pharmacist!

SYMPTOMS OF IBS

IBS is primarily a disorder of symptoms. In fact, one could question the use of the term syndrome as applied to IBS, because a syndrome is a collection of symptoms *and* signs. The most common complaints in IBS are abdominal pain and altered bowel habit occurring together, alone, or intermittently associated. So variable are the characteristics, frequency, location, and duration of the symptoms of IBS that it can present a very difficult diagnostic problem for even the most astute physician. What chance does an uninformed sufferer have of making an accurate diagnosis in a predictable manner?

The pain of IBS is most often felt in the lower left side of the abdomen, but it can occur anywhere in the abdomen and it can even be felt in the chest or back. While the pain is often mild, some individuals have even sought opiate (narcotic) drugs to relieve symptoms. Abnormal bowel habits are common in IBS with every possible combination of diarrhea and constipation. Problems do arise with the definition of *abnormal bowel habit*. In general, normal bowel function involves the opening of the bowels no more than three times a day and no less than three times a week, in most people. Stool volume and consistency, however, is variable among individuals, and it is often dependent on diet.

It is important to reemphasize the global nature of IBS. There has been a tendency to think about IBS in local colonic terms, but many studies over the past thirty years have demonstrated an association of IBS with other disorders. IBS is a can of worms when it comes to an analysis of symptoms.

TOWARD A POSITIVE
DIAGNOSIS OF IBS

Accepting that IBS is a condition characterized by symptoms, with few characteristic signs, then it becomes apparent that positive clinical diagnosis may be very difficult. This situation has led to the development of criteria for the diagnosis of IBS, based largely on questionnaires. This mode of diagnosis is based on the principle that the greater the number of non-specific symptoms of IBS that are present, the more likely that IBS is present. The most popular symptom-based criteria for the diagnosis of IBS were described by doctors Manning, Thompson, Heaton, and Morris in a classic paper entitled "Towards Positive Diagnosis of Irritable Bowel Syndrome" that was published in the *British Medical Journal* in 1978 (Vol. 2, 653–654). These Manning criteria are summarized in Table 7.1.

The Manning criteria revealed that there were six symptoms that could predict the presence of IBS (Table 7.1), but the Manning questionnaire is not a foolproof diagnostic instrument. The symptoms in the Manning criteria can be signals of serious organic disease in the guts (or elsewhere). For example, mucus in the stool can be encountered in bowel cancer and inflammation. Again, a consideration of red flag symptoms that were described in earlier chapters is necessary. The fact is that both the physician-based diagnosis and self-diagnosis of IBS are difficult tasks. I add an important caveat: Any significant change in bowel habit in an individual over the age of forty years (or thereabouts) must be investigated. My recommendation is supported by an anticipated one hundred fifty thousand new cases of colon cancer in the United States over the next year!

My dialogue must return to the notion that IBS is a diagnosis that occurs by the exclusion of organic disease in the guts. The use of multiple diagnostic interventions (medical testing) in IBS is often uncomfortable, expensive, and sometimes self-defeating. Medical testing should provide reassurance for the sufferer, but it sometimes does the opposite. Anxiety provoking medical interventions can make IBS worse!

There have been attempts to improve on the reliability of the Manning criteria by creating a series of diagnostic scores using symptoms and signs. When looking at a completely different disorder such as alcohol abuse, it has been shown that this diagnostic approach can be more accurate. Using this approach, Dr. Harvey Skinner (Head of Behavioral Sciences at the University of Toronto, Canada) and I researched the development of the Alcoholic Clinical Index in 1979,

---

Table 7.1: The Manning Criteria for the diagnosis of IBS.

See text for a discussion of the significance of these symptoms in diagnosis.

- Abdominal pain —associated with loose stools
  —associated with more frequent stools
  —eased ofter the bowel is opened

- Abdominal distension (bloating)

- Mucus in the stool

- Incomplete evacuation of the rectum or a sensation thereof

**Table 7.2: Questions the physician or patient
can use to diagnose IBS.**

Taken from Kruis et al. (Gastroenterology 87:1, 1984).

Questions to be filled out by the patient:
• Did you come because of abdominal pain?
• Do you suffer from flatulence?
• Do you suffer from irregularities of bowel movement?
• Have you suffered from your complaints for more than two years?
• How can your abdominal pain be described: burning, cutting, very strong, terrible, feeling of pressure, dull, boring, not so bad?
• Have you noticed alternating constipation and diarrhea?

Checklist to be filled out by the doctor:
• Abnormal physical findings and/or history that suggest organic disease
• ESR >20mm/2 hr
  Leucocytosis >10,000/ccm
  Hemoglobin: female <12 g%
              male   <14 g%
• History of blood in stool

where a series of symptoms, signs, and laboratory tests were assembled to predict the presence of alcohol abuse. This approach is difficult in IBS, because signs and abnormal lab tests are lacking. Dr. W. Kruis and his colleagues have prepared a useful diagnostic instrument for IBS that is valuable in the exclusion of organic disease, but again, it is not foolproof. Questions that a physician (or perhaps a patient) can use to diagnose IBS are summarized in Table 7.2. This work was published by Dr. Kruis and his colleagues in the medical journal *Gastroenterology* (87:1, 1984). Despite the recognized importance of these diagnostic instruments, they are seldom used by doctors in conventional, clinical practice.

INAPPROPRIATENESS

Some of the most impressive traditional perceptions about the patient with IBS emanate from the work of Dr. John F. Fielding and his colleagues. Dr. Fielding states in reference to IBS: "I believe that the clinical scene can be summed up in a word—inappropriateness." He refers to a common characteristic among some patients of their appearance, severity of complaints, and mannerisms that appear incongruous with the circumstances. There is no doubt that these traits are apparent in some patients with IBS, and they may be a manifestation of underlying psychosocial disturbances. However, the patient with IBS has no stereotypic behavior or presentation. We may learn later that the conscious mind may not reveal any disturbances of the mind-body connection with accuracy. Some might argue that the gut's own nervous system is acting alone to cause IBS—an intriguing possibility!

PSYCHOSOCIAL DISTURBANCES AND IBS

There are several thousand studies reported in the medical literature that examine the relationship among abnormal behavior, lack of psychological well-being, or social problems and IBS. One predictable theme seems to emerge. The individual with IBS most often has evidence of psychosocial problems in one form or another. Table 7.3

Table 7.3: Psychosocial disturbances that are linked with IBS.

These disturbances are linked in both the causes and effects of IBS. These factors definitely affect prognosis and treatment outcome in IBS.

CONDITIONS	COMMENTS
Personality problems	Dependent and overdemanding, orderly control, dramatization, suffering.
Anxiety, depression, anger	Often present (about 60 percent), linked in both cause and effect.
Stressful life events	Come in many types and sometimes hidden.
Abuse	A relationship between sexual abuse and IBS exists in females.
Conversion Reactions	So called "neurotic" symptoms without biological cause: a misnomer?
Somatoform disorders	This is the mind-body reaction—see text.
Healthcare seeking IBS	Psychosocial abnormalities appear more common in partners with IBS who seek healthcare but NOT necessarily in those with IBS who do not.

summarizes some of the more important psychosocial disturbances that may occur in individuals with IBS. However, this is not the whole story.

Landmark medical studies have shown us that individuals with IBS who visit a physician may have a greater problem with psychosocial disturbances than those who do not seek medical attention. Stated differently, the host of psychological labels that are given to the individual with IBS may not apply to a large proportion of sufferers of IBS. Only as few as one in five people with IBS may have readily identifiable psychosocial problems.

These findings or proposals may shock some healthcare professionals who have tended to approach IBS as a primary disorder of the mind. While this approach may fit some sufferers with IBS, it does not fit them all. Treatment methods have been applied generally to IBS that make the assumptions that problems are rooted in the mind and manifest in the gut. Clearly, these treatment initiatives are not universally applicable in IBS.

It may seem at first sight, that I am defeating my entire logic by emphasizing the mind-gut interaction throughout this book and then denying approaches to fix the mind as the answer to functional bowel disease. It is not the lack of a mind-gut, interaction that is the issue, these balancing acts exist! It is the way we have viewed mind-body-mind interrelationships—let me explain.

PSYCHONEUROIMMUNOENDOCRINE-PHARMACOLOGY

Please do not close this book! Modern medicine has to deal with neologisms for a time while it begins to understand the real cause of the common disorders that it has to address. The words *psychoneuroimmunoendocrine-pharmacology* have to be linked together to make a simple point. The psycho (mind) is linked with the neuro (nervous system), linked to the immuno (immune function), linked to the endocrine (hormonal controls) in a series of pharmacological (chemical) events. After all, the body is a bag of reacting chemicals and their reactions form part of the universe (Gaia). Gaia, however, is more than chemicals, it is life forces, relationships between living and innate objects, spirituality, and perhaps many other intangibles or unknowns.

MIND, BODY, AND SPIRIT

In order to understand modern misdirections in medical thinking, we need to revisit history. Founders of modern medical thought such as Hippocrates did not separate functions of the body from spirituality and superstition. Early medical philosophy was all-encompassing or holistic. Perhaps the greatest shaper of medical thought was the emergence of religion. Religion became very powerful and in many ancient cultures it ruled rulers. More cynical philosophers have proposed that the birth of Christianity and other faiths led to the emergence of an ecclesiastical deal where religion exerted an ownership of the mind, morality, and spirituality, but permitted the physician to own the domain of caring for the anatomy and physiology of the body, without daring to cross the boundary. I am not certain that I subscribe entirely to these notions, but they have some plausible connotations. In early history, the son who was too weak to tend the land as a farmer or too stupid to join the church often went to law or medical school!

Thus, the art of medicine became devoid of a responsibility for spirituality and its related issues. This approach of physicians emerged and dominated medical thinking from the third century until modern times. Religion is only one powerful influence in the evolution of medical thought. Throughout medical history, some physicians continued to focus on disease and its treatment by paying due respect to the imponderables of emotion, spirituality, and some more nebulous examples life forces. Some of these physicians were labeled charlatans or crackpots. There has been a "divorce" of medicine from these other factors that determine health and well-being. The important operant in this divorce may have been social beliefs or religion, which have always espoused antagonism to occurrences of marital divorce or dichotomy among humankind. This is an important enigma in modern medicine. Intellectual divorce has plagued medical advances.

140

BODY-MIND AND THE IBS

IBS is the archetypical example of the inefficient operation of mind-body interactions. A host of studies has shown an interaction between IBS and stress, eating, and enhanced pain perception. Among the most obvious demonstrations of the gut responses to stress is the work of Dr. Thomas P. Almy that was published in the *American Journal of Medicine* in 1951 (10:60–67).

The famous Almy experiment on a fourth-year medical student involved the recording of direct observations of the movement and color of the lining of the gut. Dr. Almy introduced a proctoscope (instrument to examine the lining of the rectum) into the anus of this student in relative circumstances of no stress. The scientist then played a hoax on the student by telling him that he had detected cancer of the rectum. This falsehood caused observable increases in contractions in the bowel and engorgement of the lining of the bowel with blood (due to enhanced blood flow). After the hoax had been explained, the rectum returned to its earlier state of tranquility, with a more normal color of its lining. There are many experiments on humans that have examined the effects of the mind on gut function with much more sophisticated recordings. More investigation of the nature and characteristics of the complex neurohormonal connections between the mind and gut have merely served to exemplify the importance of the mind-body.

It is difficult to summarize the mind-gut research in IBS because there has been so much of it! In general, patents with IBS (and other types of functional gut disease) seem to have an altered sensation in their guts with a tendency for hypersensitivity. This means that events in the gut (or the mind) are more amplified in people with IBS. For example, some individuals with IBS appear to have a much lower threshold to pain.

In IBS, this concept of amplification of gut-mind activities is in evidence by observations of an increased reaction to simple events like eating. In addition, the bowel in IBS seems more reactive to mechanical events like distension and to its own messengers (hormones) that normally orchestrate gut function. If one examines the act of distension of the guts, one may now understand why failure to handle even normal amounts of gas in the gut can give rise to unpleasant symptoms, because of amplified responses. Not only is amplification a problem, but evidence exists that normally coordinated mind-gut interactions are out of sync in IBS. There is dysregulation. Furthermore, the abnormalities in the complex messenger network that controls the mind and gut are not often located in one area of the gut. Patients with IBS appear to have abnormal responses in both the small and large bowel, and often elsewhere in the guts.

If we accept more holistic types of approaches to IBS, then mind and body must be perceived as one connected by an enormous communications highway (terminology borrowed from Vice President Al Gore) that is composed of chemical messengers and nervous impulses. The influences on these messengers and their triggers are located within or outside the body. I coin the term, *mindgutbodyenvironment* to move towards the thinking of "Gaiaguts." Please allow me this neologism to make my point.

GAIAGUTS

Earlier, I introduced the concept of Gaia, without explaining this term that is used in New Age medicine. I am *not* necessarily embracing the concept of the Gaia Hypothesis, but it is a useful example of the concept of oneness and the inextricable linkage of life, body, mind, environment and universe.

The Gaia Hypothesis describes a "oneness" of human life but extends the concept to a oneness of the biosphere of the earth, and, to some, the universe. This personalization of the earth as oneness is part of the theories of planetary consciousness, and it has been labeled Gaia by New Age scientists, after the Greek Earth goddess.

The concept of Gaia is shrouded in neopaganism, atmospheric biochemistry, and other esoterica. It may seem that the concept of Gaia is a far cry from IBS, but I propose the holistic consideration of functional gastrointestinal disease (or functional disease of any organ). Complete thinking about all aspects of life may result in major advances in therapy or prevention of disease. However, one has to accept the incomplete nature of our understanding of life forces in this framework of presumed completeness. My proposals may meet resistance, especially in conventional medicine, and therefore I must digress into the work of the pioneers of modern biology and medicine to support my approach. I doubt that this support will satisfy some people's skepticism.

THE DYNAMIC INTERCONNECTING NETWORK

The concept of bodyminds is supported by neuroscience experiments that show the presence of receptors of various types for transmitter molecules throughout the body. A very enlightened account of this information highway is found in Dr. Pert's book titled *Molecules of Emotion*. Pert indicates that the areas of neuroscience may have been perceived formerly as distinct. However, they are connected to each other in a sophisticated network of communication. The evidence for this is compelling and is based on the demonstration of receptor sites for neuropeptides (chemical messengers) that are common to different types of tissues.

Dr. Pert and her colleagues defined the presence of many types of receptors on different tissues. Her striking observations concern the ubiquitous nature of the opiate receptor. The observations have been extended to gastrointestinal hormones. The term *gastrointestinal hormone* may be a misnomer. It is argued that many of these hormones are probably mislabeled as gastrointestinal, because they act frequently at sites outside the gastrointestinal tract (e.g., the brain and nervous system).

One of many examples of the information network and its complex communications involves the role of cholecystokinin (CCK). CCK is a hormone that is released during eating and causes gallbladder contraction, which then results in bile flow to assist in digestion. It is known that CCK receptors, and therefore the actions of CCK, are apparent in the brain and immune system as well as the gastrointestinal tract. The neuropeptide CCK is known to govern the feelings of hunger and satiety. Relatively recent research shows that the presence of receptors for the hormone CCK are present not only in the guts but also in the brain and spleen. By lateral thinking, Dr. Pert refers to the spleen as the "brain of the immune system." This is lateral thinking that is to be strongly commended, in my opinion.

Dr. Pert has drawn attention to what is quite well known about the role of CCK release during eating and its effects on satisfying feelings of hunger and causing movements in the gut, especially in relation to the gallbladder. However, she proposes an interesting simultaneous role for CCK on immune function; her opinion being that to have your immune system revved up shortly after eating is a bad idea, because your immune system might mount an attack on the undigested meal! For this reason, her conjecture is that it would make sense that the same CCK system that creates a sense of satiety in your brain and makes your gallbladder go to work is also able to signal the immune system to slow down.

The neuropeptide CCK is one example of an information substance that occurs on the complex, interconnecting information highway that forms the basis of the concept of bodyminds. This concept is quite different than isolated, cause-and-effect views of the functions of the body. Information systems with nervous impulses and neuropeptide connections add intelligence to body functions and further add the concept of "molecules of emotion," which has been well described by Dr. Pert. IBS and other functional gut disorders appear to fit into these notions of a biopsychosocial constellation (bio-life, psycho-mind).

EXTENDING THE CONCEPT OF "MOLECULES OF EMOTION"

Our understanding of signals and their coordination and meaning remains incomplete. When one looks at unknown forces that may shape body function by acting on the bodymind, the situation becomes somewhat indecipherable given our current level of knowledge.

The radical-thinking biologist Dr. Rupert Sheldrake has proposed that there are certain energy fields that are not made up of identifiable energy or matter. Dr. Sheldrake postulated further that there is a phenomenon of morphic resonance such that these fields organize energy into matter. This hypothetical occurrence implies that if something has already been done (created), the knowledge on how it was done is available, because it has been recorded in a kind of morphogenic field. These morphogenic fields are energy systems that may cause structural occurrences by recordings of activity, and it is proposed that they can result in the development of a kind of memory system, akin to a genetic code.

The thoughts and concepts that I propose are not embraced by conventional medicine, and they may not be universally accepted by practitioners of alternative medicine. In order to further our understanding, we can examine ancient medical disciplines such as Ayurvedic medicine where these concepts are not examples of alien thinking. Dr. Deepak Chopra talks about the unity of matter and spirit, body and soul. In popular writings, Dr. Chopra refers to the "field of intelligence" that connects mind, spirit, and emotions. In a foreword to Dr. Pert's book, Dr. Chopra indicates that receptor experiments and the mapping of the information network in the body provides a science-based explanation for awareness and consciousness and its profound influences. Dr. Chopra states, "The body is not a mindless machine, the body and mind are one." I believe that many people must now be inclined to believe this aphorism, especially in relationship to the gutmind or mindgut. My extensions of reasoning may offer credence to the idea of Gaiaguts.

THE IRRITABLE "ANYTHING" SYNDROME

One is impressed by the body of literature on IBS and the careers in medicine that have been built on the research of this disorder. While conversations about IBS are common in medicine, one hears very little about the irritable heart syndrome, the irritable brain syndrome, the irritable kidney syndrome, etc. Does this irritable "anything" syndrome really exist? I believe it does. Its overt occurrence, however, is linked in part to simple anatomy. The greater the nervous innervation (or communication) of an organ of the body, the more likely it is to be irritable. In the case of the gut, the nervous system of the digestive tract is so large that it has been described as having its own brain (or lots of little brains). In addition, the degree of communication with "molecules of emotion" (discussed in chapter 12) determines the manifestation of organ irritability.

One could be bold and say that disturbances of the intelligent information network that constitutes, in part, the bodymind could manifest themselves in many organs. Are the psychological disturbances or nonspecific ancillary complaints that are so common in IBS merely part of a more global disorder of the bodymind? I believe that they are!

I could attract criticism by those who would adopt the notion Ca ne dit rien ("it means nothing"). On the contrary, if it meant nothing, then the constellation of functional visceral disorders, like IBS, would not exist. Perhaps more important is that the acceptance of the bodymind concept could alter treatment approaches and result in more effective interventions or disease-prevention strategies. This situation may then lead to a reversal of the pessimism that is sometimes expressed by physicians who have to treat IBS and other functional disorders of the gut.

To quote Dr. John F. Fielding, the physician who excelled in his knowledge of IBS: "The prognosis, in so far as cure is concerned, is not good; very few people become and remain symptom-free, but many, none the less, obtain subjective relief." Although one can attribute this statement to Dr. Fielding in 1977, things have not changed much in the treatment of IBS over the past twenty years. At least, recognition of this circumstance may spur a search for alternatives.

Medical thinking about functional disease has turned the wheel at least twice over the past couple of millennia. Hippocrates and Galen did not divorce the mind from disease. The scientific basis of a mind-body interaction was discovered later by great scientists like Pavlov. This contributed to a dissociation of thinking between spirituality or emotion and body to some degree. This basis was explored throughout the last two centuries by Cannon and Beaumont (referred to earlier), and subsequently others through recent times. In recent times, the wheel may have turned again as the scientific explanations start to incorporate the issues of emotion, spirituality, and unknown forces to reinforce the concept of bodymind—now the idea of Gaiaguts may seem plausible. Insulting the guts insults the emotions, and insulting the emotions insults the guts in a never-ending and complex union by intelligent, nervous, and chemical interconnections. These events do not occur in isolation of the environment to which humankind is exposed—or creates for itself.

MANAGEMENT OF IBS

The vast array of suggested treatments for IBS in conventional medicine could be accepted as reasonable evidence that few of them are effective. Standard textbooks of medicine or gastroenterology contain suggested treatment approaches to IBS that can leave an informed reader with a sensation similar to looking through ground glass. Few options are presented in a concise and clear manner for application in the therapy of IBS, but many of these options are questioned in terms of effectiveness.

The outcome of treatment in IBS is a function of both the physician's and the patient's expectations. Perhaps more important is the doctor-patient relationship. Dr. D. A. Drossman and Dr. W. G. Thomson have stressed the importance of the doctor-patient relationship. The components of an optimal physician-patient interaction in treating IBS includes cost-effective testing, reassurance, patient education, continuity of care, and the establishment of realistic treatment goals.

Ignorance creates fear when it comes to any medical disorder. Many studies have reinforced the importance of patient education in the successful management of IBS. Knowledge is important and can be transmitted by the physician or allied healthcare professional. Some studies suggest that this does not often happen in routine clinical practice. An efficient and cost-effective practice is to encourage patients to read books that permit an understanding of functional gut disease. Of course, this is one prime reason for the writing of this book. Several excellent and scientifically credible books are available that tend to take a more "conventional approach" to functional gut disorders than this book.

In my opinion, the two most important books on IBS written for patients are: *Gut Reactions: Understanding Symptoms of the Digestive Tract* by Dr. W. G. Thompson, (New York: Plenum Press, 1989), and *Irritable Bowel Syndrome: A Practical Guide* by Dr. G. Watts (London: Mandarin, 1990). These books (Table 7.4) do not delve in detail into the popular, alternative, and complementary options that patients are exercising increasingly these days.

Table 7.4: Four books on IBS and functional gastrointestinal disorder that are valuable in self-help tactics.

These books are among the most valuable in the author's opinion.

Gut Reactions: Understanding Symptoms of the Digestive Tract
W. Grant Thompson (Plenum Press, NJ, 1989)
> An excellent treatise on symptoms with an emphasis in conventional medical options

Relief from IBS
Elaine F. Shimberg (Ballantine Books, NY, 1988)
> Very simple and readable description of IBS alone

Irritable Bowel Syndrome
Nigel Howard (Element Books Ltd., 1995)
> A short book that explains holistic approaches and steers towards alternative approaches

Seven Weeks to a Settled Stomach
Ronald L. Hoffmann (Pocket Books, NY, 1990)
> A holistic approach with specific dietary recommendations

FIBER SUPPLEMENTS

The first reaction from almost every physician in the treatment of IBS is to recommend an increased intake of dietary fiber. Despite the popular support for this therapy, its efficacy remains in doubt in some cases of IBS. Fiber in the diet is very healthy for many reasons, including regulation of bowel habit, the potential prevention of colon and other cancers, and a reduction of blood cholesterol. There have been many protagonists of the health benefits of dietary fiber. Dr. H. Trowell and Dr. N. Painter, the modern pioneers of these thoughts, have provided compelling arguments that fiber in many forms has versatile health benefits.

Some studies of fiber supplements have led to opinions that fiber like bran, methylcellulose, or ispaghula are merely placebo treatments for IBS, with effects of enhancing stool volume and frequency. Sometimes a patient with IBS may actually make his or her symptoms worse by supplementing fiber in the diet. This increase in symptoms is usually overcome by combining the use of a bulk fiber laxative (e.g., Metamucil) with the introduction of a high-roughage diet containing at least approximately 25 grams per day and liberal fluid intake. The fiber supplements should be gradually increased in the diet to avoid a shock to the system. Enhanced fiber intake has significant effects on absorptive function in the bowel, and it changes the ecology of the gut by complex actions, including effects on the bacterial flora of the colon.

There are many different types of dietary fiber, which are summarized in Table 7.5. A skilled dietician or healthcare giver can use combinations of both insoluble (e.g., bran) and soluble (e.g., pectin) fibers to balance the effects of fiber on the bowel. For example, bran can cause softening and bulking of the stool, but it can sometimes result in diarrhea. This latter untoward effect can sometimes be counteracted by the administration of pectin or other soluble fibers.

Supplementation of dietary fiber in IBS is quite useful at relieving symptoms of incomplete evacuation of the bowels, but it is often ineffective for the control of abdominal pain. The relative lack of ben-

Table 7.5: Fiber supplement ingredients.

Preparation	Description	Contact with water
Bran fiber	Fibrous outer layer of cereal grains, usually wheat	Poorly soluble with water holding dependent on particle size
Plantago species (*Ispaghula*) *P. ovata* *P. psyllium* *P. indica*	Small dried ripe seeds; cellulose-containing walls of endosperm and mucilage-containing epidermis	Colorless transparent mucilage forms around insoluble seed
Ispaghula husk	Epidermis and collapsed adjacent layer of *Plantago* species	Swells rapidly to form a stiff mucilage
Sterculia gum	Gum obtained from Sterculia species	Forms a homogeneous adhesive gelationous mass
Methylcellulose	Methyl ester of cellulose	Slowly soluble, giving a viscous colloid solution
Soya fibers	Insoluble and soluble cotyledon and pulp	Universal beneficial properties

efit that can be encountered in some patients with IBS should not lead to a lack of recommendation of fiber supplementation. Dietary fiber is a general promoter of health, and it has benefits beyond the control of symptoms of IBS.

THE FIBER STORY

Dietary fiber comes from the supporting structure of plant foods and generally resists digestion in the human gastrointestinal tract. Although there are many types of fiber, they are generally described as belonging to either of two broad categories: soluble and insoluble. Soluble fiber tends to disperse in water and form a gel, but it is not absorbed into the bloodstream. Insoluble fiber also holds water (hydroscopic), but it travels through the digestive tract virtually intact, to the colon where it is fermented to a variable degree. Soybeans and legumes in general contain significant amounts of soluble fiber. The husks of soybeans contain an insoluble fiber called lignin, as well.

In 1980, two scientists, Neil Painter, M.D., and Denis Burkitt, M.D., proposed that a lack of adequate fiber in the diet may be a key factor in predisposing many individuals to some of the common chronic diseases that affect Western societies. They found that societies in which fiber intake is high—that is, societies that are largely vegetarian—have a much lower incidence of several chronic diseases, including colon cancer, heart disease, and most digestive disorders, than industrialized Western societies.

The change in diet—and resulting rise in certain diseases—among mobile populations also added credibility to the hypothesis of Painter and Burkitt. For example, Japanese people born in Hawaii have diverticular disease and colon cancer with a frequency similar to that of white Americans, while Japanese people living in Japan have a relatively low incidence of these colonic diseases.

Once it was recognized that fiber had a therapeutic role in preventing and treating many digestive disorders, the work of Burkitt and Painter became a hot topic in the West. From high-fiber cereals to wheat bran supplements to oat bran muffins and simple advice to add more fresh fruits and vegetables to the diet, fiber quickly became a focus of both the medical and the lay communities.

Many people think of bran as the most valuable source of fiber, primarily because it has been superbly marketed as promoting regularity of the bowels. In fact, insoluble fibers are sometimes referred to as bulk laxatives. However, the soluble fibers found in soybeans also regulate bowel action. They are fermented in the colon to produce short-chain fatty acids, which stimulate colonic activity, but the insoluble fiber found in soy does not make the stool too bulky. My love for soy as a promoter of general health is most apparent in my book "*The Soy Revolution*," Dell Publishing, Random House, New York, 2000.

ADDING FIBER EVERY DAY

Most people consuming a Western diet have a deficient intake of fiber, often amounting to less than 10 grams of fiber per day versus 20 to 25 grams a day for those eating the recommended Western diet. If we consider only the benefits of fiber for digestive health, it is not surprising that vegetarians tend to have far fewer digestive complaints than omnivores. Existing research suggests that increasing fiber intake can relieve or assist in control of the symptoms of diverticulosis ("pockets" in the bowel) and some cases of functional bowel disease and inflammatory bowel disease. Equally important, adequate fiber has been shown to reduce blood cholesterol, and the soluble type of fiber found in soybeans is particularly up to this task.

It is ironic that, until fairly recently, individuals with gastrointestinal complaints were often advised to reduce their fiber intake. Some people believe that they must reduce fiber as they age because their systems can no longer handle whole grains and raw foods. However, reducing fiber often exacerbates several symptoms such as the stubborn bowels and "abdominal aches" that commonly affect mature individuals. Recommendations within the medical community have changed as data confirming the value of including fiber in the diet accumulate.

A common mistake among individuals who "get religion," so to speak, about fiber, is to increase dietary fiber intake too quickly. Some abdominal bloating and excessive gas formation are inevitable during an initial period of adjustment to added fiber in the diet. For this reason, it is best to add fiber to the diet gradually over a period of weeks, rather than try to increase intake to the optimal amount within a day or two. It is best to work through the transient unpleasantness that commonly occurs in the early stages of the healthful inclusion of fiber in the diet. Fiber induces changes in the function and inhabitants of the gut in a slow but beneficial manner.

Vegetarians have little difficulty consuming adequate fiber in their diet because the variety of grains, beans, legumes, fruits, and vegetables in their diet tends to provide a good, balanced mixtures of soluble and insoluble fiber. Because it contains both soluble and insoluble fibers, soy is an ideal source of fiber, especially when taken in a traditional Asian format. Unfortunately, the "refining" of soybeans to match the appeal of the Western palate has led to many commercially available soy foods that are deficient in soy fiber.

Agreement exists about a desirable level of fiber intake among several major health organizations, including the America Diabetes Association and the National Cancer Institute, both of which set their recommendations at 20 to 35 grams a day. The Reference Daily Intake (RDI) of dietary fiber proposed by the FDA for nutritional labeling purposes in the United States is 25 grams a day. This recommendation matches those of several European countries and those made by the Department of Health in Australia.

The World Health Organization (WHO) has been more specific in defining dietary fiber requirements by expressing recommendations in terms of nonstarch polysaccharides. Expressed this way, their recommendation for nonstarch polysaccharides is 16 to 24 grams a day, which is consistent with estimates of 27 to 40 grams of total dietary fiber a day.

MUSCLE RELAXANTS

Many drugs that can cause relaxation of smooth muscle and prevent spasm are prescribed in IBS. These drugs can be partially effective in relieving pain in IBS, but clinical studies have shown variable results. I believe that these drugs should be avoided where possible. They are often limited in their use by the occurrence of side effects. For example, anticholinergic drugs can cause a dry mouth, blurred vision, and urinary problems. I believe that one of the best agents for dealing with bowel spasm is enteric-coated peppermint oil. This therapy is discussed in detail later in this chapter.

PLACEBO RESPONSE

Studies of drug therapies in IBS show placebo responses to be very common. These responses are variably present in up to four out of five people with IBS. This makes it very difficult to show the benefit of any treatment for IBS. The placebo-reacting phenomenon makes the IBS an ideal target for safe and gentle interventions, such as remedies of natural origin. Alternative medicine describes many techniques that can affect the gutmind e.g., Yoga, biofeedback, music therapy, prayer, chiropractic, touch therapy, exercise, etc.

I am decidedly unimpressed with drug therapy in many patients with IBS. Table 7.6 summarizes current drug therapies and therapies

Table 7.6: Drugs used in the therapy of IBS or under investigation.

The listed therapies for pain, diarrhea and constipation are ineffective or of marginal benefit in the author's opinion.

Therapy	Example
Pain	Analgesic
	Antispasmodic agents
	Opioidlike agents
Diarrhea	Loperamide
	Cholestyramine
Constipation	Fiber*
	Laxatives
	Cisapride
	Misoprostol
	Nonabsorbed solutions (Golytely)*
Newer interventions	Hormone antagonists
	Calcium-channel-blocking drugs
	Antagonists of visceral pain
	Psychotropic drugs

*recommended by author

under investigation. To date, no startling clinical outcomes in IBS have been described with any drug therapy.

ESSENTIAL OILS AND GASTROINTESTINAL ACTIONS

Essential oils of several plants, e.g., peppermint, fennel, dill, and caraway are natural antispasmodic agents (interfering with bowel contractions) that cause spasm. In addition, Dr. Mowrey, a distinguished alternative physician, announced that "more than 30 pathogenic microorganisms have yielded to the influence of peppermint." The broad antimicrobial action of peppermint indicates possible uses in suppressing enteric microbes in several conditions, including travelers' diarrhea and opportunistic infections of the gastrointestinal tract in HIV disease (AIDS/ARC). Peppermint oil may also inhibit Helicobacter pylori, which is the most important cause of acid-related disease in the stomach. Other oils, such as oil of oregano, have similar effects. In his book, Dr. Mowrey reviewed the research of Maksimenko and Pasechnik (1966), in which choleetric, antiulcer, and anti-inflammatory properties of peppermint were proposed. If peppermint oil or oregano has an antiulcer effect, it is possible that it exerts this effect by interference with the growth of *H. pylori*, which is the key focus of current treatment regimens to cure peptic ulcer disease.

Fennel contains aromatic or essential oils that are very similar in chemical structure and biologic effects to peppermint oil. Fennel was listed officially in the U.S. pharmacopoeia for many years, and this herb is still officially recognized for its medicinal properties in more than twelve foreign pharmacopoeias worldwide.

The effects of essential oils such as fennel and peppermint are localized in the gastrointestinal tract. In contrast to other antispasmodic medications that are used to treat functional gastrointestinal disturbance, peppermint exerts a local gastrointestinal effect, whereas synthetic compounds exert pharmacologic effects as a consequence of their systemic bioavailability and activity. The general systemic effects of synthetic antispasmodic medications, such as mebeverine or dicyclomine, may limit their use and cause adverse effects.

It has been hypothesized that the carminative effect of essential oils may be related, in part, to their action on intestinal foam. Peppermint, cinnamon, orange, dill, and caraway oils have been shown to be highly effective in disrupting gastrointestinal foam as a consequence of the stimulation of gastric and intestinal secretions. Foam is generally found in the upper gastrointestinal tract, and it is not perceived to be a problem in the large intestine.

It is believed that the disruption of the bubbles in gastrointestinal foam may lead to a collapse of the foam resulting in the release of gas that can then be eliminated by belching or by the passing of flatus. The buildup of foam and its retention in the lumen of the gastrointestinal tract is believed to give rise to abdominal discomfort due to intestinal spasm and colic. This gas buildup may give rise to dyspepsia or lower abdominal pain. It has been well-recognized that antifoaming agents are useful in the facilitation of the passage of gas from the gastrointestinal tract, and they are associated with general relief of the symptoms of functional gastrointestinal disease.

Several clinical studies have shown the beneficial effects of essential oils, especially peppermint oil, on a variety of gastrointestinal disorders. Rees et al. (1979) undertook a double-blind crossover trial of the effects of peppermint oil on the relief of symptoms in the IBS. In this multicenter study, there was a significant improvement in the relief of symptoms of IBS compared to placebo. These results were confirmed in a further multicenter trial, performed by Dew et al. (1979), where twenty-nine patients from seven hospital centers entered into a double-blind crossover study to examine the effects of peppermint oil on symptoms of IBS. In a critical review of the use of peppermint oil in the treatment of IBS, Dr. M. H. Pittler and Dr. E. Ernst, of Exeter, England, examined several published studies and concluded that evidence exists to support the use of peppermint oil in IBS. However, they did report concern about the construction of some of the trials and expressed some doubts about efficacy (American Journal of Gastroenterology, 93: 1131–1135, 1998).

In the study by Dew et al. (1984), patients received either peppermint oil or placebo capsules and, during each treatment period of two weeks, patients were requested to record the severity of abdominal symptoms, stool frequency, and side effects of the medication on a daily basis. The overall assessment of the patients showed that the patients' symptoms improved significantly while taking peppermint oil capsules as compared to placebo and that the patients considered peppermint oil to be better than placebo in relieving abdominal symptoms. Patients who received peppermint oil had a much lower daily symptom score than those receiving placebo. It was concluded that peppermint oil was a potent agent for the relaxation of gastrointestinal smooth muscle. This latter study confirmed the earlier findings of Rees et al. (1979) and clearly demonstrated the benefit of peppermint oil in treatment of IBS in a multicenter, controlled clinical trial.

Essential oils are very safe, and they are ubiquitous in foods. Peppermint is used as a flavoring in a variety of beverages and foods. No systemic toxicity of peppermint oil or fennel oil is known in modest dosage (0.2 ml for peppermint) despite many years of use. If further studies can confirm the benefit of essential oils in a delayed-release (enteric-coated) format, then these natural products will be very useful first-line, nontoxic options for many people affected by functional bowel symptoms, in the absence of organic gastrointestinal disease.

OTHER OILS ARE GOOD

Certain oils (fats) are health-giving, especially, the omega 3 fatty acids (fish oils). Indeed, there are many fats that cause ill health, but there are other dietary fats that are obligatory to promote good health. While saturated fat of animal origin is associated with cardiovascular disease and colon cancer, certain types of unsaturated fats are associated with the prevention or treatment of cardiovascular disease and cancer. This is a relatively poorly understood enigma. The many effects of essential fatty acids and their role in the production of prostaglandins is summarized in Table 7.7. Prostaglandins are hormones that control many body processes.

There are two important categories of essential fatty acids, which include the omega-6 series and omega-3 series fatty acids. Omega-6 series fatty acids are ubiquitous in the diet and are found to a major degree in vegetables, whereas omega-3 fatty acids are found largely in fish and marine mammals. There are interesting exceptions. Certain legumes (e.g., soybeans) contain significant amounts of precursors of

Table 7.7 The protean effects of essential fatty acids and prostaglandins on body function

- The normal function of the immune system
- Formation of substrates for hormone production and effector properties
- Regulation of blood pressure by involvement in vascular tone and collateral circulations
- Regulation of responses to pain, inflammation, infection, and cancer
- Controlling glandular secretions and their composition
- Regulation of smooth muscle and neural function
- Effecting cell membrane structure and mitosis of cells
- Regulation of cell oxygenation and nutrient intake
- Providing energy substrates for key organs

omega-3 fatty acids. The two most important omega-3 fatty acids with health-giving benefits are eicosapentanoic acid (EPA) and docosahexanoic acid (DHA).

FISH OIL AND THE GUT

Several studies imply that omega-3 fatty acids are important for normal gut function. A recent study of enteric-coated (delayed release) fish oil (Beluzzi et al., *New England Journal of Medicine*, 1995) in the prevention of relapse in Crohn's disease (a form of inflammatiory bowel disease) showed excellent results. Further studies are underway with enteric-coated fish oil for inflammatory bowel disease, and this option seems to be particularly attractive in children who may suffer growth retardation from treatments and results of the disease. I believe that fish oil in an enteric-coated format is one of the most exciting options for the treatment of inflammatory disease of the bowel—and although not studied in a controlled manner, it is effective in some cases of IBS for reasons that I cannot explain.

HYPNOTHERAPY AND IBS

Only the most hide-bound skeptics have difficulty accepting that hypnosis works for many disorders. It provides a pathway of relaxation and suggestion that can work in the treatment of functional gastrointestinal disease. Why? A great deal of time has been spent discussing the nature of the mind-body interaction in functional disorders, and the placebo response in IBS is known to be very high. Without resorting to scientific studies, the history of the development and contention that surrounds hypnotism is probably enough for most people to take this form of therapy seriously—at last!

Conventional physicians have focused on recent experiments with hypnotism and IBS as laying the groundwork for its application. Hypnotism or its major component of suggestion has been used for several millennia, and records of its use are found in ancient Greek, Persian, Chinese, and Ayurvedic medicine. It is noted in ancient Greek medical practice that the induction of trancelike states (hypnotism) was often used for presumed hysterical or emotional disorders. Unfortunately, until the last century or so, many previously labeled emotional states can be found to have a physical basis. Remnants of hypnotherapy are alleged to be found in ancient Druid culture in England. The Druids referred to hypnosis as a form of magical sleep. It was used to treat common ailments and even to cast spells on the unwary!

Hypnotherapy uses the power of suggestion during relaxation to cause positive changes in the bodymind. It has to find its greatest application in clear-cut disorders of the bodymind, such as functional gastrointestinal disease.

Dr. R. F. Harvey and his colleagues were permitted to report their open-label (uncontrolled experiments) experiences with hypnotherapy (*Lancet*, 1984, 1: 424–425). These researchers selected individuals with refractory (not responding to acceptable therapy) IBS for group hypnotherapy sessions. There were thirty-three patients with troublesome, unresponsive IBS who received four sessions of hypnotherapy, alone or together with others. After approximately two months, it was found that one-third of the patients were free of symptoms, about one-quarter experienced measurable improvement, and the remainder (39 percent) achieved no benefit. This study started chins wagging in modern medicine and paved the way for Dr. P. J. Whorwell's use of hypnosis in the treatment of IBS, a use of hypnosis that he had proposed in 1984, before the work of Dr. Harvey and his colleagues.

WHORWELL'S STUDIES

Dr. P. J. Whorwell of the University of South Manchester in England has engaged in the research of gut-directed hypnosis. In 1984, Dr. Whorwell and his colleagues published the results of a controlled trial of hypnotherapy in the treatment of patients with severe IBS (*Lancet*, 1:1232–1234). In this study, the use of hypnotherapy was compared to psychotherapy, and the hypnosis-treated group had a better outcome of therapy.

The treatments applied by Dr. Whorwell and his colleagues were more than hypnotherapy. They involved an educational process where the patients were given explanations about the physiology (workings and functions) of the guts. The subjects were then asked to attempt to modify these functions. A form of self-touch therapy was included where their own hands were positioned on their abdomen to transmit a sensation of warmth that could provide relief of the patient's symptoms of colic, bloating, and pain. For some patients, the therapy took several weeks before a significant response was obtained.

The question remains whether or not this form of therapy is practical in most clinic locations. Furthermore, very few physicians have training in hypnotherapy or relaxation techniques. The interesting observation is that deep hypnotic trances are not required for the therapy to be effective, and a large part of this procedure appears to involve education and relaxation. The important factor is that the education, relaxation, touch, and hypnosis should be targeted to the bowel for IBS.

How does this therapy work? It is known that patients with functional gastrointestinal disease have increased sensitivity in their guts. For example, their response to gut distension and the presence of gas is often heightened. The components of the treatment applied by Dr. Whorwell may modify the sensitivity of the bowel in patients with IBS. Certainly, studies have shown that the rectum may be very sensitive in certain patients with IBS. Dr. Whorwell and his colleagues have measured pressures and assessed sensitivity in the rectum in two separate studies, and their results imply that hypnotherapy alters these processes.

One important issue is the knowledge that educational approaches with hypnosis and relaxation can be used to treat other diseases or functional disorders of the gut other than IBS. Some studies have shown that hypnosis can reduce the recurrence of symptoms in patients with peptic ulcer, and there is no reason to doubt its benefit in a variety of other circumstances. In fact, hypnosis (and acupuncture) can alter gastric acid secretion by the stomach.

Despite the favorable outcome of these studies, very few patients receive hypnotherapy for IBS or other functional bowel disease. Why? I believe the answer rests in the belief by many conventional physicians that these treatment methods border on fringe medicine, and this belief is reinforced by the average physician's uneasiness with the application of therapy about which they know very little. The same may be true about other treatment modalities that move into the realm of alternative medicine.

EDUCATION AND IBS

The recognition that the prescription of antispasmodic drugs, stool softeners, dietary fiber, antidiarrheal drugs, and psychotropic agents (mind-altering drugs) gives quite limited relief in IBS has led physicians in conventional medicine to reexamine their management approach. The simplest approach is to let the individual attempt to manage his or her own problem by education, which steers them to lifestyle changes that may promote health. This approach is certainly cost-effective in the days of escalating healthcare costs. There have been several studies that have attempted to elucidate the potential benefits of education in IBS, but only in recent times has the importance of this approach been finally recognized by conventional medicine.

A groundbreaking study of the effects of patient education in the lifestyle domains of diet, exercise, and psychological well-being was performed recently at the Mayo Clinic. Dr. L. J. Colwell and colleagues reported a very favorable outcome of an educational class on health-promoting behaviors for the reduction of symptoms in the IBS. The introductory remarks in the report of this study in the *American Journal of Gastroenterology* in 1998 (93, 6:901–905) are very striking. The Mayo Clinic research discusses how patients may "manage their symptoms holistically through lifestyle changes." I draw attention to the use of the term "holistically" by the Mayo researchers. Clearly, we may be witnessing an example of the change in the treatment pardaigm, where holisitic interventions (the basis of alternative and complementary medicine) are emerging at centers of medical excellence (i.e., conventional medical excellence).

In an eloquent editorial in the *American Journal of Gastroenterology* (93, 6:860–861, 1998), Dr. G. F. Longstreth stresses the value of "teaching patients with IBS to care for themselves." One has to believe that knowledge has the power to heal. In his editiorial, Dr. Longstreth asks why the educational protocol used by the Mayo Clinic researchers was effective in the management of IBS. He discusses the importance of the strength of the physician-patient relationship (or physician-health-care worker relationship) and the use of self-help material. Self-help can be delivered in many formats such as audiovisual aids or written material. Of course, this is one of the principal reasons why several individuals have written books on IBS or functional gut disease.

SELF-HELP BOOKS AND MATERIALS

Self-help materials for functional digestive disorders have been grossly underutilized in medicine. This is a serious cost containment issue, and I am surprized that the third-party payors in medicine (HMO's and insurance companies) have not woken up to this valid and ethical approach to saving money in medicine. The most accessible information is in bookstores, and Table 7.4 lists some of the books available on the subject. This book differs in its attempt to examine both the conventional approach and the ever-popular alternative or complementary medical therapies, many of which require much further reassessment for their safety and implied efficacy.

The most interesting recent observations of the effects of education on IBS is the previously described work by Dr. L. J. Colwell and his colleagues from the Mayo Clinic. These researchers set up a special educational class, which included many recommendations for change of lifestyle, identification of food intolerance, nutritional activity, exercise, etc. Stress management and behavioral strategies were included in this approach. Overall, this study showed significant improvements in many symptoms of IBS, but not all health-promoting behaviors were adopted by the patients and some symptoms were persistent. Compliance with alternative medical interventions may be an issue of the future!

EXPANSION OF THE WORK OF THE ROME GROUP

From the original meetings in Rome in 1988, there has been a continuing international effort to classify and diagnose IBS in a more positive manner. This resulted in the formation of the Multinational Working Teams to Develop Diagnostic Criteria for Diagnosis of Functional GI disorders. The initial Rome criteria used for classification and diagnosis of functional gut disease have been revised from the basis of the Rome II documents, which include a new book (available on the Internet at www.romecriteria.org). This international effort has paved new ground that may result in changes in disease code classification for functional gut disorders and lead to the more widespread use of symptom-based diagnostic questionnaires—which are not without limitations.

For the healthcare professional, a new book entitled *Functional Disorders of the Gut* was recently published (edited by Dr. S. F. Phillips and D. H. Wingate). This multi-author book is one of the most complete series of documents on modern research in functional gut disorders. I recommend it highly.

CHAPTER SUMMARY

There have been recent changes in how functional disorders of the gut—especially IBS—have been perceived by modern medicine. Physicians are moving away from single causation, disease-based models of medical disorders to a more integrated conceptualization. This integrated approach permits a better understanding of the many dimensions of functional gut disorders. These changes are congruent with a holistic medical approach and the idea of the unity of body function. Dr. Douglas A. Drossman, one of the world's leading experts in functional gut disorders, states in an editorial in the *American Journal of Gastroenterology* (94:2803–2807, 1999):

> The biopsychosocial model provides the structure to understand the multidetermined nature of IBS (e.g., as the integrated product of altered motility, enhanced visceral sensitivity, and brain-gut dysregulation, as modified by psychosocial influences), and to treat the patients using multicomponent methods (e.g., diet, intestinal and centrally acting medications, psychological/behavioral treatments).

I applaud this approach, but comments about alternative medical strategies are conspicuously absent, but implied! The boundary between the conventional and alternative approaches to the management of fuctional digestive disorders is now blurred.

CHAPTER EIGHT

CONSTIPATION, DIARRHEA, AND PAINS IN THE BUTT

WHAT GOES IN HAS TO COME OUT

Control of bowel function occurs with an important gatekeeper mechanism. This mechanism is facilitated by the normal function of the anorectum (lower portion of the bowel and the anus with its intricate controls). Continence of stool is an important milestone in childhood development, and problems with bowel control may often have their roots in aberrant parent-child relationships.

In this chapter, I shall examine aspects of the gatekeeper function of the anorectum and relate this to bowel habit. The act of passing stool is determined to a major degree by a balance between the rates of movement of fluids through the guts and the absorption of these fluids by certain areas of the gut. In some states of disease, the guts may secrete fluids and cause diarrhea. This is termed secretory diarrhea. Secretory diarrhea is not functional, it spells the presence of disease or perhaps excessive purgative use.

It is important to understand that altered bowel habit, in the form of diarrhea or constipation, can reflect a disorder at almost any region of the tubular digestive tract, or it may result from other factors that affect the psychoneurohormonal control of the guts. Again, we revisit the holistic concept of Gaiaguts. Before specific causes of anorectal dysfunction are addressed, it is important to visit the developmental aspects of bowel control in childhood and its relevance to bowel action and control in adult life.

ANAL BEHAVIOR AND ITS ORIGINS

Behavioral psychologists are often besotted by the child within. The "inner child" is a complex concept, and I wish to broaden this concept by stressing the important relationships between bowel function and developmental phases of childhood. Dr. Sigmund Freud (the famous Viennese physician who was considered by many of his peers to be a pervert) described phases of childhood development from early infancy. One of the first signals of the presence of the gutmind is the characteristic sequence of feeding followed by bowel actions—the eat, poop routine of the infant is known to all.

The eat, poop routine has been mislabeled as the gastrocolic reflex (gastro-stomach, colic-bowel). Although there is a notable increase in movements of some segments of the colon (especially the sigmoid colon) when the stomach is distended, the response of small and large bowels to food involves a highly complex neurohormonal response. This response is influenced greatly by diet, posture, exercise, and psychological factors. Again, one has to ponder the information highways of the gutmind or bodymind. Some of the events that happen in the guts during eating have phylogenetic significance. In the chapter on IBS, I discussed certain molecules of the information network in the guts that may switch off immune function during eating, but other examples of intelligent evolution of gut function are apparent. The value of the upright posture in humans for the facilitation of bowel movements can result in a welcome, facilitated exodus of the contents of the bowel. However, squatting rather than sitting facilitates the dumping of stool.

GUT RESPONSES ARE SUBJECT TO LEARNING

The well-defined associations of eating and gut function become the subject of lessons for developing children. A parent can readily identify the occurrence of the eating-pooping sequence and this is the cue that is used for potty training in most children. So powerful is this lesson that the eating-pooping reflex can persist throughout adult life in a format that is infrequently extinguished (or greatly modified).

The recognized rush to the bathroom in states of stress is allegedly related to the gastrocolic reflex by virtue of its commonality in certain phases of sociobehavioral development. It has been proposed that both the gastrocolic reflex (eating-pooping sequence) and the "stress stool" phenomenon are explained by the linkage that occurs between the acts of a mother nursing a baby (or a father bottle feeding) and the emotional interactions (bonding, etc.) that occur between parent and infant. These links between physiological events of feeding, stooling, and emotional events are firmly imprinted on the developing mind. This is a kind of psychophysiological fingerprint of the gutmind. Rupert Sheldrake may see it differently in "fingerprint behavior."

How does this dialogue relate to abnormal bowel habits? Unfortunately, a full explanation is not completely available. It is well known that during periods of stress or fright, a sense of helplessness or fear (or negative emotion) surfaces and the molecules of emotion drive the information highways of the gutmind. These negative emotions can cause a regression to the gutmind fingerprinting that relates to the relief of helplessness or fear that was associated with feeding, nurturing, and the eating-pooping routine.

An individual who is stressed and unable to exercise coping mechanisms regresses to the protective state of the mother-infant relationship. These people can run to the bathroom with stress and even gallop to the pot with abdominal gurglings, release of gas, and untimely discharges of stool. These imprinted psychodynamic responses of the gutmind can become chronic, intermittent, modestly troublesome, or incapacitating. There is looming evidence that we can teach the organs of the gut to behave in the ways we want them to—this is called visceral learning.

This situation is known as nervous diarrhea, but it is really one of a mixed group of heterogeneous (different) disorders that we have considered generally to be part of IBS. Some physicians have tried to argue that emotional linkage and its manifestations such as nervous diarrhea are a distinct entity. I do not subscribe to this notion because the emotional linkage may not be overt or detectable, but it may still be present, or absent. Similar kinds of psychodynamic linkages occur between the mind and other areas of the gastrointestinal tract.

CONSTIPATION

The most common type of constipation in some societies may be a figment of imagination. The idea of the ritual exodus of fecal matter has preoccupied people from time immemorial. Many factors in the gutmind determine bowel patterns and an accurate definition of constipation defies definition. In general, if the bowel does not open at least once every three days, then constipation may exist for most people, but not for all! There are some of individuals who open their bowels infrequently but who remain healthy and often content, unless the seed of compulsive regularity is planted in their mind.

Constipation most often conjures up the idea that the bowel is lazy. Although this may be the case in examples of atonic (lazy) constipation, sometimes delays in evacuation are experienced in hypertonic (spastic) types of bowels. We are discussing the movements of the bowel where atonic constipation implies an inactive, lazy bowel and spastic constipation (hypertonic) refers to an overactive bowel with excessive contractions.

The recognition that constipation may be of the lazy type (poor motor function of the bowel) or hyperactive type (spastic contractions) is important in a search for ways to correct the problem. People often take laxatives to facilitate movement of the bowel (e.g., senna) but if the bowel is already hyperactive, the laxative can make the bowel even more erratic in its behavior with occasional tendencies to enhance constipation. The same can be true about loading a lazy bowel that is already loaded with dietary fiber that holds water. Lazy bowels do not tend to deal with excessive fiber loads. The result of fiber in a lazy bowel can be the same as concrete that sets in a concrete mixer, especially if insufficient fluid is around in the colon to keep the fiber mushy.

There are some ways to distinguish atonic constipation from spastic constipation on clinical grounds. A carefully taken patient history that identifies the associated symptoms with constipation can be valuable. Talking to patients or examination of patients, however, does not reliably separate the atonic from the spastic type of constipation. Hence, tests are often required, but they are sometimes inadequate, may not result in the right advice for treatment, and are frequently avoided by the patient.

ATONIC BOWELS

Lazy bowels are most often encountered at the extremes of age. They sometimes cause incontinence with overflow of watery diarrhea and can masquerade as a primary complaint of diarrhea or soiling, especially in the elderly or very young. This incontinence and stool overflow is sometimes linked to a condition called encopresis. Studies of the clinical characteristics of encopresis have been surprisingly few and far between in the medical literature. The whole idea of lazy bowels, colon inertia, sluggish colons, etc., requires careful definition. The afflicted may go a month or more without opening their bowels, and over the period of evolving constipation, the individual often becomes stressed, irritable, or emotionally distraught. Why?

The emotional disturbances that are often encountered in constipated individuals are frequently explained in terms of their reaction to the physical symptoms (abdominal fullness and pain) that results from constipation. I suspect other factors operate. These other factors of considerable importance include the change in bacterial flora of the guts, which control general health, and the variable presentation of unwanted toxins to the body from the bowel contents, that may start to putrefy and ferment. The idea that the bowel is a source of toxins for the body is one of the most argued topics in conventional and alternative medicine. I believe that these extremes of opinion stand in the way of symptom relief for many patients who have ill health from constipation!

BOWEL TOXINS

We do not need to explain in detail the biochemistry of putrefying stool in the colon. Logic dictates that volatile compounds including gases and organic acids that can have negative effects on the body may be generated in the colon. Some types of conventional medical thought imagine that the colon is merely a boring conduit or receptacle for stool, but elegant experiments show the contrary. The colon is a dynamic organ that handles fluids in a regulated way. It has a very active lining, and it is capable of absorbing a lot of substances, including drugs that may be administered in suppository or enema format.

We return to the concepts of balance, not only in the colon but also in our thoughts about the colon (or its "thoughts" about itself). The healthy colon does not need to be washed out, cleansed, or purged, but the unhealthy or unbalanced colon may require this kind of attention on an intermittent basis. Therefore, the medical benefits of colon cleansing are not always redundant. Circumstances determine its beneficial application. Kings, queens, and aristocrats of old times who purged themselves to oblivion were tipping the scales of regular behavior, a mistake sometimes made by the modern colon therapists.

HEALTH AND DIGESTA

Maybe we can agree that we are what we eat (diet) or even that we are what we absorb (gut function). I propose a missing and important issue in this line of reasoning. We are also a function of the contents of our guts, especially the colon. These gut contents are best referred to as the digesta. The digesta is an inextricable linkage of the diet and gut function that controls both gut and general body health.

The digesta is an ever-changing component of the Gaiaguts. The importance of the digesta has been proposed in an elegant manner by Dr. Andreas M. Pappas, Ph.D., especially in relationship to the antioxidant status of the body. The concepts that I propose extend the importance of the digesta to general health.

The digesta is the sum total of the contents of the gastointestinal tract and its composition in the colon is particularly relevant to health. The contents are determined by ingested food and drink, modified by additions or deletions by the gut (digestive enzymes, mucus, gases, bile), and largely determined by the gut microflora (bacteria, yeasts, molds, protozoa, etc., or unwanted guests such as parasites).

The gut contents form a very active biological soup (or slurry) that solidifies during its passage through the colon. These contents are exposed to a large surface area of the gut, and therefore a large surface area of the body. The chemical status of the body is usually defined in context of blood and tissue contents without due consideration of the role that the digesta plays in determining this chemical status.

There is a large number of chemicals or metabolic products present or produced in the digesta, including food additives, nutrients, organochemicals, end products of bacterial metabolism, oxidation products of food, ingested chemicals or bile, and free radicals produced from bacterial metabolism—to name a few. In the presence of gut disease, different chemicals or products are produced, such as reactive nitrogen species and modified proteins that can act as potential allergens.

One area of particular interest is the oxidation status of the digesta. The benefits of an array of antioxidants in the digesta is of particular importance and this antioxidant status is largely determined by food eaten, but it is like all contents of the gut that are modified by the ecology of the gut. In general, the antioxidant status of the digesta is a key regulator of health, and it is particularly important in the development of colon cancer or bowel inflammation. Perhaps more important, the digesta has been all but ignored in its potential role in functional gut disorders, especially IBS.

Antioxidants such as vitamin E or its analogues (especially gamma-tocopherol) and phytochemicals (especially isoflavones) may be important in disease prevention and antiaging. Many phytochemicals and some phytonutrients and end products of the processing of botanicals by the gut are absorbed in the colon or act on the colon—contrary to popular belief among conventional medicine practitioners.

COMMON CONSTIPATION HAS NO IDENTIFIABLE CAUSE

We have learned that medical jargon sometimes resorts to the diagnosis of the destitute by the use of the term *idiopathic* (of no readily identifiable cause). We mention the occurrence of imaginary constipation, fueled by the media or old wives, (or husbands') tales. Imaginary constipation has a cause—it is imagined. If not recognized, these individuals with creative thoughts can reach for laxatives to abuse their colon and do even greater damage by inflicting their imagination on other family members. It may shock some readers to learn where the billion dollars, worth of laxatives go on annual basis. While many are presented to a deserving colon, a large number become examples of substance abuse.

Misconceptions about what constitutes a normal bowel habit can cause a lot of bowel problems. The brain and the body (together with the many tiny brains in the bowel) may decide on normal bowel patterns. We know that behavior or interventions can change body functions (e.g., psychotherapy, changes in brain chemistry). When the normal bowel is given an unnecessary stimulus to act, it starts to learn to act only in the presence of the stimulus. This is an easy way to create a vicious cycle for the bowel. In fact, the bowel may desire an increasing threshold of stimulation over a period of time. This situation is an example of a type of self-inflicted bowel disorder. It is an effective way of inducing psychosis of the second brain(s) (or enteric nervous system) that is modified by the master regulation of the main brain.

We need to think not only about the bowel itself but the residents within the bowel that are affected by our attempts to bring the colon's function under control. Purgatives, strange food preferences, and other rituals can alter the microflora of the bowel, which controls our health and well-being.

THE ROLE OF POTTY TRAINING (PRIMARY PREVENTION)

Parental influences during toilet training of young children can have long-lasting effects on bowel habits. The neurotic parent who is obsessed with his or her own idea of bowel regularity can shape an individual's life-long toilet habits. Fear of public toilets is so common that it contributes to stool holding that can reduce the body's normal call to stool. Stressful life events during toilet training in children can cause enduring constipation, which is sometimes attacked by the zealous use of purgatives by parents. Most readers may recognize these circumstances as examples of extreme behavior. However, bowel patterns and habits can be modified to varying degrees by varying degrees of misguided thoughts and social influences. Understanding the pernicious effects of poor potty training is a key to primary prevention to several types of functional bowel disease.

MENTAL ILLNESS AND THE COLON

Some of the most extreme examples of atonic constipation can be found in developmentally disabled persons or in individuals with serious mental illness. In these circumstances, for example, the colon can blow up like a huge inflated tire. This is called a megacolon.

While ballooning of the colon is often thought to result from failure of individuals to act on urges to open their bowels, some authorities argue that other factors operate. We have learned that depression ("the common cold of psychiatry") alters bowel function, but changes in the nervous system and its highways of communication (hormones and neurotransmitters) are believed to be important. Mind-altering drugs used in the treatment of significant psychiatric illness also have a profound effect on the bowels.

These factors apart, bowel problems are very common in mental institutions and in people with psychiatric illness. This situation raises the possibility that the changes in the bowel can contribute to (or perhaps cause) psychiatric illness. If one was to inquire about the daily work of healthcare personnel in psychiatric institutions or long-term care facilities, one would appreciate that as much time is spent dealing with bowel or digestive problems as is spent dealing with mental or psychiatric disorders.

Accepting that digestive disorders are a key issue in diseases of the central nervous system, a great deal of work has been performed to examine the role of bowel disease in the cause of mental disease. Conventional medicine will not embrace the notion that derangements in the bowel cause psychiatric disease or contribute to nervous system disabilities. I find this surprising because much precedent exists in the medical literature to link bowel disorders with the brain.

An obvious example of a gut-brain disease link is the absorption of ammonia from the bowel of patients with advanced liver disease. Under these circumstances, highly complex neuropsychiatric disorders can occur, ranging from confusion to incoordination to permanent brain damage, to stupor, to coma to death. The site of maximal absorption of ammonia in this disorder, known as hepatic encephalopathy, is the colon. The source of the ammonia is the digesta!

The idea that disorders of the bowel cause brain disease is deeply rooted in several traditional medical disciplines. Chief Two Trees of the Cherokee Nation, who was a well-known medicine man practicing in the Carolinas in 1970s and 1980s, believed that mental illness was clearly linked to unwanted inhabitants of the bowel (most notably parasites of diverse type). Many examples of the successful treatment of mental disorders by Chief Two Trees have been related by Talking Bear (John Roberts, N.D., an English naturopath who worked with Two Trees). Traditional North American Indian medicine, like Ayurvedic medicine, invariably uses body cleansing techniques for health with a focus on parasite removal—whether or not there is hard evidence of their presence.

Sporadic reports linking bowel parasitosis and brain disease exist in the medical literature. In these reports, brain disorders are not related to the presence of the parasites in body tissues. Coincidentally, the occurrence of bowel parasites in institutionalized patients (especially mental patients) is strikingly high. The mechanism of the association (brain and bowel disease) is not known (or often acknowledged). The vast array of "molecules of emotion" and sharing of receptors among living organisms (e.g., single-celled protozoans have opiate receptors) may imply that parasites could communicate not only with each other but also with the body and the brain—at least indirectly. This area of medicine seems farfetched but is underexplored.

I am not suggesting that ridding the bowel of unwanted inhabitants is a panacea for neurological or psychiatric disease. I am, however, suggesting that it may be more important than we care to recognize.

HYPERACTIVE BOWELS (SPASTIC CONSTIPATION)

Spasm of the bowel acts to prevent the efficient forward movement of the gut contents. Excessive or incoordinate contraction of smooth muscle is possible at any site in the tubular portions of the digestive tract. For example, the sigmoid colon (in the lower left quadrant of the abdomen) is a frequent site for spastic contractions. In contrast to the lazy bowel, spastic types of constipation are encountered usually in adolescence, maximally in young adulthood with a persistence to middle life—especially in females. The lifetime pattern of spastic constipation is characterized by waxing and waning of symptoms, and it often resurfaces with a vengeance in the perimenopausal period (period of one to two years) around the menopause (the point in time when menstruation ceases). These symptoms appear to be hormonally determined and they may respond quite well, on occasion, to soy intake or topical progesterone cream.

Spastic constipation is most often a component of IBS. Excessive contractions that occur in a sporadic, uncoordinated manner can be demonstrated often in portions of the left colon in people with spastic constipation. Some sufferers have an exaggerated "gastrocolic reflex" in the early time period following a meal (sometimes during a meal), with the result that a person may have abdominal cramp and run to the bathroom. In these circumstances, the person with spastic constipation is seldom rewarded by a satisfying bowel movement. The stool of the spastic bowel is sometimes like sheep or rabbit droppings. Small pellets of stool covered with mucus are delivered, often after much straining and cramping that can remain unrelieved. Tenesmus (the sensation of incomplete emptying of the bowel) is another hallmark of spastic constipation.

RITUAL STOOL GAZING

Practically everyone may, at one time, or another visually inspect their own stool. Variations in stool color, content, and odor are normal occurrences, but major deviations of stool shape, size, contours, or color can be alarming for some people. A lot can be learned from studying the morphology (structure) of stool. Little pebbles of stool (rabbitlike) imply constipation, and the person who eats a good amount of roughage can usually present a large, soft, easily passed stool. The latter type of stool is a gratifying event for many and an ambition for the person with IBS, spastic constipation, atonic colon, or diarrhea of any type. The idea of examining the morphology of stool (gross appearance) has not found space in modern medical textbooks. A lot is to be learned from the general appearance of fecal matter. One must not forget the red flags of blood in the stool, but stool structures and dimensions can be very revealing signs of digestive health.

The perfect stool has an end with a flat head that is sausagelike with a tapering tail. The flat head of stool is a response to the brakes that are applied to the exit of stool by the lower rectum and anal margin. When the brakes of the anal margin are lost, the head of the stool is lost. Dumping of stool from the anus modifies the tail of the stool, perhaps implying that the anus closed after passage of the stool in an abrupt manner.

The examination of stool in gastroenterology practice is unpopular for the gastroenterologist, the patient, and the laboratory technician who can make a diagnosis by examining stool contents and characteristics. Laboratory reports on stool are limited to comments on content rather than appearance, perhaps because it takes a relatively long time to get a stool specimen to the lab.

Some scientists have taken the examination of stool to extremes. Scanning electron microscopy (very high powered microscopic examination) of stool is quite revealing. The topical geography of the stool (observed at microscopy) derived from a high-fiber diet is very impressive, in comparison to the flatlands or featureless surfaces of the rabbit pellets that are sometimes produced by the person on the average Western diet!

Stools can be hard, watery, fragmented, tubular, etc. The floating stool can signify malabsorption of nutrients (e.g., contains fat) but solid floaters are those stools that have a high gas content. Bacteria in the colon (the microflora) ferment stool and produce gas. The floating solid stool is distinguished by its gas content and odor. In the absence of a special event (e.g., bowel infection), a stool clad in an overcoat of slime, mucus, or blood is never found in a state of health.

SPASTIC COLON, SPASTIC BRAIN

A number of studies draw attention to aberrations of personality in patients with spastic constipation, usually as a part of IBS. The person with a spastic colon has been labeled obsessive, compulsive, neurotic, anxious, stressed —and you name it! The application of questionnaires to these patients to assess their psychological makeup can produce weighted scores that conjure up the idea that their disorder is related to events in the mind (psychosomatic). Two questions arise.

The first is, "Did the bowel upset cause the neurosis, or was the neurosis responsible for the bowel upset?" This is a classic chicken-and-egg argument. The second question is, "Which mind or brain is involved—the many little brains in the gut or the big brain (and mind) in the head?"

THE SECOND BRAIN(S)

The idea that the gut has its own brain, or lots of little brains, is not a new idea. These concepts have grown out of early observations in the nineteenth century that isolated segments of the gut can carry on their own movements and activities without an external nerve supply. A classic example of the cutting-off of an external nervous supply without having profound effects on gut movements is the act of vagotomy (cutting connections of the vagus nerve, which provides a rich supply of nervous fibers to the gut). While the nervous system of the bowel has a rich and highly developed network of nerves that connect it to the nervous system, in some segments of the gut (most notably the colon), the nerves within the gut that form relay stations (ganglions) far outnumber the supply of nerves from "outside" the gut.

The well-developed nervous system of the bowel shows an ability to act alone, without the influence of nervous control from the central nervous system. The function of the nervous system within the gut is referred to as the enteric nervous system (ENS), which has its own agenda (mind, function, activity). This activity, however, can still be influenced by the master brain (the brain and mind of the body).

The ENS can be considered simply to have two components or networks of nerve cells and fibers. The first network has one location (Meissner's plexus) and the second has another (Auerbach's plexus) within the wall of the tubular digestive tract. These two networks of the ENS have their own sensory nerves (nerves that deliver sensations), and they have links to other nerves (modulating neurons) that can cause even more neurons (motor nerves) to cause the guts to move. These nerves act on smooth muscle of the bowel and cause contractions.

If we add to our understanding of this network of nerves the knowledge that they are controlled by a whole host of messages in the form of neurotransmitters and hormones, the idea of a second brain (or many little brains) emerges. Chemical messengers are well known in neuroscience as important components of the transfer of signals in the main central nervous system. These chemical messengers include acetylcholine, norepinephrine, 5 hydroxytryptamine, serotonin, substance P, vasoactive peptides, dopamine, enkephalins, and somatostatin.

Neurotransmitters are made from nutrients taken in through the diet: in particular nerve cells are largely composed of essential fats. Certain surprises exist in nature. For example, capsaicin (a substance found in pepper plants) blocks substance P, which is involved in pain control, and common drugs used to treat psychiatric disorders (e.g., Prozac) work through an effect on serotonin (a chemical that affects bowel function). We may have to rethink approaches to gut health and well-being in terms of natural agents or environmental influences. Our thoughts may have to expand into the realms of psychoneuronutrition or neuropsychogastroenterology (or other disciplines with neologistic names). Perhaps we must consider whether or not we should direct our therapy against the brains of the guts or the brains of the body. New directions in the treatment of functional disease of the gut are researching drugs that affect receptors in the ENS.

The idea of giving the guts psychotherapy should not prompt a call for psychiatric help for the physician who is enticed by this option; after all, what is hypnosis or biofeedback training in gastroenterology, other than supportive psychotherapy for the gut (including its own brains and the brains of its master, the central nervous system)?

NETWORKS WITHIN THE ENS

There are well-developed networks of neurons (nerve cells) within the ENS that convey messages that make the walls of the bowel move. This area of communication within the *autonomous* ENS (independently working nervous system) is an active area of research. Much effort has been expended on trying to understand how the external nerve supply of the bowel controls motor (movement) functions, but attention is now being focused on the ENS.

The connecting nerve fibers or relay stations (referred to as interneurons) in the ENS use a variety of chemicals and peptides (small proteins), and they are examples of neurotransmitters within the ENS. Modern authors who have attempted to explain the scientific basis of body-mind connections (e.g., Candace B. Pert, Ph.D., and Michael D. Gershon, M.D.) have discussed these messenger molecules in great detail. Dr. Pert describes these chemicals as "molecules of emotion" that help explain "why you feel the way you feel!"

There are many messenger molecules. Examples include serotonin, substance *P*, bradykinin, somatostatin, and enkephalins. Dr. Gershon, in his book *The Second Brain* (referring to the brain(s) of the gut) illuminates the role of serotonin, whereas Dr. Pert focuses on opiate receptors. The precise mode of action of all of these messenger compounds is a matter of complex research, and it is beyond the scope of our discussion to describe the known (or unknown) actions of each agent. For example, substance *P* is known to contract the circular layer of smooth muscle in the bowel, and the actions of substance P are effectively blocked by natural agents such as capsaicin. I mention this information because it forms one of many examples of the scientific basis for remedies of natural origin for gut disorders.

THE BIG STRAIN

During defecation, the anus and rectum work together in a coordinated manner to permit stool to pass with ease. The anus and its attachments form a complex gatekeeper mechanism that prevents incontinence of stool; but when the events that control defecation occur in an uncoordinated manner, the exit of stool can be obstructed. This results in the common occurrence of straining in vain.

There are several symptoms that suggest the presence of obstructed defecation. Individuals with this disorder invariably strain to open their bowels, often to no avail. There is often a pronounced descent of the anal margin during defecation and a sensation of incomplete evacuation of the rectum is quite common. Afflicted individuals may insert their fingers into their rectum to remove stool, and some learn to strain while pushing against the resistance of folded toilet tissue. Occasionally the lining of the lower anal margin (and even rectum) can prolapse and appear during straining.

It is surprising how the coordinated events that occur during defecation remain underexplored in spite of the recognition of incomplete relaxation of the anal sphincter in many people with constipation. A century ago, Dr. L. von Frankl-Hochwort and Dr. A. Froehlich defined the importance of the tone of the anal sphincters in defecation in a classic scientific paper entitled "Ueber Tonus und Innervation der Sphinkteren des Anus." Modern gastroenterologists may have one believe that the phenomenon of obstructed defecation is a relatively new discovery, and some ascribe it incorrectly to the work of Dr. L. A. Buie and Dr. W. L. Butsch in the 1930s, following the publication of their classic paper entitled "The Importance of Recognizing the Contracting Anus."

Obstructed defecation is one of the most common causes of constipation, and it is frequently mismanaged. All the laxatives in the world, straining, and dietary modifications will not facilitate normal evacuation of the bowels in the presence of a gross disorder of the gatekeeper mechanism of the anorectum. Obstructed defecation of a varying degree may occur in about one half of all people with chronic constipation. It is suggested that obstructed defecation is most often due to an inability of an individual to relax the external anal sphincter but other mechanisms involving contractions of the rectal wall, movements of muscles within the pelvis, and alterations in rectal sensations may all operate to cause obstructed defecation.

MANAGING GATEKEEPER OBSTRUCTION

Understanding the sequence of events during defecation is the key to correcting obstructed defecation. The act of defecation is triggered by distension (pressure) in the rectum due to the presence of stool. Normally, it is an act under voluntary control where pressure in the abdomen rises from contraction of the abdominal muscles and descent of the diaphragm. Contraction of the abdominal wall occurs in concert with pelvic-floor and anal-sphincter relaxation. The pivotal event is relaxation of the pelvic floor in coordination with the increase in pressure with the abdomen. Under normal circumstances, the sling of muscles around the anus relax and stool slides by with ease.

Understanding these events facilitates a process of pelvic-floor retraining where individuals who are afflicted can relearn the correct sequence of events to overcome the incoordinate muscle actions during defecation. One simple method that can overcome obstructed pooping is the adoption of an extreme squatting position. Some people may notice that a low-set toilet pedestal facilitates defecation and perhaps the most facilitative position for defecation is squatting over a hole in the ground. Southern European and Eastern Asian public lavatories are often equipped with squatting holes, in contrast to the "throne" of Western society. Extreme squatting is a simple and effective cure for some people with obstructed defecation.

The process of complex pelvic-floor retraining has been detailed in several scientific articles in the last decade. In brief, breathing exercises are often taught with simultaneous contraction and relaxation of the abdomen. Sophisticated biofeedback training can be used where pressures are measured in the rectum and at the anal margin. The recordings can be displayed on a screen and the patient can be instructed to engage in the correct maneuvers to coordinate pelvic-floor movements, This is a form of simulated defecation. The two main principals of therapy are sensory conditioning, such as making the subject more aware of rectal detention, and coordination training.

The use of biofeedback and pelvic floor retraining requires sophisticated instrumentation and highly specialized personnel, and it is probably necessary only in recalcitrant (difficult to treat) cases. Many individuals benefit from perineal exercises alone, where the rectal margin can be elevated by voluntary pelvic muscle contractions. This exercise is similar in principal to Kegels, which are used to tighten vaginal musculature especially when laxity occurs following childbirth. Focused attention on the bowel and anal margin may be enough to cause considerable improvement in the symptoms of constipation in many people.

DIARRHEA

The word *diarrhea* can be easily understood from its derivation in the Greek language, but it defies an easy definition. The Greek word dia means "through" and rhein (rrhea) means "flow." In simplistic terms, we are talking about a "through flow" of stool that is more voluminous, frequent, and less well formed (liquid) than normal. A precise definition is very difficult. Many factors control the weight of stool— the weight of the stool is often related to its water content and it is a rough guide to the presence of diarrhea, but it is not the whole story.

Studies of stool weight, water content, and solid content have been performed on "normal" people, and the ranges of these components are very variable. One of the most frequently quoted studies in the United States. (performed in Dallas, Texas) indicates an average stool weight of 142 grams per day in "healthy" men and 55 grams per day in "healthy" women. This compares with 107 grams per day for "healthy" men and 50 grams per day in "healthy" women in Edinburgh, Scotland. It is striking to compare these figures with stool weights of Bantu natives in Africa, where average stool weights are alleged to be about, 1000 to 2000 grams per day. What accounts for the difference?

The characteristics of stool (weight, solid content, water content etc.) in states of apparent health are most often related to differences in fiber intake in the diet, hormonal factors, and psychosocial factors. One key to the recognition of diarrhea is the frequency of

---

Table 8.1: The four major mechanisms of diarrhea.

Sometimes diarrhea is caused by a combination of factors.

MECHANISM	COMMENT
Exudative diarrhea	A kind of discharge of stool and inflammatory contents from the bowel, as seen in infections and serious inflammation
Osmotic diarrhea	An unabsorbable component of the diet draws fluid out of the bowel e.g., lactose, salts of magnesium
Secretory diarrhea	Increased secretions by the gut overwhelm the balance of the gut e.g., medications, toxins from bacteria, hormonal problems
Diarrhea due to motor disturbances (dysmotility)	The normal movements of the bowel are disrupted e.g., IBS, following surgery to the gut, etc.

bowel actions. A hypothetical range of normality of stooling is between three times per day and three times per week.

There are hundreds of listed causes of diarrhea in modern textbooks of gastroenterology. This has led to an attempt to classify diarrhea and its causes by the mechanisms that operate to cause the diarrhea. The four broad categories of mechanisms of diarrhea are listed in Table 8.1. Exudative and secretory types of diarrhea are most often associated with serious diseases, but any type of diarrhea can be caused by illness. In this book, we have focused on functional disorders of the gut or lifestyle factors that bring us to a more focused consideration of osmotic diarrhea and diarrhea due to motor problems in the bowel. We must consider the possibility that more than one mechanism that causes diarrhea can operate at the same time.

OSMOTIC DIARRHEA

There are many agents that will tend to draw in and hold water in the bowel. These agents interfere with the normal function of the colon, which is to absorb water from stool. Water holding (osmotically active) agents interfere with the formation of solid stool. Diarrhea will occur when the amount of water in the cavity of the colon exceeds the capacity of the colon to absorb water. This event most commonly occurs when undigestible material, that is osmotically active (water drawing and holding), enters the colon. Fiber and certain carbohydrates in the diet are common causes of this situation. One of the principal offenders is lactose (milk sugar), which creates osmotically active ingredients in the colon that have the added properties of irritating the colon. As common as this situation is, it is frequently overlooked.

LACTOSE INTOLERANCE

Lactose is a simple sugar (disaccharide) like sucrose (table sugar). These simple sugars are split by enzymes (disaccharidases) in the small intestine into single sugar units, which are rapidly absorbed into the body and used as fuel. The enzymes that split disaccharide sugars (e.g., sucrose, lactose, and maltose) are located in the surface areas of the cells that line the small intestines. These enzymes are called disaccharidase enzymes.

If the lactase (the dissaccharidase) enzyme that splits lactose into its component units (galactose and glucose) is deficient or absent, then the lactose taken in the diet can spill over into the lower bowel to a variable degree, where it creates havoc in the colon. The havoc created is due to its osmotic activity and the actions of bacteria on the lactose that produce compounds (e.g., short-chain fatty acids) that trigger diarrhea. Deficiency or absence of the enzyme lactase, which splits the sugar lactose into its component sugars, is called lactose intolerance.

Lactose in the colon attracts water in the colon, causing distension of the bowel, and it stimulates movements of the bowel to clear the water (diarrhea ensues). We shall learn that the colon is teaming with friendly bacteria that seize the opportunity to ferment sugars like lactose. This fermentation process causes the release of more water, gases, and organic acids. Organic acids (short-chain fatty acids) can be utilized by the colon as an energy source to some degree, but they are osmotically active. The extra gas and water produced by lactose fermentation is a further burden to the colon and havoc occurs.

If large quantities of lactose are consumed or if the enzyme lactase is deficient or absent, then urgent and explosive diarrhea can occur. Some individuals can have extreme symptoms such as incontinence of stool in an unpredictable manner.

Other sugars or compounds may cause osmotic diarrhea, and their activity is often more covert and less well recognized as a cause of diarrhea. The quest for sweeteners that do not add too many calories has led to the use of sorbitol in candies and dietetic foods. Sorbitol is a well-defined cause of osmotic diarrhea, and its presence has been associated with conditions that have been called chewing gum diarrhea, popsicle diarrhea and dietetic food diarrhea. Candies that are labeled "sugar free" may frequently cause diarrhea for this reason.

Perhaps surprising for some is the presence of nonabsorbable carbohydrates in fruits and vegetables. Many types of fiber are really complex molecules of non-absorbable carbohydrates, but other complex, nonabsorbable sugars are present in our diet. One special example is the presence of nonabsorbable sugars (carbohydrates) in soybeans. The carbohydrates stacchyose and raffinose found in soybeans are not absorbed by humans (and some animals to whom soy is fed). These carbohydrates enter the colon and are acted on by bacteria (friendly types) to produce gas and water, thereby loosening the bowel. While the actions of stacchyose and raffinose sound nefarious, these carbohydrates work to our benefit by promoting the growth of friendly bacteria in our colon that promote general health. The presence of the right type of bacteria in our bowels can help protect against colon cancer and contribute indirectly to important body functions such as general immunity.

Stacchyose and raffinose make crude soy an unfriendly food for the digestive tract, but studies of people who live a long and healthy life in Japan link the presence of these carbohydrates in the diet to longevity. For more details, readers are referred to the author's book *The Soy Revolution*.

THE ORIGIN OF LACTOSE INTOLERANCE

Deficiency or absence of the enzyme lactase that splits lactose into its component sugars presents itself by three mechanisms (Table 8.2). In many people, genetic programming seems to cause a decline in lactase with maturity. The body of opinion that perceives milk (dairy products) as dangerous in adults stresses the argument that nature did not intend adults to use milk as a source of food. I do not accept this reasoning. Dairy products are useful foods when consumed in moderation, but allergy to dairy protein is very common, especially in infants and young children.

Lactose creeps into our diet in many foods in addition to milk (Read food labels!). Estimates of the occurrence of lactose intolerance vary. Table 8.3 quotes some averages. In their excellent book *The Milk Sugar Dilemma*, Dr. Richard A. Martens, M.D., and Sherlyn Martens, RD, provide excellent advice for the person with lactose intolerance. I recommend this book highly. Intolerance to lactose is managed generally by dietary adjustments and the addition of the enzyme lactase (available as Lactaid).

Table 8.2: Types of lactose intolerance.

TYPE	COMMENT
Congential, familial, hereditary,	Rare and life-threatening, it is genetic associated with other types of disaccharide intolerance (e.g., maltose, sucrose) and is found in premature infants.
Acquired lactose intolerance (programmed by genetics)	All mammalian milk contains lactose. Lactase enzyme activity has peak activity within a couple of days after birth and then declines variably throughout life. This phenomenon is thought by some to be tied to theories of maturity in animals, being associated with food sources alternative to dairy milk. This is the common type of lactose intolerance.
Acquired lactose intolerance	The lactase enzyme is "knocked (secondary to disease usually)out" of the small intestine by infections (sometimes transient), inflammation, cancer, malnutrition, and diseases associated with malabsorption.

Table 8.3: Approximate occurrence of lactose intolerance.

Based on data supplied by the National Institutes of Health.

Caucasians	15%
African Americans	75%
Mexican Americans and Hispanics	75%
Eastern Asians (Orientals)	90%

The fuss relates to the fact that lactose intolerance is very common and often overlooked. Lactose intolerance seems benign but it must not be forgotten that it can be a manifestation of more serious digestive disease, for example malabsorption or inflammatory bowel disease. The advice and guidance of a physician and dietician are recommended in cases any of doubt.

> ## Table 8.4: Medications or food additives that can cause diarrhea—not all are listed.
>
> - Laxatives—all kinds
> - Food sweeteners—e.g., fructose, mannitol, and sorbitol
> - Chemotherapy for cancer—many examples
> - Drugs for asthma—e.g., aminophylline
> - Fat substitutes—e.g., Olestra, and some food additives
> - Arthritis medications—e.g., all NSAIDs, colchicine
> - Diuretics (water pills)—e.g., furosemide, thiazides
> - Drugs for CNS disorders—e.g., L-Dopa, prozac
> - Cardiovascular drugs—e.g., digoxin, quindine
> - Blood-pressure-lowering drugs—e.g., propanolol, guanethidine
> - Cholesterol-lowering drugs—e.g., lovastatin, gemfibrizol
> - Antisecretory drugs—e.g., H2-receptor antagonists, proton pump inhibitors

DRUGS AND DIARRHEA

Laxative use and abuse is quite a common cause of diarrhea—often expected and sometimes wanted. Less obvious drug-induced causes of diarrhea are summarized in Table 8.4.

Table 8.4 shows that a great number of drugs or additives to our diet can cause loose bowels. The advice of a pharmacist is recommended in regard to the connection between these drugs and diarrhea.

PAINS IN AND AROUND THE ANUS

Nonspecific discomfort around the anal margin is a common problem. Many people have hemorrhoids (piles) of variable severity, which can give rise to many symptoms or signs including pruritus ani (itching sensation), anal pain, and bleeding. A number of natural therapies are used with success to treat hemorrhoids, and piles are aggravated or caused by adverse lifestyle habits. Exercise and balanced nutrition can help prevent and treat this problem. The application of witch hazel can be soothing. Dietary fiber may be preventive for hemorrhoids, but advanced cases may require surgery. Natural inhibitors of angiogenesis (new blood vessel growth) have found a role in the management of hemorrhoids. Shark cartilage cream, made with the patented angiogenesis form of 100 percent pure shark cartilage (Cartilade) has been used successfully in open-label experiments to treat hemorrhoids.

Beyond the induction of common anal problems due to tight-fitting underwear, poor anal hygiene, and anal sex, there are two intriguing conditions that affect the anus and rectum that remain beyond the boundaries of explanation. The first is a condition called proctalgia fugax which gives rise to short-lived (fleeting), sometimes very severe rectal pain, and the second is pruritus ani (anal itch) of unknown cause.

Proctalgia fugax tends to occur in early adulthood and midlife and it seems to affect people who are quite healthy. It sometimes occurs in association with straining or after coitus, and it may be related to spasm of pelvic floor muscles. This disorder has been labeled unpleasant and incurable but quite harmless. Psychiatric disturbances are not the hallmark of this condition, which sometimes responds to chiropractic intervention, hydrotherapy (external), and simple upward pressure applied by the fingers to the anal margin.

Pruritus ani is one of the most common problems affecting almost everyone at some stage to a variable degree. It is often a symptom alone from any other problems. Although it can be caused by colonic inflammation, hemorrhoids, or parasites, these conditions are frequently absent. The common advice given by physicians (or relatives) not to scratch is easier to say than do. Sufferers may make matters worse by douching the anal margin with irritants.

Alternative medicine affords some options for this problem of chronic anal itching but few research studies have been performed to confirm any benefits of the various interventions. Sitz baths are very useful, but this condition often responds very well to probiotic therapy with lactobacilli. The use of lactobacilli is said to be more valuable if the stool is markedly alkaline (high pH). Hundreds of topical creams and ointments are available, including local anesthetics, antihistamines, and cortisone-containing creams. Topical ointments containing calendula are particularly valuable, as is the use of the astringent witch hazel. Unfortunately, additives to these creams, ointments, and lotions may make the itching worse, and local anesthetics and antihistamines are capable of causing sensitization. Many physicians engaged in alternative medicine link pruritus ani to food allergy, but this relationship is not clear.

SEROTONIN

The concept of the gut and its second brain or brains has percolated through mainstream medicine only in the past five years or so, as pharmaceutical companies research the value of serotonin antagonists in the regulation of bowel function. Serotonin (5-hydroxytryptamine) is a messenger molecule (molecule of emotion) within the network of nerves of the ENS and the autonomic nervous system that is connected to the central nervous system (CNS).

There are multiple receptors (target sites of action) of serotonin in the ENS and the CNS. Scientists are now unravelling the importance of blocking serotonin sensory reception (sensations from the gut). For example, blocking certain serotonin receptors in the vagus nerve and the fourth ventricle of the brain (CNS) has found a major role in the control of serious nausea and vomiting that is induced by chemotherapy for cancer.

There are different types of serotonin receptors that can be stimulated (agonist drug) or inhibited (antagonist drug). The drug tegaserod, for example, can produce significant relief of symptoms in individuals with constipation due to IBS. While these findings are promising and complex for a layperson to understand, it is notable that practioners of alternative medicine have been using supplements that are precursors of serotonin or serotonin itself for several years to regulate CNS and bowel function.

The story of serotonin pharmacology is an example of the blurring of identity between alternative and conventional medical approaches. Medical pluralism is a heartbeat away!

USE OF PRECURSORS OF NEUROTRANSMITTERS (MOLECULES OF EMOTION)

Many of the molecules of emotion have nutrient precursors that are converted into active messengers. For example, tryptophan (an amino acid) starts a precursor chain with conversion to 5-Hydroxytryptophan to serotonin and tyrosine is converted to norepinephrine to epinephrine. The idea of giving the nutrient precursor(s) to make neurotransmitters more available is a natural approach to the correction of excesses or deficiencies of molecules of emotion.

Although the administration of precursors can often result in enhanced synthesis of neurotransmitters, it is not clear if it results in release of these molecules of emotion at their site of action. Administration of precursors, for example, L-tryptophan, can actually affect the function of connections in the ENS—especially the firing of neurons that use serotonin as a principal transmitter. Perhaps the pivotal issue is the lack of knowledge concerning the ability of increased release of molecules of emotion to result in ongoing stimulatory or inhibitory effects in the ENS and its attachments within the gut. The whole circumstance is clouded by the knowledge that feedback mechanisms (brakes) exist when levels of molecules of emotion are simply adjusted.

Feeding nutrients, especially supplement amino acids, that are precursors of transmitter molecules appear to have promising therapeutic (treatment) properties; but there is need for more definition of their effect. These areas are of great importance in alternative medicine where nutrient precursors and "medicalized foods" are embraced as treatments. Among other things, this approach forms the basis of a scientific approach to psychoneuronutrition.

CHAPTER SUMMARY

Functional disorders figure highly as a cause of bowel upset, but drug side effects and adverse lifestyle are important. The role of the ENS is becoming increasingly apparent in bowel control, and new neurohormonal-regulating agents afford promise of a more rational approach to the elimination of constipation and diarrhea. Natural approaches to bowel regulation are often to be generally preferred to drug therapy.

CHAPTER NINE

FOOD
INTOLERANCE AND SENSITIVITY

TERMS AND MISUNDERSTANDINGS

If ever there was a subject that is veiled in controversy, it is the definition and management of adverse reactions to food. The body can react in many ways to food; and terminology about clinical reactions to food becomes very important when discussing lack of tolerance to certain substances in our diet. A couple of definitions are in order so that we can clear the fog of controversy about food allergies. I subscribe to the notion that food allergies and intolerances present real problems for some individuals.

Food allergy: In its true form (according to conventional medicine), it involves the actions of the immune system against dietary components that act as allergens (antigens). The term *allergy* is thrown around in common language, but food allergy involving immune mechanisms is much less common than other adverse clinical reactions to food.

Food intolerance: This is a lack of acceptablility by the body of food components for a variety of reasons, other than as a consequence of an immune reaction in the body. Some foods have druglike actions on the body (e.g., histamine in fish or tyramine in cheese or red wine), some contain toxins (e.g., organic chemicals, herbicides, or pesticides), some can release chemicals in the body that cause inflammation (e.g., histamine release by strawberries), and some foods are irritants to the guts (e.g., capsaicin in peppers). A common cause of intolerance to food is deficiency of enzymes required for digestion of the sugar lactose, found as the principal sugar in milk products.

The above distinction between food allergy and intolerance (or idiosyncratic response to food) is in itself a controversial issue. Orthodox medicine makes this distinction but alternative (ecological) medicine proposes many grey zones in adverse clinical reactions to food. Perhaps the term *food sensitivity* is useful because clinical reactions to food may often have an uncertain mechanism or be associated with immunological mechanisms that are not detectable in standard clinical practice.

ADVERSE RESPONSES TO FOOD, NOT READILY EXPLAINED

There are countless reports of patients who respond to the elimination of certain agents from the diet, where there is no clear evidence of true allergy (immune mechanism) or an identifiable factor that determines intolerance to the food. Accepting this proposal—which is not accepted generally by conventional medicine—other mechanisms operate. These other mechanisms are ill defined or unknown. Researchers have claimed other mechanisms of food intolerance. These have been termed false food allergies. False food allergies are believed to be related to a nonspecific mechanism involving the release of histamine (an inflammatory mediating chemical) in the body. Histamine release is not the only potential mechanism of adverse response to food. Other molecules that are produced in the body and cause inflammation can be released by certain foods or food additives. These molecules include types of prostaglandins that are proinflammatory and leukotrienes. Perhaps some of our molecules of emotion are tied up in this process.

Illnesses with varied symptoms (headaches, skin rashes, nausea, aches and pains) can be caused by histamine release. This release can be precipitated by food components such as tyramine (present in cheese, Brewer's yeast, soused herrings, red wine), phenylethylene (chocolate), sodium nitrite (sausages, cold meats, Dutch cheeses, canned fish), and starchy foods (fermentation in the bowel can produce histamine). The latter example of starch in foods causing adverse reactions to food can be considered one real example of the phenomenon of autointoxication an issue that has been hotly debated in medicine.

The phenomenon of autointoxication involves the concept that toxic substances can be produced in the bowel by fermentation of food. Conventional medicine has argued strongly against this occurrence, based on the reasoning that the colonic lining is very efficient at preventing the passage of toxins into the body. When starch-containing foods are eaten excessively, especially those that contain cellulose, fermentation by colonic bacteria can produce histamine that can be absorbed into the body and provoke inflammatory responses. This mechanism of false food allergy has been proposed by Professor D. A. Moneret-Vantrin, a French physician who has published his work extensively in the peer-reviewed medical literature.

FOOD INTOLERANCE—A FORGOTTEN CAUSE OF ILLNESS

Early in my career, I was convinced that food allergies were the diagnosis of the destitute physician, but now I believe that adverse effects from food appear to have more to do with common reality than with quackery. Perhaps the biggest problem in the study of food allergies or intolerance is the varied, and often contradictory, opinions expressed among the medical profession about the value of existing diagnostic tests for food allergies. In the clear-cut type of food allergy, circulating levels of antibodies may be raised to certain food components. Skin testing is a common practice to detect food allergy, but skin tests can be quite unreliable. Perhaps the best diagnostic approach is elimination of the offending dietary agent that is identified by careful history-taking, together with challenge-testing of the offending food. Challenge-testing involves the administration of the offending agent under carefully controlled circumstances, preferably in a manner where both the doctor and the patient are unaware of the agent used in the challenge (double-blind testing). Testing for food allergies is expensive, cumbersome, and often insensitive.

ARROGANCE PREVAILS: DICHOTOMY EXISTS

On the one hand, there is a small group of physicians that denies the significance of food allergy or intolerance in disease, whereas on the other a minority of zealots claims that food allergies are the universal cause of illness. The vast majority of physicians falls somewhere between these polar opinions, with a tendency for conventional medicine to downplay food allergies and intolerance. Polar opinions cause divisions in medicine and two intransigent schools of thought have appeared in the arena of adverse reactions to foods.

These two groups have referred to themselves as immunologists (or allergists) and ecologists. I believe in the concepts proposed by both, and the blended (integrated) approach seems most prudent based on current knowledge. Conventional medicine demands that the ecologist (a healthcare giver who studies the way in which environmental factors cause illness) provide evidence for the many claims about "allergies" that are commonly adopted by the general public. Evidence appears to have accumulated that food allergy and intolerance is a real problem in society. Beginning with the classic work of A. H. Rowe in 1931 (*Food Allergy: Its manifestations and Diagnosis and Treatment*), every decade has witnessed a renaissance in the study and treatment of food allergy. Medical interest in this topic seems to wax and wane.

Perhaps the most unfair criticism of the ecologist's approach to clinical reactions to food involves the argument that this discipline of medicine fails to distinguish between true allergy to food and food intolerance (or idiosyncratic responses). The problem in providing this distinction is that the mechanisms of common adverse reactions to food remain poorly understood, and where a certain mechanism of food allergy is suspected its demonstration is very difficult. For example, the accepted occurrence of false food allergies due to histamine release can probably be confirmed only by complex testing such as intraduodenal histamine challenge (giving histamine through a tube placed in the upper intestines) performed in a double-blind manner. This land of testing has no role in routine clinical practice.

DISEASES AND FOOD ALLERGY

Disorders where a clear link has been shown to food components include rhinitis, conjunctivitis, asthma, angioedema, eczema (and other skin rashes), migraine, and celiac disease (gluten enteropathy) and its variant disorder of dermatitis herpetiformis (a relatively uncommon condition in the United States). Less clear but quite convincing associations have been made between food allergies and rheumatoid arthritis, multiple sclerosis, inflammatory bowel disease (ulcerative colitis and Crohn's disease), and certain psychiatric disorders. Multiple allergies are believed to occur in some individuals, and one extreme form of clinical reactions to food and the environment has been called the total allergy syndrome: In this condition, an individual may be perceived to be so sensitive to their environment that they must adopt a cloistered existence. If total allergy syndrome exists, it must be very rare and caution must be exercised in reaching or accepting this diagnosis.

THE GUT AS A COMPLEX IMMUNE ORGAN

The gastrointestinal tract contains a large amount of tissue that is involved in immune function. It has very complex and still poorly defined mechanisms for dealing with antigens (allergens) taken in food and antigens present in its normal or abnormal residents (viruses, bacteria, and yeasts). The digestive and immune functions of the gut are inextricably linked. For example, in cases of deficiency of certain enzymes (e.g., enzymes from the pancreas that digest protein) more protein may be present in the gut in a format that can act as an antigen that challenges the immune function of the bowel. The study of the immune functions of the gut has been hampered by its relative inaccessibility—gut immunologists are a rare breed of physician.

Clumps of lymphoid (immune) tissue are interconnected in the intestines by a complex arrangement of lymphatic channels, and immune-competent cells are scattered throughout the walls of the bowel. Antibodies (especially immunoglobulin type A, IgA) are found in intestinal secretions. These antibodies appear to play a role in blocking hypersensitivity (immune) reactions in the bowel, and they function to reduce the uptake of large molecules by the gut, thereby preventing their access to the body. A deficiency of IgA is associated with immune disorders in the body.

THE BOWEL LETS ANTIGENS INTO THE BODY

Some physicians are surprised or fail to recognize that the gut permits antigens to penetrate its lining and gain access to the general circulation in the body. These antigens can initiate various types of immune reactions such as those involving lymphocytes (T cell, delayed hypersensitivity) or antibodies (immune complex formation). Certain diseases or conditions can cause antigens to move freely across the gut wall by enhancing the permeability of the intestines. This condition of free access of large molecules through the gut is the principal feature of the leaky gut syndrome (discussed in detail in chapter 11). Enhanced permeability of the intestines is well recognized in the presence of parasitic infections and certain states of immune deficiency (e.g., IgA deficiency and AIDS).

When an allergen (or antigen) crosses the gut wall it can cause hypersensitivity reactions (immune damage) as a result of antigen and antibody reactions or cell-mediated immunity, involving T lymphocytes. These reactions can change the movements of the bowel (gastrointestinal motility effects), cause swelling of the bowel wall, and increase secretion of mucus in the gut. Several researchers have cautioned about the assumption that altered gastrointestinal motility is often caused by food allergy. In most cases of the common IBS, true allergic reactions do not exist. Nevertheless, some cases of IBS are reported to respond to certain food exclusions.

FOOD "ALLERGY" IS UNDERDIAGNOSED

The term *allergy* was coined in the early 1900s by Dr. von-Pirquet, an Austrian physician who believed that the phenomenon of allergy was "an acquired specific altered capacity to react to physical substance on the part of the body." Dr. von-Pirquet was not focused on immunogical mechanisms when he made his inferences about allergy (immunology was not a developed area of medical knowledge in 1906). Modern physicians who are engaged in the practice of conventional medicine exhibit a consistent desire to reserve the term allergy to cases where evidence of immunological hypersensitivity is demonstrable. Again, modern medicine seems to cling to the explainable. What was in Dr. von-Pirquet's mind cannot be gleaned with hindsight, but his observations were empiric and it is doubtful if considerations about specific mechanisms of allergy clouded his thoughts. Reactions to food components, other than immunologically mediated, cannot be dismissed. They are real, frequently reported in the scientific literature, and often overlooked in clinical practice. Everyone knows the term food allergy, but few distinguish immunological factors from other factors that cause adverse reactions to dietary ingredients.

We have recognized that some food antigens cross the wall of the gut and enter the general circulation where they can provoke a variety of responses in the body, including immune responses. Accepting this phenomenon readily explains certain types of "food allergy" and raises the question why overt food allergy is not more common than generally identified, or more of an overt, serious problem for the body?

In early life, the gut is much more permeable to food antigens than in adulthood. A newborn baby may receive macromolecules from milk in the early period following birth, but "closure" of the gut occurs within a couple of weeks. When food antigens enter the body in early life, antibodies are formed, usually IgA. In adult life, much smaller amounts of food antigens enter the bloodstream due to complexing of the food antigen with IgA (blocking antibodies that attach to the food antigen) and other defense mechanisms exist that constitute the gut barrier.

THE SIGNIFICANCE OF ABSORBED ANTIGENS

In states of health, the body appears to deal with potentially absorbable antigens in the diet in an efficient manner. It has been supposed, quite erroneously, that antigens are digested completely or that the gut wall presents an impermeable barrier to potentially noxious agents that could be absorbed from the gut contents. In fact, the digestive tract is a potential source of all sorts of potential toxic agents, including food antigens, bacteria, breakdown products from bacterial actions, toxins (endotoxins and exotoxins from bacteria), and a whole range of digestive enzymes. If set free on body tissues, enzymes in the gut could potentially digest cells and cause untold harm. When unwanted toxins are absorbed, they can play a role in the causation of a variety of diseases, certainly if immunological mechanisms are activated.

KEEPING UNWANTED MOLECULES OUT

The walls of the intestine have to let in the components of the diet that are required for healthy nutrition, but keep out the unwanted substances. The mucosa (lining of the intestines) acts like a highly sophisticated sieve with great powers of discrimination under normal conditions. These mechanisms operate like the doorman at an exclusive club.

The newborn intestinal tract is capable of taking large particles and passing them across its lining cells by a process of engulfment and transport. In this process, the molecules are taken up at the cell surface, package in a little envelope (bubble) made from the cell membrane itself, and discharged from the opposite side of the cell. This engulfment and transport across the cell and discharge at the opposite side of the cell is termed endocytosis (into the cell) and exocytosis (out of the cell). In contrast, many simpler molecules derived from food pass through the cells by diffusion around the cells through "junctions." This is the sievelike action of the lining of the bowel.

The process of uptake of large molecules appears to be particularly important in newborn infants where factors, such as antibodies, in mother's milk can be transferred to a newborn child to confer immunity to infections. This phenomenon of transfer of large-sized, "marker" molecules (e.g., horseradish peroxidase—an enzyme) has been demonstrated in laboratory experiments in animals. The same process, however, occurs in humans until a time in maturation occurs where this uptake becomes much less—a process of "closure."

The closure of the gut wall to big molecules does not seem complete. Evidence exists that this occurs to a variable degree in the intestines of adults. The process of transport of big molecules sometimes occurs between cells, but the spaces between cells are normally kept closed by structures called tight junctions. There is evidence of specialized transport in certain cells in the adult bowel. These cells are called *M* cells and they are found lying on top of lymphatic tissue (called Peyers patches). These *M* cells seem to be specially placed close to lymphatic tissue to present antigens to the immune functions that are exerted by the lymphoid tissue. Other mechanisms of uptake of antigens (big molecules) exist, including special ways of absorbing immune complexes (antibodies combined with antigens). When disease occurs or the bowel ages, the sieve becomes less efficient and more leaky, in both directions. The leakiness of the gut in adults is variable from person to person.

OTHER DEFENSES TO ENTRY OF UNWANTED MOLECULES

It is clear that the immune system plays a major role in controlling the uptake of antigens from the gut into the body. However, other factors that do not involve the immune system play a major role in keeping unwanted molecules or antigens out of the body. The processes that are important alone or in combination in excluding unwanted molecules are summarized in Table 8.5. Note the involvement of digestive factors and immune function in controlling these processes.

The role of normal flora in the gut in the maintenance of health in the gut and the entire body is reviewed in detail in chapter 10. The presence of desirable collections of certain types of bacteria in the

Table 9.1: Factors that operate together to prevent the absorption of unwanted molecules or antigens from the gut into the body.

IMMUNE MECHANISMS
- The actions of antibodies, e.g., IgA (or other immunoglobulins)
- Cell-mediated immunity due to actions of T lymphocytes

NONIMMUNE MECHANISMS (DIGESTIVE FUNCTIONS)
- Gut secretions (e.g., enzymes, mucus)
- Microflora of the bowels
- Mucosal (lining) cells have special barriers to penetration
- Movement of the guts (peristalsis)
- Filtering functions of the liver

intestines has many advantages for health, including an indirect action in controlling antigen absorption (especially toxic or damaging antigens). Good bacteria have to be present to maintain a healthy balance of the population of "bugs" in the normal bowel. This balance occurs by competition among bacteria for food and alterations in the climate in the bowel (e.g., pH—acidity or alkalinity). Secretions from the guts contain antibodies that can block antigen absorption (IgA) and sticky fluid called mucus that traps antigens or bacteria. Mucus contains chemicals called glycoproteins that can prevent the attachment of bacteria to the lining of the gut, so they are washed away and destroyed by enzymes.

The function of the stomach is very important in preventing the penetration of bacteria, viruses, yeasts, and other organisms through the guts. Gastric acid presents a hostile environment for any living organism. It serves to sterilize food to some degree. A number of studies have shown that in the absence of gastric acid, certain bacteria (especially gram-positive types) may increase within the gut (notably the small intestine).

GASTRIC ACID—ESSENTIAL?

The medical profession has been obsessed with the study of gastric acidity for several centuries. However, most of the research performed on gastric acid has focused on excess of gastric acid and its control by drugs or mutilating surgery. Absence of gastric acids (known as achlorhydria) has received some attention, but the health implications of lesser degrees of reduced acidity (hypochlorhydria) remains relatively underexplored. This situation is surprising in view of the massive and widespread use of drugs (H_2-receptor antagonists and proton pump inhibitors) that lower gastric acid. We learned that these acid-lowering drugs are among the most commonly used medications in Western society, and within the past five years, H_2receptor antagonists have become freely available as over the counter medications (see chapter 3 for a more complete discussion of acid-lowering drugs).

Gastric acidity is sometimes referred to as the principal gastric barrier because of its powerful protective functions. Although acidity plays a major role in killing micoorganisms that contaminate the diet, it is also involved in the development of hypersensitivity reactions to antigens (big molecules in the diet).

Notable studies in the 1960s (Drs. S. C. Kraft, R. M. Rothbert, and C. M. Kramer, *Journal of Clinical and Experimental Immunology* 2:321–326, 1967) showed that protein molecules (in this case bovine serum albumin) gained access to the general circulation; but, in the absence of gastric acid, they provoked antibody production. This study and others imply that gastric acid (and the digestive actions of pepsin— stomach enzymes) create a barrier to the entry of a variety of unwanted molecules (antigens) into the body. Such unwanted molecules include microorganisms or their fragments, toxins, and food antigens.

It is accepted that these unwanted molecules could potentially cause a variety of diseases, e.g., bowel disease or autoimmune disease. Whether reducing gastric acidity predisposes people to other coexisting illnesses has received relatively little attention—except perhaps in the study of causes of gastric cancer. Many physicians will argue that surveillance studies of acid-lowering medications do not show a trend for an enhanced incidence of other diseases, but the area of enhanced food-antigen absorption in association with varying degrees of reduction of gastric acidity has not been examined in detail. For example, it may not occur to a physician that someone who has low acidity in his or her stomach and develops inflammatory skin or joint conditions could have food allergies. If food allergies are not considered (or investigated thoroughly), they may not be detected. Throughout conventional and alternative medical literature, the occult nature of food allergies continues to be discussed. I think the jury remains out on whether long-term gastric-acid suppression could cause an increased occurrence of food allergy that may not have been recognized. Clearly, further study is required.

If insufficient stomach acid represents a potential risk to health, then replacing this acid might be expected to be of some benefit. The administration of dilute hydrochloric acid, betaine, or acidic foods is commonplace in the treatment of low stomach acidity in alternative medical practice, and it is a special part of the practice of naturopathy.

Naturopaths emphasize a wide range of signs and symptoms that can be perhaps attributed to low stomach acidity. In his excellent book entitled *Total Wellness*, Dr. Joseph Pizzorno, N.D., a well-respected naturopath, stresses that many more disorders are caused by too little gastric acid than too much stomach acid. This opinion is questionable but intriguing. Conditions that have been associated with low or absent stomach acid are summarized in Table 9.2, but clear evidence that replacing acid can ameliorate symptoms or signs of diseases associated with low-acid status does not seem to exist in the medical literature. It is important to note that an association between the presence of low acidity and a disease does not imply that the disorder is directly caused by low stomach acidity, but there may be an indirect relationship. One example of an association is occurrence of autoimmune disease or food allergies in states of low stom-

---

Table 9.2: A list of disorders associated with low stomach acid.

Please note that a direct causal association between low acid and these disorders often does not exist. Modified from Dr. J. Pizzorno, *Total Wellness*, 1996.

SYMPTOMS ASSOCIATED WITH LOW GASTRIC ACID
- Dyspepsia
- Nonspecific digestive upset
- Adverse clinical reactions to food
- Itching—especially anal
- Skin disorders, e.g., acne
- Poor digestive function

DISEASES ASSOCIATED WITH LOW GASTRIC ACID
- Autoimmune disease (many types)
- Food allergies
- Diabetes mellitus
- Skin disorders, e.g., eczema, vitiligo
- Osteoporosis and inflammatory arthritis
- Parasites

ach acidity. The common cause of achlorhydria is the disorder pernicious anemia, which is characterized by autoimmune attack on the
stomach—thus, a misleading chicken-and-egg argument exists.

CAUTION ON ASSOCIATIONS AND CAUSES OF DISEASE

The difference between an association with a disease and an occurrence must be distinguished from a clear-cut cause-and-effect relationship. Relationships between diseases can be very indirect. One of
the best examples of a spurious or tenuous relationship between diseases is the bona fide reports of an increased incidence of suicide in
people with peptic ulcer. Does this mean that peptic ulcer causes suicide? Of course not, but there are some studies that point to an
increased occurrence of suicide in people with peptic ulcers.

What is the link? It is known that excessive alcohol consumption
can predispose to peptic ulcer disease, and excessive drinking is more
common in some people with peptic ulcer. People with stress or psychiatric disease tend to drink excessively. The relationship between
peptic ulcer and suicide may be more explained in terms of a relationship between suicide and alcoholism or psychiatric disorders—
circumstances where clearer cause-and-effect relationships exist!

THE SEARCH FOR THE IMMUNOLOGICAL FRILLS IN FOOD ALLERGY

This chapter started with a definition of terminology and the distinction between food allergy (reserved by some for immune reactions)
and food intolerance (a reaction to food other than as a consequence
of an immune mechanism). The proposed compromise of the use of
the term *food sensitivity* can be heavily criticized because it fails to
bring us closer to an understanding of clinical reactions to food, if no
care is taken to define the mechanism.

Dr. Anne Ferguson, a famous immunologist from Edinburgh,
Scotland, has drawn attention to the slow development of research into

the clinical immunology of the gut, in comparison to investigations of general immune functions in the body. She reasoned that the principal cause of this lack of progress was the relative inaccessibility of gastrointestinal tissues, secretions, and bowel contents. Much of her excellent work demonstrated that the immune reactions of the lymphoid tissue (immune tissue) of the gut and other lymphoid tissue associated with mucosa in the body (e.g., lungs and genital tract) have different reactions to antigens than the general immune system of the body. In other words, just as the gut has its own little brains involved in its nervous control, it appears to have an immune system that can function somewhat differently than general immunity elsewhere in the body.

We have learned that the gut has its own geography, ecology, and inhabitants, which are separated from the body itself (compartmentalized) in an effective way, but communication exists. Communication between the gut and the body is rather like political ideation in nondemocratic societies—it has to be controlled! While scientists have tended to focus on the small intestine as the key part of immune reactions in the gut, the ability of the gut to mount an immune response is spread throughout its entire length. After all, the civilization of the guts stretches from mouth to anus and communication control (especially immune functions) must be available to control the dynamic activity resulting from the interactions of the bowel inhabitants (bugs) and foods or ingested materials (the digesta).

The complexity of immune interactions in the guts and the inextricable linkage of immune functions with the physiology of digestion explain why simple and reliable tests of food allergy (sensitivity or intolerance) are few and far between. This situation is confounded by a persistent lack of knowledge of the mechanisms of clinical reactions to food. Therefore, the contentious debate about the value of certain diagnostic tests for food allergy or intolerance may take many more years to resolve.

DIAGNOSIS OF FOOD ALLERGIES, SENSITIVITIES, AND INTOLERANCES

The diagnosis of food allergy or intolerance is embroiled in mystery and controversy in the mind of many healthcare givers. In medical

Table 9.3: Some types of food reactions defined.

ADVERSE REACTIONS NOT DUE TO IMMUNITY

• Food intolerance or idiosyncracy or toxins in food, e.g., diarrhea and bloating from lactase deficiency, food toxins from bacteria or molds, etc.

REACTIONS DUE TO IMMUNE MECHANISMS

• Reaginic reactions are mediated by IgE (rarely by IgG)—types of antibodies. Symptoms occur shortly after or within hours of eating the offending food, but may last for days. Symptoms include: abdominal pain, vomiting, nausea, diarrhea, skin rashes (urticaria or "wheels"), soft-tissue swelling, rhinitis (sinusitis), and wheezing (asthma). Severe reactions cause anaphylaxis—shock, low blood pressure, loss of consciousness, and, rarely, death.

• Nonreaginic reactions cause an inflammatory response including tissue swelling and vascular changes. Symptoms occur 6–24 hours after exposure to the offending food antigen. Early or delayed reactions occasionally occur by this mechanism (within 4 hours or after 24 hours), and results can be severe, e.g., iron deficiency, malabsorption, gastrointestinal blood loss, skin rashes, lung disorders, etc., especially in children.

practice, there comes a time when general symptoms of ill health have to be explained—doctors feel very inadequate if they have to say they do not know (an understandable but problematic reaction). I have reiterated that this circumstance can result in the "diagnosis of the destitute." Conventional medicine has shown an unwillingness to acknowledge disease states that are not readily explainable in scientific terms. The diagnosis of food allergy is to many conventional physicians, a diagnosis of the destitute.

Other disorders fall into this category of questionable diagnoses (labels that are not always considered tenable). To name a few contentious diagnoses —at least according to orthodox medical thinking—we have: chronic fatigue syndrome, yeast overgrowth (Candida), fibromyalgia, and Gulf War syndrome. It is no coincidence that alternative medicine figures strongly in the management of these disorders. When conventional medicine fails to manage or even to acknowledge the disorder, the doors to alternative medicine open. Some types of adverse reactions to foods are defined in Table 9.3.

THE DIAGNOSTIC TESTS

When a physician orders a diagnostic test for food allergies, he or she thinks about the accuracy of the test. This phenomenon is referred to in simple statistics as the sensitivity and specificity of the diagnostic tests. It is the ability of a test to provide an accurate diagnosis. To understand this further, a diagnostic test is of dubious value if it has false positives or false negatives. In fact, the terms *sensitivity* and *specificity* refer to the number of times a person who is truly negative, for the disease in question, shows up a negative result on the test and the number of times a person who is truly positive shows up a positive result on the test.

Table 9.4 describes a number of commonly used diagnostic tests for food allergy with some comments about their advantages, disadvantages, or limitations.

Table 9.4: Diagnostic tests applied in clinical reactions to food.

TEST	COMMENT
History taking	By far the most important diagnostic approach, includes family history.
Elimination diets and food challenge	See text—eliminate the offending food and reintroduce it to show that the food is the real cause of the problem.
Skin tests	Three techniques: scratch, prick, or intradermal. Expensive, require high-quality reagents and skilled interpretation. Intradermal tests rarely needed. All these tests should be confirmed by diet elimination.
Radioallergasorbent Test (RAST)	RAST measures antibodies to food antigens. Expensive and limited accurracy.
Other tests	• Eosinophil count in blood • Complement activation • Hemaglutinating antibodies • Serum Ig's (immunoglobulins) • Immune complex detection • Lymphocyte function tests • Leucocyte or blood histamine • Intestinal permeability

By far the most important aspect of diagnosis of food intolerance involves careful history taking to define the dietary miscreant or allergen (type of food causing the problem) and a process of elimination testing and diet reintroduction to show that the dietary factor in question is causing the problem.

Much work has been done on the subject of diagnostic testing for food allergies, and some advances have been made. Dr. R. St. C. Barnetson, M.D., and Dr. M. H. Lessof, M.D., are two of Britain's foremost authorities on food allergy. In their chapter in the book *Clinical Reactions to Food*, these doctors consider food allergy and intolerance in the context of a challenge to "medical orthodoxy." The following quotation from their work summarizes problems with mythical and magical thinking in the area of reactions to food. They state:

> The pseudo-scientific approach is not without danger. While it would be arrogant for doctors to think that all fringe medicine is therapy by lunatics for lunatics, some critical examination is essential in order to avoid misleading the public and—even more so—some of the more gullible and sensation-seeking publicists of press and television. The fact that no scientific explanation is available at present does not alter the fact that some of the unorthodox phenomena described in books on subjects such as food allergy may well have some scientific basis. It is necessary, however, to outline some of the unacceptable facets of fringe medicine, so that the patient is not positively harmed.

THE ELIMINATION CHALLENGE ROUTINE

To confirm that a certain component of the diet (e.g., food antigen or additive to food) is causing the problem, a careful elimination of the offending agent can be undertaken, followed by its reintroduction. This type of maneuver in diagnosis must be performed by an expert. Various elimination diets have been described, and it is generally desirable to exclude many known, common food allergens from the diet for at least two weeks.

Without the offending agent in the diet, symptoms or reactions should go away. However, to clinch the diagnosis, the problems should reappear when the offending agent is reintroduced into the diet. Provoking reactions to food by reintroduction of offending agents requires careful supervision, and it should never be undertaken in an outpatient setting when people who have had serious reactions to food are studied. People with a history of anaphylaxis (shock) to food should not be rechallenged.

The most convincing, scientific approach to challenges involves the double-blind challenge. The recipient and the donor of the suspected food antigen are both unaware of whether the putative antigen is being used in the test. This approach is very time consuming, but it is regarded as a sure way to make unbiased observation that can confirm or refute the presence of a clear, clinical reaction to food.

SYMPTOMS AND DISEASES ASCRIBED TO FOOD REACTIONS

A number of popular books on food allergies might have one believe that reactions to dietary antigens are the universal cause of disease. There is no doubt that the range of symptoms and disease that is associated with or can result from food allergies is extremely diverse, but direct causal links often defy clear definition. Despite the common nature of clinical reactions to food, their presence is often doubted, sometimes ignored and frequently questioned by conventional medicine—sometimes in an irrational manner! In routine medical practice, the consideration of food allergies is frequently a last resort—if the consideration even surfaces.

Table 9.5 summarizes the multisystem nature of the symptoms of food allergies. Many of the more severe types of food reactions are encountered in childhood, but some can persist into adult life.

FOOD ADDITIVES, DYES, AND CHEMICALS

Food taste is one thing but preference is another. In order to increase the appeal of foods, drinks, drugs, and dietary supplements, modern manufacturers have reached for a whole host man-made chemicals

Table 9.5: The symptoms or signs of food allergy (or intolerance or sensitivity).

These can be found in many body systems. Please note these manifestations are not specific to clinical reactions to food. Arguments prevail about cause and effect relationships in medicine.

BODY SYSTEM	CONDITION
Skin	Eczema
	Redness, vascular change
	Dermatitis
	Urticaria
	Angioedema
Blood	Anemia
	High white-cell count
	Eosinophilia
	Thrombocytopenia (low platelets)
Gut	Nausea, vomiting
	Abdominal pain, distension
	Diarrhea
	Malabsorption
	Blood loss, overt or occult
	Loss of body protein
Airways	Rhinitis, sinusitis, croup
	Sneezing, coughing,
	Bronchial spasm (asthma)
	Lung inflammation (pneumonitis)
	Otitis media
Brain and nervous system	Behavioral problems
	Irritability
	Hyperactive disorders
	Fatigue
	Migraine (other headaches)
Miscellaneous	Sudden infant death syndrome
	Bedwetting
	Fibromyalgia
	Arthritis
	Bone and joint pain

and food additives. While improvements in the presentation of these consumer items can be expected from these artificial additives, the long-term safety of a number of these man-made substances is questionable. Further incentives to add chemicals to food or ingested goods are to increase food stability, alter taste, and prevent spoilage.

Table 9.6: Examples of disorders caused by food additives.

CONDITION	COMMENT
Recurrent skin rashes, urticaria and angioedema	Certain foods or drinks are identified by almost one half of all people with these conditions as a potential cause. Azo dyes and tartrazine can cause these problems.
Respiratory disorders	Aspirin sensitivity is associated with cross reactivity to tartrazine dyes. Sodium benzoate and azo dyes are frequent culprits.
Attention deficit disorder and hyperkinetic disorders	Feingold postulated that dyes, food additives and preservatives cause these common disorders. Elimination diets give inconsistent results.

In some circumstances, there's a price to pay for these additions. There are many detailed reference books on food additives and their potential adverse effects:

The whole issue of food additives as a cause of disease is controversial. In general, consumers are advised to read labels, and a good rule of thumb is to avoid food additives, colorants, and so on, if you can.

ORAL TOLERANCE

The immune phenomenon of oral tolerance is of much interest in the potential treatment of chronic inflammatory diseases such as arthritis (rheumatoid disease) and inflammatory bowel disease (ulcerative colitis, Crohn's disease, and their variants). If a body tissue that is often the site of chronic inflammation (or a component of the tissue) is injected directly into the body, it will cause a chronic inflammation, induced by an immune reaction affecting similar tissues in the body. However, if the tissue in question is fed by the oral route at the same time that it is injected directly into the body, the occurrence of inflammation in the similar body tissue of the host can be avoided.

While the mechanism of immune tolerance (or its basis) has not been known generally to traditional medical systems such as traditional Chinese or Korean medicine, the idea of feeding animal cartilage that contains collagen foreign to the person with arthritis has been practiced for centuries with good effects. Current research in conventional medicine is identifying the possibility of using the phenomenon of immune tolerance in treating idiopathic (of unknown cause) inflammatory bowel disease. Again, the idea of giving hog (colonic or intestinal) mucosa to treat bowel disease is not a secret restricted to alternative medicine. Crude, powdered hog colonic mucosa is quite effective in the adjunctive management of inflammatory bowel disease. This is an example where modern immunology—a well-accepted component of conventional medicine—is reinforcing the treatment methods of alternative or ancient forms of traditional medicine.

CHAPTER SUMMARY

Food sensitivities appear to be commonly reported by patients, but they are often difficult to pinpoint and verify. Alternative medicine may have overstressed the importance of food allergy, but conventional medicine may have given this subject little justice. In general, food sensitivities, allergies, and intolerance are best handled by an expert.

The immunological function of the gut is inextricably linked to overall gut function. Traditional (ancient) medical systems have used interventions for centuries that are now increasingly explained by modern immunology research. The overlapping of disease states reinforces the notion of Gaiaguts.

CHAPTER TEN

GUT FRIENDS
AND FOES

THE ENVIRONMENT WITHIN

Nowadays, people are more concerned about the environment than they have ever been. We think about pollution and destruction of our ecology, but often little thought is given to the environments within our body. One such environment with its own ecology, geography, and life is the guts. Just like the different civilizations, climates, and topography of the earth, the gastrointestinal system has its own regions that are colonized by bacteria and other microorganisms. A wide range of citizens occupy the guts, including yeast, bacteria, viruses, and sometimes free-living organisms like worms and other parasites. We have in our guts both friendly and unfriendly microorganisms.

The normal world of the guts has an array of bacteria that occupies the entire gastrointestinal tract. In regions of the guts where the climate is hostile, such as the acidic stomach, few bacteria are to be found. However, in the colon, which processes digestive waste and stool (the digesta), the environment is teaming with bugs. In states of health, these bugs function together in the guts, especially the colon, to maintain balance and general well-being of the body. If ever there was forgotten territory for modern medicine, it is the flora and fauna of the guts.

The friendly microorganisms in the gastrointestinal tract constitute what is called the microflora of the gut. This microflora is part of a highly complex but integrated ecosystem in the mouth, distal (terminal portion) small intestine (ileum and lower jejunum), and the colon. Many of the bacteria in the gut are welcome visitors because they assist the body in digesting material and support gut functions. Some bacteria actually produce essential vitamins and many can detoxify products in the diet. However, some bacteria are unwelcome visitors that can cause severe gastrointestinal upset, contribute to vitamin deficiency, and produce toxins that damage the body.

For more than one hundred years, scientists and medical researchers have recognized the occurrence of friendly bacteria, but only in the past decade has interest been reactivated in the possibility of promoting the growth of friendly bacteria in the guts. Using these friendly bacteria to promote general health and well-being is a branch of medicine called probiotic medicine (pro – for, biotic – life). Probiotic medicine is regarded as complementary medicine, but it has enjoyed a limited role in treatments used by conventional medical practitioners. Naturopaths refer to probiotic therapy as alternative medicine, but probiosis is a classic example of pluralistic medicine.

FRIENDLY BACTERIA

Of the four hundred to five hundred different types of bacteria that are found in the guts, several types have been researched and identified as being particularly important in promoting both a healthy gut and a healthy body. Examples of these types of bacteria include *Lactobacillus bulgaricus*, *Lactobacillus acidophilus*, *Bifidobacteria bifidus*, and *Streptococcus faecium*.

Bacteria generally have two names. The first name starts with a capital letter and denotes the type (genus) of bacteria, for example, *Lactobacillus*, and the second starts with a small letter and describes the species, in other words, *acidophilus*. Just to make matters a little more complicated, there are different strains of certain species of bacteria, and different strains can have different effects on health because of their different properties. An example of an important, health-giving strain of the friendly bacterium *Lactobacillus acidophilus* is the DDS-1 strain. The DDS-I strain of *Lactobacillus acidophilus* is used frequently as a dietary supplement to promote health. A range of bacteria are used in human and animal food supplements, and examples are given in Table 10.1.

THE FLORA OF THE GUT
DETERMINES GENERAL HEALTH

It is known that gut flora play a role in digestion by releasing nutrients from food after the food has entered the large bowel and already traversed the principal site of absorption of nutrients in the small bowel. Bacterial enzymes (glucosidases) remove sugars from phytochemicals and render them capable of being absorbed. The soy isoflavones genistein and daidzein (examples of phytochemicals) are known to be very important health-giving compounds found in soybeans. Their availability to be absorbed into the body depends on the ability of bacteria in the colon to remove sugars from these isoflavones. The free isoflavones are then absorbed and able to exert versatile biological effects that are beneficial for health.

Friendly bacteria can metabolize (chemically transform) hormones, drugs, bile acids (secreted in bile from the liver), and dietary carcinogens (cancer-causing chemicals) in an advantageous manner for health. Unfriendly bacteria can do the opposite. The microflora play an important direct role in nutrition of the lining of the colon. Bacteria synthesize short-chain fatty acids (e.g., proprionate, acetate, and butyrate). These short-chain fatty acids produced by bacteria in the bowel can provide about three-quarters of the energy requirements of the lining cells of the colon. In addition, these compounds have the added advantage of preventing the growth of bacteria that

Table 10.1: Examples of friendly bacteria that are available for use in human and animal food supplements as probiotics.

HUMAN FOOD SUPPLEMENTS	ANIMAL FEED SUPPLEMENTS
Lactobacillus acidophilus DDS-1	Lactobacillus acidophilus DDS-1
Lactobacillus brevis	Lactobacillus plantarum
Lactobacillus bulgaricus	Lactobacillus casei
Lactobacillus casei	Streptococcus faecium
Lactobacillus casei spp Rhamnosus	Streptococcus lactis
Lactobacillus caucasius	
Lactobacillus plantarum	
Lactobacillus salivarius	
Bifidobacterium bifidum	
Bifidobacterium longum	
Streptococcus faecium	

cause infectious types of diarrhea. Furthermore, they assist in stimulating the maturation of the immune response in both the bowel and the body in general. It is not obvious to everyone but the gut has a very large immune system. It has many lymph nodes and connections with the spleen. In fact, the gut comprises a large fraction of the mass of the immune tissues that are present in the body; and this immune organ responds to molecules of emotions.

TOXINS AND THE GUTS

The idea that the bowel can be a source of toxins is now a generally accepted, but often challenged, concept in conventional medicine. Every day we encounter toxins in our diet that have to be dealt with by the gut or adjacent organs such as the liver, which detoxifies many toxic substances. The bowel itself can be a source of toxins. However, the bowel as a source of toxins tends to be thought about in conventional medicine in very specific disease circumstances, such as the presence of chronic liver disease. In liver disease, such as cirrhosis of the liver, liver insufficiency (impaired function of this organ) can occur. Impairment of the function of the liver due to a variety of diseases results in a loss of the ability of the liver to detoxify chemicals in the body. In states of serious impairment of liver function, the liver cannot handle protein in the diet. In this circumstance, ammonia, produced from protein in the diet, enters the circulation and causes serious problems such as mental confusion and loss of consciousness. This is called hepatic coma. The liver acts as a filter for bacteria that can enter the bloodstream, and this is one of several reasons why blood infections and abdominal infections are common in people with severe liver disease.

Part of the conventional, medical treatment of liver impairment that results in this condition of hepatic coma (or precoma) is to cut down on protein intake to reduce ammonia production in the body, by the administration of nonabsorbable sugars, like lactulose, which can inhibit ammonia absorption. In some cases, physicians use preparations of friendly bacteria such as *Lactobacilli* to crowd out bacteria that can metabolize protein to ammonia. However, in clinical trials of the efficacy of *Lactobacilli* supplements in this situation, the results have been varied and, on occasion, disappointing. Although friendly gut bacteria can play a useful role in this situation, the real problem is the untreatable nature of advanced liver disease.

The reason why I've discussed this problem of liver failure and its frequent lack of response to friendly bacteria treatment is because relatively poor treatment experiences with the giving of friendly bacteria (Lactobacilli) are sometimes used as evidence that this practice is not generally effective. I believe that this specific example of the limitation of therapy with probiotics (friendly bacteria) has stuck in the mind of many doctors and has colored their general thinking about treatments with friendly bacteria. In addition, colonization of the bowel with friendly bacteria generally takes a long time (weeks) before real benefit is seen. Patients and doctors do not always have the luxury of time and when they do, they are often impatient for immediate benefits of therapy. We want the "quick fix" that natural medicine rarely delivers.

SEEDING THE GUTS: PREBIOSIS AND PROBIOSIS

The process of reseeding the intestines with friendly bacteria found in healthy intestines is called probiotic therapy. Probiotic therapy has not evoked much interest among conventional (and even some alternative-thinking) physicians, and it falls under the category of witchcraft to less well informed doctors. There is an ancillary method that can be used to assist in the seeding of friendly bacteria in the intestines, and this involves the use of specific foods (complex sugars) that feed the health-promoting bacteria. This type of treatment is called prebiotic therapy, and it involves the use of complex carbohydrates (oligosaccharides) that are foods that are preferentially utilized by the good bugs such as *Lactobacilli* and *Bifidobacteria*. Particularly good sources of oligosaccharides (FOS) that promote the growth of *Lactobacilli* and *Bifidobacteria* are bananas and onions, which contain a lot of fructooligosaccharides (FOS), and soy beans and soy flour, which contain the complex sugars stacchyose and raffinose. Also, good bacteria love dietary fiber.

Although prebiosis and probiosis as treatments have not become popular in conventional medicine, there is increasing evidence of their potential benefit.

LACTOBACILLI AND BIFIDOBACTERIA

Lactobacilli and *Bifidobacteria* differ in their structure and the conditions under which they grow, colonize and attach in the bowel. *Bifidobacteria* and *Lactobacilli* are used very often in the dairy industry to produce fermented dairy foods such as yogurt, fresh cheese, desserts, and buttermilk. In addition, these bacteria have enjoyed widespread use in the manufacturing of infant foods and pharmaceutical preparations.

It is not possible to enter into a discussion about (or even to point out) all of the friendly bacteria that are found in the gut; and it is even less possible to discuss their different effects. There are many that we know very little about and some that have probably not even been recognized. In states of health, the bacterial populations in the gut remain surprisingly constant in their types and numbers. The flora (microorganisms) of the guts have a high metabolic activity (vigorous chemical and transformation reactions) and they have a major effect on several important components of healthy gut and body function.

Normal gut bacteria promote the normal structure and function of the lining of the intestines, and they prime the immune system in the guts. In this regard, some of the friendly bacteria are particularly important in enhancing the body's resistance to disease by simulating immune function and exerting interference with organisms that infect the bowel and cause infectious diarrhea. Friendly bacteria in the microflora of the bowel are one of the most important constituents of the digesta, which plays a major but underestimated role in health.

YOUR FRIENDS FIGHT YOUR FOES

It is well recognized that *Lactobacillus acidophilus* and *Bifidobacteria bifidus* are able to interfere with the growth of a variety of other bacteria, including bacteria that cause serious infections, diarrhea, or dysentery (e.g., pathogenic *E. Coli*, *Typhoid bacillus*, *Shigella*,

Salmonella, and *Bacillus cereus*). In several clinical trials, Bifidobacteria or *Lactobacilli* or combinations of these bacteria, plus or minus other friendly bacteria, can have favorable results in the prevention and treatment of bacillary dysentery (bacterial infections causing diarrhea) in infants and adults.

There are certain types of bacteria that can putrefy food and produce toxic products. Examples are the bacteria called *Clostridia* and other types of coliforms (bacteria commonly found in the bowels). Putrefaction of food by these bacteria can result in the production of toxic products from protein in the diet, called toxic amines. It is known that both *Lactobacilli* and *Bifidobacteria* can prevent the formation of these toxic amines.

Some individuals may recognize this occurrence in themselves when they eat a heavy animal protein load in their diet, such as a large steak. Red meat can cause foul gas in some individuals, and this occurs as a consequence of the action of bacteria that putrefy protein. Animal protein contains a generous amount of sulfur-containing amino acids, which can form sulfur-containing gases that have a foul smell (like the odor of rotten eggs). This type of foul gas with animal protein (and egg yolk protein) in the diet can be corrected to a varying degree by oral supplementation with friendly *Lactobacilli*.

Preparations of *Lactobacilli* and *Bifidobacteria* have been shown to be beneficial in the prevention and treatment of travelers' diarrhea especially when it is related to bacterial causes. In addition, these friendly bacteria are particularly useful when used together to prevent the overgrowth of harmful bacteria following antibiotic therapy. There are several organisms that can be a problem as a result of their emergence or overgrowth when antibiotics are used. The condition of antibiotic-associated colitis (sometimes called pseudomembranous colitis) can be quite severe with diarrhea and acute illness. This condition is associated with the overgrowth of the bacterium *Clostridium difficile*. Broad-spectrum antibiotics may cause suppression of normal flora and overgrowth with the yeast *Candida albicans*, especially in infants and in individuals who have diminished immune function, such as the elderly, and in people who are infected with HIV or AIDS. The administration of friendly bacteria such as *Lactobacilli* and *Bifidobacteria* may help prevent and treat many of these circumstances.

Table 10.2: Proposed major benefits of probiotic therapy.

- Assistance with digestion
- Alleviation of digestive disorders, e.g., colitis, IBS, peptic ulcer
- Enhancement of the synthesis of several vitamins (especially B complex)
- Enhanced mineral absorption, especially calcium
- Protection against pathogenic bacterial infections, e.g., *E. coli* infection
- Reduction of symptoms of lactose intolerance, permits limited reintroduction of dairy products
- Reduction of yeast overgrowth (candidiasis), notable reduction in vaginal thrush
- Improvement in immune function, "primes" the gut immune system
- Anticarcinogenic effects, some good evidence
- Prevention of *Helicobactor pylori* infection and its association with peptic ulcer, dyspepsia, and gastric cancer
- Acne prevention?
- Cholesterol reduction, modest and unpredictable

The mechanism of the antagonistic effects of friendly bacteria against unwanted visitors (pathogenic bacteria and yeast) is complex. *Lactobacilli* are known to produce several substances that are inhibitory to pathogenic bacteria. *Lactobacillus acidophilus* can produce compounds such as acidophilin, lactocidin, and acidolin, which can help fight intruding bacteria. *Bifidobacteria* produce products that inhibit the growth of infectious bacteria like *Salmonella*. These *Bifidobacteria* tend to produce acetic acid (vinegar), in contrast to lactic acid produced by Lactobacilli. Acetic acid with small amounts of formic acid inhibits the growth of *Salmonella* bacteria.

Several reviews of the beneficial effects of *Lactobacilli* and *Bifidobacteria* have appeared in the medical literature. The overall potential benefit of these organisms is summarized in Table 10.2.

CHOOSING FRIENDLY BACTERIA IN DIETARY SUPPLEMENTS

The bacteria most often favored in probiotic regimens include: *Lactobacillus acidophilus*, which is found in the lower small intestine and colon; *Bifidobacteria bifidum,* which is a friendly citizen of the colon; and two more transient guests, called *Lactobacillus bulgaricus* and *Streptococcus thermophilus*.

Certain strains of *Lactobacillus acidophilus* have been investigated and proposed to be the most desirable and versatile in their health-giving benefits. These types of preferred *Lactobacillus acidophilus* are the DDS-1 strain that was developed at the University of Nebraska and the NAS super adhesion strain. The NAS super adhesion strain is found in a dairy-free source, and this strain is quite desirable because it attaches to the intestinal mucosal lining. The DDS-1 strain was named after the Department of Dairy Science (DDS) at the University of Nebraska, but this strain has been propagated in outside labs and arguments about the quality of all the DDS variants prevail.

Lactobacillus acidophilus strains share a lot of benefits. There are a couple of types of *Bifidobaceria* that are proposed as desirable for use as health-giving supplements. These include *Bifidobacteria infantis* (NLS Super Strain) and *Bifidobacteria bifidum* (Malyoth Super Strain). I accept that supplementation of the adult diet with *Bifidobacteria* is safe, even when not medically supervised. However, I believe that probiotics, such as *Bifidobacteria infantis*, when used in babies should be used only under the supervision of a qualified healthcare giver. I accept that benefits can accrue by the use of probiotics in infants, but this is not an area for the amateur to meddle in. I reject recommendations for the unsupervised use of probiotics in babies and infants that have appeared in popular literature. In addition, I caution against the use of probiotics in an unsupervised manner in pregnancy, without denying that they may have some benefit.

Lactobacillus bulgaricus tends to be only a transient in the gastrointestinal tract, but it has a good record in some studies for the management of dyspepsia, heartburn, and even excessive appetite. This record is somewhat anecdotal in studies of natural medicine, but clusters of cases have been reported to have definite benefit from *L. bulgaricus* for a variety of functional gastrointestinal disturbances. One strain of *Lactobacillus bulgaricus* that has been extensively researched is the LB51 strain, known to synthesize a natural antibiotic substance that can ward off pathogenic bacteria. In addition, this strain of *Lactobacillus* has been associated historically with longevity, and it is reported as effective in Eastern European medical literature for the treatment of inflammatory bowel disease. More research is required with this organism that appears to afford promise in the treatment of some gastrointestinal diseases.

CHOOSING A PROBIOTIC SUPPLEMENT IN A HEALTH FOOD STORE

For probiotic supplements to be effective, they need to be viable (living) when swallowed and sufficient in number to colonize the gut. Friendly bacteria can be encouraged to grow in the guts if they are given with the medium in which they were grown. This is sometimes called the supernatant or "jungle juice" that the bacteria make from the food that they were presented during their growth period. Stomach acid can kill friendly bacteria and seriously reduce the number of viable bacteria that can enter the bowels and establish themselves. To avoid this, friendly bacteria have been suspended in oil matrices (e.g., safflower oil) or presented in coated capsules, which afford varying degrees of protection for the bacteria or the probiotic

Table 10.3: Reasons why individuals use probiotics.

CONDITION	COMMENT
Yeast infection	Assists in reduction of *Candida* overgrowth, but action not immediate and recurrence common with cessation of probiotics.
Antibiotic therapy	Broad spectrum antibiotics "knock out" friendly and unfriendly bacteria. An advantage from reseeding the guts with probiotics.
Digestive disease	Uncertain benefits in some disorders, e.g., *Helicobacter pylori* infection, but a real advantage in *Clostridium* overgrowth is documented.
Acne	Possible benefit.
Hypercholestrolemia	Unpredictable effect.
Colon cleansing.	The idea of cleansing and reseeding is interesting, but its attributed health benefits require research.
Immune dysfunction	An underestimated potential for probiotics. Promising research data.

Table 10.4: Summary of some of the reported benefits of friendly bacteria (*Lactobacilli* and *Bifidobacteria*) and comments about the implications of the benefits.

BENEFIT	COMMENT
Synthesize vitamins	Not all strains of *Lactobacilli* have this advantage. *L. acidophilus* synthesizes folic acid, vit. B6, B12, niacin, and riboflavin.
Enhances digestibility of foods	*Lactobacilli* and *Bifidobacteria* produce enzymes that can split food and reduce some symptoms of sad guts.
Helps lactose intolerance	Lactose is the milk sugar that is broken down by lactase. Lactase is secreted by *Lactobacilli*.
Suppresses gut pathogenic organisms	Natural antibiotics and resistance factors suppress unwanted bacteria and the yeast *Candida albicans*.
Reduces blood cholesterol	*Acidophilus* produces antilipidemic factors.
Functional disorders of the gut	More research required but studies are promising, e.g., halitosis, irregular bowel habit.
Traveler's diarrhea	Good trial results.
Gut infections	Strong evidence for benefit emerging.

products from the otherwise lethal effects of gastric acid.

In order to facilitate the growth of some friendly bacteria, certain substrates (foods) that are used by the bacteria can be given at the same time. Soy flour containing the nonabsorbable sugars stacchyose and raffinose is used by some individuals to promote the growth of *Bifidobacteria*, but several manufacturers of probiotics have started to use FOS that are derived from chemically treated sugarcane. Some protagonists of probiotics argue against the use of FOS on emotional, economic, or pseudoscientific grounds. The fact is that FOS, whether synthetic or natural, are useful for providing fuel for friendly bacteria to colonize the gut or to exert a desired metabolic effect as a consequence of their use by friendly bacteria.

The most frequently used probiotics are combinations of *Lactobacillus acidophilus* and *Bifidus longum* (with FOS) or *Bifidus infantis* and *Lactobacillus acidophilus* (with FOS). Common reasons why people use probiotics are listed in Table 10.3. Much more research is required to confirm the many alleged benefits of probiotic therapy. The general lobby in conventional medicine has been directed toward antibiotic use to eradicate unwanted bacteria in the gut, rather than the use of potentially health-giving bacteria—the friends that fight the foes!

Probiotic and prebiotic treatments have many alleged benefits that are summarized in Table 10.4.

SELECTING A PROBIOTIC DIETARY SUPPLEMENT

Dr. S. K. Dash, a researcher in probiotic therapy, has made many significant contributions to the development of bioactive probiotic supplements. He proposes that the use of names like *Acidophilus* or *Probiotic* means very little unless the product fulfills certain criteria. Table 10.5 is derived from the excellent work of Dr. Dash on the selection of an optimal probiotic, dietary supplement. Enteric coating of probiotic supplements is always a good thing because it protects the friendly bacteria from acid and digestive enzymes.

DO BACTERIA IN PROBIOTICS SURVIVE?

One of the biggest problems in probiotic therapy is the retention of the viability of the organisms for their desired site of colonization of the gut in the intestines. It is known that bacteria are destroyed by gastric acid or digestive enzymes, but some strains appear to be more resistant to destruction in the harsh, acidic climate of the stomach. For example, one study performed at the Veterans Administration Hospital in Minneapolis implied that one particular strain of a nondairy probiotic (DDS-*Acidophilus*) showed significant survival characteristics when given by the oral route. This strain was shown to implant in the bowel and multiply in a range of one-hundred-fold to two-hundred-fold.

The precise dosages of probiotic therapy required to achieve a desired effect remain unexplored. Therefore, treatment is somewhat empiric, and to be effective it is best applied and monitored by a

Table 10.5: The features of an optimal probiotic dietary supplement.

From the work of Dr. S. K. Dash. One key issue is the ability of the probiotic agent to implant and survive in the colon.

- Contains the right strain(s). Genetically one can be more effective than others.
- Is viable. Viable or live probiotics are effective.
- Remains stable and viable for long period.
- Has the ability to survive in the intestines.
- Produces beneficial effects in the intestine.
- Probiotic products sitting on the shelf (without refrigeration) lose potency first. For this reason, refrigerated, viable probiotic products are recommended.
- Nondairy probiotic products are recommended by health professionals for persons allergic to dairy products and for persons with yeast infection.
- Nitrogen-flushed packaging of probiotics enhance the stability and shelf life of the probiotics.
- Fortification of probiotics with prebiotic fructooligosaccharides (FOS) enhance the value of probiotics. FOS feed probiotics selectively and enhance their growth in the gut.
- Combinations of unknown and undesirable bacteria in probiotic products can even be harmful to the human body. Also, combinations of known and friendly bacteria in disproportionate manner can alter balance of the flora in the gut.

knowledgeable healthcare practitioner. It is known that probiotic therapy is effective, only if it is taken on a daily basis.

Probiotic capsules, tablets, or powders that supply at least two billion live organisms (colony-forming units) are desirable. Several products contain two billion to five billion colony-forming units in desired dosing schedules. However, in established problems, such as yeast infection, higher numbers of viable probiotic organisms may be required. I support the use of enteric-coated (delayed release) probiotic capsules.

WHY DO PROBIOTICS MAKE SENSE?

It is recognized widely that food may contain a variety of friendly organisms. There is no doubt that the reliance on wholesome food, such as high-quality yogurt, as a source of probiotics is preferable to taking supplements. However, much food in Western societies is processed or contains pesticides and chemicals that will destroy desirable bacteria. A major problem has existed with the feeding of antibiotics to animals that are used in the food chain, but this practice has been largely curtailed in Western society. These circumstances have led to the rational proposal that the average American diet does not provide the probiotics needed to maintain normal flora in the guts.

Probiotic therapy makes sense in providing one of the many complex factors that can promote healthy gut function. Other factors, however, must be considered alongside the use of probiotics. The use of food that is raw and alive with enzymes may have real advantages. Increasing evidence exists that organically grown food provides the best source of plant nutrition.

Organically grown food has been shown in some controlled studies to be more nutritious than conventionally grown food. These studies imply that fruit and vegetables grown under organic conditions generally contain less heavy metals, less organic residuals, and a higher content of essential minerals and some phytonutrients. Clearly, attention to the sources of food is important in achieving optimal nutrition and this knowledge has led to growing interest in organic food and the substitution of processed foods by foods made from scratch.

The main bar to the adoption of more healthy forms of food, for example, organic or home processed, is economics. Junk food containing refined sugar and hydrogenated oils is cheap and readily available. There is no doubt that education in traditional culinary arts and home economics may greatly assist digestive health. Probiotic therapy has been practiced (unknowingly) for many years. Good examples are the use of fermented milk and soy.

IT HAS TO BE HOMEMADE YOGURT

Many individuals who are familiar with the potential advantages of probiotics often consume yogurt. Unfortunately, most commercially produced yogurts lack useful probiotic organisms. In order to overcome this problem, some companies have added *Lactobacilli* to yogurt. However, when the yogurt with added *Lactobacilli* is left to stand for a few hours, the added probiotic does not survive. Furthermore, this probiotic addition to yogurt can produce excessive acidity, resulting in unpleasant taste and further killing of bacteria in the yogurt (including the probiotic).

If individuals who wish to take probiotics are able to make fresh yogurt, then they can derive a desirable amount of viable, probiotic organisms. This situation usually means a commitment for the person to make fresh yogurt at home using well-controlled and meticulous preparation techniques. Without special preparation techniques, even homemade yogurt can fall short as a source of probiotics. For these reasons, many physicians avoid using probiotics in food sources, and they most often opt for probiotic dietary supplements (or prescriptions of probiotic capsules).

Table 10.6: Further summary of some of the reported benefits of friendly bacteria (*Lactobacilli* and *Bifidobacteria*) and comments about the implications of the benefits.

BENEFIT	COMMENT
Synthesize vitamins	Not all strains of *Lactobacilli* have this advantage. *Lacidophilus* synthesized folic acids, vit. B6, B12, niacin and riboflavin.
Enhance digestibility of foods	*Lactobacilli* and *Bifidobacteria* produce enzymes that can split food and reduce some symptoms of sad guts.
Help lactose intolerance	Lactose is the milk sugar that is broken down by lactase, which is secreted by *Lactobacilli*.
Suppress gut pathogenic organisms	Natural antibiotics and resistance factors suppress unwanted bacteria and the yeast *Candida albicans*.
Reduce blood cholesterol	*Acidophilus* produces antilipidemic factors.
Functional disorders of the gut	More research required but studies are promising, e.g., halitosis, irregular bowel habit.
Traveler's diarrhea	Good trial results.
Gut infections	Strong evidence for benefit emerging.
Gallstones	Likely benefit, no good trials.

PROBIOTIC THERAPY FOR DISEASES

The use of friendly bacteria to treat disease is not alien to conventional medicine. However, alternative and complementary medicine appear to have claimed this therapeutic intervention in their armamentarium. There are many disorders that can be treated allegedly by probiotic therapy. A conventional medical practitioner might gaze in disbelief at the purported versatility of probiotics that are listed in Table 10.6.

In January of 2000, the *American Journal of Gastroenterology* produced a supplement on the functional significance of the bowel microflora. This supplement reported the proceedings of a round table discussion of fifteen of the world's leading experts on bacteriology and its associated specialties. These scientists from centers of medical excellence echoed the comments of many practitioners of alternative or naturopathic medicine who have regularly practiced the art of probiotic therapy for more than three decades.

I recommend this journal supplement (*AMJ Gastroenterology*, No. I, Vol. 95, Jan. 2000), which provides clear definitions of effective probiotic agents, and presents evidence for the efficacy of probiosis in the prevention and treatment of gastrointestinal diseases. In addition, it reinforces my notion that probiosis can be used to help combat immunodeficiency states (e.g., HIV). It is also emerging with a role in the treatment of functional gut diseases. Clearly, the bacterial components of the digesta are an important factor in IBS, functional dyspepsia, and functional, global gut disorders.

CHAPTER SUMMARY

This chapter attempts to provide an opinion about the credibility and/or science available to support the various disease-state applications for probiotics. On balance, conventional medicine may do well to examine the potential health-giving benefits of friendly bacteria. These benefits can be very valuable in gastrointestinal diseases that are difficult to treat.

CHAPTER ELEVEN

TIPPING THE
BALANCE:
PURGATION, DYSBIOSIS,
LEAKY GUT, AND
TOXICITY

THE BALANCE

In states of health, the gastrointestinal tract goes about its complex business of digesting food in a quiet manner. I have characterized the gut as an individual within us in some circumstances, but I have acknowledged the concept of unified body and gut function (Gaiaguts: unity influenced by its environment and predetermined in its function and well-being by genetics). There is a state of natural balance of gut function, where the gut is at ease with itself and its contents, thereby acting as both a beneficiary of and benefactor for the body. The healthy gut lives in quiet contentment and channels this pleasure to the body.

It has become apparent that tipping the balance in the ecology of the bowel has far-reaching consequences. The simplistic viewpoint that the guts can be a common source of toxins for the body is not a new concept, but it is gaining increasing popularity in the theories of integrated (alternative, complementary, natural or pluralistic) medicine.

EMERGING PRINCIPLES IN ALTERNATIVE GASTROENTEROLOGY

Several principles, or beliefs, are clung to by the unorthodox gastroenterologist. They can be highlighted:

- Body cleansing is necessary because of environmental toxins, particularly those "toxins" that enter the body from the bowel.
- The presence of toxins requires an active process of detoxification or the opening up of blocked pathways of detoxification.
- Toxins get into the body through a leaky gut. The phenomenon of enhanced intestinal permeability is more common than recognized, and it causes a wide variety of diseases.

The conventional physician often raises an eyebrow to the above ideas or claims. Pooping one's way to health by purgatives, the use of natural means to detoxify the body, and the universal explanation of many diseases as a consequence of a leaky gut are not prominent conventional medical thoughts; but these thoughts are dawning on patients!

A large segment of the population has linked its feelings of well-being to bowel regularity, and the approaches of alternative physicians seem to make sense to many patients. Physicians cannot continue to ignore the "environmental medicine group," a group that draws attention to ubiquitous environmental toxins. Conventional medicine tends to reject the notion of the importance of the gut as a source of toxins per se. This environmental movement in thought gained momentum in the 1920s, and it has been resurrected recently with a new sense of credibility.

POOPING FOR HEALTH, ILL HEALTH, OR PSYCHOLOGICAL GAIN

The conventional medical way is to partially recognize the role of the bowel and its inhabitants as a source of toxins for the body. After a long period of belief in the phenomenon of intestinal autointoxication, Dr. W. C. Alvarez led the modern, conventional medical perception by publishing his classic paper "Intestinal Autointoxication" in *Physiological Reviews* (4:352–393) in 1924. Dr. Alvarez stressed the notion that the mucous membrane of the colon is very efficient in preventing the passage of toxins into the general circulation. The defenses of the lining of the intestine are much more complex than was realized by Dr. Alvarez in 1924, but his work drew attention to the presence of many toxins in the gut. Alvarez, partially shut out our thoughts about the gut "letting in" toxins.

Modern research has shown us increasing evidence that the lining of the guts is variably permeable to unwanted agents. Several of these agents are present in the digesta, including infectious organisms, toxic chemicals, bacterial degradation products, etc. In fact, the colon may be a site where some agents are actually transformed and absorbed into the body, especially when transformation is by bacteria. Examples of this phenomenon include the cleavage of conjugated phytochemicals such as isoflavones, by enzyme activity in some gut bacteria.

On a simple basis, the residence time of stool in the colon is an important issue. If stool stays around too long, more fermentation or other types of biotransformation of chemicals or undigested food may occur. Increasing residence time of unwanted chemicals increases the time available for the unwanted absorption of these toxins by the bowel.

There appears to be good reason to facilitate bowel emptying, and this is ideally undertaken by correct lifestyle adjustments (adequate roughage, fiber in the diet, balanced nutrition, avoidance of toxic chemicals, exercise, etc.). On a selective or intermittent basis, purgation is often a pleasurable experience that is refreshing—real or perceived. When purgation becomes a regular preoccupation, however, many problems can ensue.

LAXATIVE USE AND ABUSE

Temporary disturbances in bowel habit are common. Extensive travel and a change of diet or environment can easily disrupt a toilet routine. On these occasions, occasional use of purgatives is probably prudent and quite safe. Significant change in bowel habit in mature individuals cannot be ignored. The epidemic nature of colon cancer—which frequently presents with a change in bowel habit—is a concern that should be well known to the public. I reiterate that any significant change in bowel habit in an individual over the age of forty years should raise a suspicion of bowel cancer.

Purgatives (cathartics) are among the most commonly used medicinal agents and the magnitude of consumption of purgatives far outstrips any occasional application for minor irregularities of bowel function. The birth of medicine carried recommendations about the healthy nature of regular bowel habits, and this concept persists among the public and many physicians. On occasion, the concept is perceived as so important that it precipitates the ritual or even obsessive use of laxatives.

The importance of ritual purgation in medicine was highlighted by Dr. L. J. Witts (*Lancet*, 1:427–430, 1937). Despite the loss of interest in the gut as a source of toxins in the 1920s, a significant proportion of the medical profession linked lingering stool in the bowel to many afflictions. The strong and enduring belief that bowel evacuation determines general health (a fact not a myth) has led to a common modern-day problem with excessive laxative use by many people. The modern renaissance in the role of purgation for health in alternative medicine may be fueling this problem.

There are many overt abusers of laxatives who may have suffered with constipation for many years. In these individuals, chronic use of laxatives is a way of life, and it contributes to a lazy bowel, often increasing the degree of constipation over a period of years. These overt abusers can graduate from the gentle aperient to the chronic use of potent purgative products.

Chronic laxative abuse leads to serious medical problems more often than is generally detected in clinical practice. Laxatives promote electrolyte and water loss (especially potassium), often cause direct damage to the nerve supply of the colon, and sometimes result in body organ toxicity (e.g., oxyphenisatin and liver injury). These physiological effects of laxatives can result in a wide spectrum of symptoms and signs including: diarrhea, dehydration, low potassium, cardiac arrhythmias, abdominal pain, etc. Less obvious consequences of severe laxative abuse include bone disease (osteomalacia and osteoporosis), unhealthy weight loss, swelling of body extremities (edema from low blood proteins), impaired immune function, skin pigmentation, permanent damage to the bowel (cathartic colon), and occasional death!

TYPES OF LAXATIVES

Many early disciplines of medicine introduced their own botanicals, herbals, and methods for inducing the exodus of the contents of the bowel. In general, the four different types or categories of laxatives are:

- irritant or stimulant laxatives
- osmotic laxatives
- bulk-producing laxatives
- lubricant laxatives

The most effective—but also the most potentially toxic—laxatives belong to the stimulant or irritant group. The list of stimulant laxatives is very long but commonly features anthraquinones (e.g., senna and cascara), castor oil (active constituent ricinoleic acid), polyphenolic compounds and others that are somewhat obsolete (e.g., bisacodyl, phenolphthalein, and oxyphensatin). These potent purgatives are all capable of inducing a laxative-abuse syndrome of variable severity when used repeatedly. Some of these laxatives have been removed from the U.S. market but are for sale in several third world countries—travelers please beware.

Osmotic laxatives tend to work by retaining water and electrolytes (especially sodium and potassium) within the bowel. Examples include magnesium salts (Epsom salts, Glauber salts, Milk of Magnesia etc.), nonabsorbable sugars (lactulose, laevulose, sorbitol), and nonabsorbable solutions taken in large volumes (e.g., Golytely). Lubricant laxatives and stool softeners masquerade under the identity of gentle purgatives, but the stool-softener dioctyl sodium sulphosuccinate inhibits fluid absorption, and mineral oil both lubricates and stimulates the colon.

Alternative medicine sometimes promotes the notion that the

natural way may often be the safe way, but this is not always the case. Nowhere is this more apparent than in the case of "natural" laxatives. A whole host of natural herbal laxatives or bowel astringents have a disturbing toxic effect on the bowel when used in excess or with inappropriate frequency. In general, purgation is best undertaken on an occasional basis using osmotic laxatives and bulk fiber products. In the absence of any contraindication, a good dose of natural magnesium sulphate (Epsom's salts) with fiber addition has few rivals in terms of safety, efficacy, or cost.

PURGATION AS THERAPY: MYTHS AND MAGIC?

It is a myth that the majority of people need regular and frequent purgation to avoid accumulation of body toxins from the bowel. Equally, it is a myth that toxic accumulation (autointoxication) in the body from the bowel is unimportant. It is probably more important than hitherto supposed in current conventional medicine, and it should not be rejected as a useless intervention in health maintenance in selected circumstances. It is possible to construct an endless series of myths and countermyths in alternative and conventional medical practice. The key to the correct initiative is the balanced point of view. The truth often lies between the two extremes of opinion—especially in the case of purgation for health.

The concept of the myth in medicine is easier to spot and understand than the more pernicious occurrence of magical thinking in medicine. Magical thinking in medicine takes a variety of forms but the most significant type is the *belief* of the doctor that his or her thoughts or opinions, in and of themselves, may *cause* certain events (cures, wellness diseases or health disorders). The *belief* of the doctor may be transmitted in the physician - patient relationship, but nowadays we see the increasing strength of the patient's *belief* impacting the physician's practice. Rather than a traditional focus on physician-patient relationships, new thoughts of the patient's "Bill of Rights" determines greater consideration of the patient-physician relationship. Treatment has fortunately become more of a two-way street.

Magical thinking in medicine is a function of naïveté (or perhaps ignorance). The child thinks in a magical manner when anxiety is created by an idea that something occurred (e.g., illness or death) because the thoughts of the event came to consciousness. Conventional medicine might argue that "magical thinking" is a function of ignorance or naïveté on the part of the alternative healer—especially common among those without formal biomedical training. The alternative healer will defend this by projecting the thought of magical thinking as part of the spiritual mind-body connection. After all, oneness in the function of the body is an increasingly accepted concept, and we all recognize the concept of the self-fulfilling prophecy.

Magical thinking has undoubtedly entered the realm of alternative medicine and it should not be encouraged in disease-management strategies, even though it may be encouraged in understanding spirit mind-body connections. Alternative medicine has crossed the boundary of magical thinking in gut diseases, but conventional medicine will not take off its blinders. These arguments are quite important and will not be readily resolved. Physicians must listen to patients who are taking more time to listen to their bodies. Whatever the prevailing medical opinion, patients are increasingly seeking natural alternatives and demanding that modern medicine provide them.

WHO CAN BENEFIT FROM COLON CLEANSING?

Ask an alternative-thinking physician this question and the answer will be, generally, "almost everyone." Ask an orthodox physician and after a common expression of sarcasm, generally, they will not even address the question. Throughout this book, contrary points of view have been discussed, but many physicians, including myself, are tired of medicine at the crossroads. Balanced approaches of pluralistic medicine (what works) seem prudent because integrated medicine (blends of alternative and conventional medicine) is not readily within our immediate grasp—despite some claims to the contrary!

The idea of cleansing the body—by elimination of toxic reservoirs (e.g., stool or intestinal parasites) and the promotion of detoxification—is neither novel nor new. Cleansing and detoxifying the body is deeply rooted in Ayurvedic medicine, traditional Chinese medicine, and North American Indian medicine.

In the words of William Wood, a seventeenth-century settler in New England, North American Indians were described as free of "health wasting diseases"—with "straight bodies strongly composed"—and "small waisted, lanke bellied and well-thighed" (Wood 1633, cited by Barbara Griggs in *Green Pharmacy*, 1991). In her book entitled *Green Pharmacy*, Ms. Griggs emphasized the use of emetics and purges by the North American Indian healers, based on their belief that all disease was introduced into the body through the gastrointestinal tract. Commenting on American native medicine, Griggs states in her book: "The sick man was thoroughly purged and vomited—early observers spoke of vomits strong enough to kill a horse—before a preparation of healing herbs was given to him. Then he was fasted before being put on a light diet of gruel made from grain and roots, until recovery was complete."

The approach of purging, fasting and the introduction of a nutritious diet with cleansing herbs is the mainstay of not only Native American medicine, but it is a fundamental approach of Ayurvedic medicine and modern-day alternative medicine. This treatment algorithm persists today among naturopathic physicians, with claims of increasing substantiation for its health benefits. It has been argued that medicine in early cultures was designed to treat parasites, which were a dominant cause of disease and therefore are not relevant in modern times. We will learn, however, that gastrointestinal parasites are still a very common and overlooked cause of suboptimal health in modern society. If one accepts all unfriendly microorganisms as examples of intestinal parasitosis, then a universal health problem emerges.

LESSONS FROM AYURVEDA

The term Ayurveda is a combination of two Sanskrit (an ancient Indian-Asian language) words. The word *Ayur* means "life" and *veda* refers to "knowledge" or "science." Ayurveda is often referred to as the "science of life," and it has its origins five millennia ago on the Indian subcontinent. This science of life has been practiced in a well-developed format for about three thousand years. It has influenced the development of many other traditional medical systems in countries far afield, such as Japan, Egypt, Europe, and Russia. Ayurvedic medicine has been mistakenly perceived as primarily a form of herbal medicine, but it is regarded as one of the most comprehensive medical systems available that covers all disciplines of modern medicine—of course with a different approach!

Several modern accounts of Ayurveda fail to represent the expansive nature of this medical discipline, perhaps to capitalize on its herbal pharmacopoeia for the manufacture of dietary supplements. The fundamental principles of Ayurveda still remain largely unknown to many practitioners of Western medicine, some of whom wish to classify it as some form of quasi-religious superstition. Interested readers are referred to the excellent book on the subject by Swami Sada Shiva Tirtha entitled, *The Ayurveda Encyclopedia*, Bayville, NY: Ayurveda Holistic Center Press, 1998. Some basic management concepts of Ayurvedic medicine are highly relevant to the current widespread interest in body cleansing.

Ayurveda teaches that the main cause of illness is poor digestive function. Undigested foods are believed to sit in the colon and become a source of toxins as a consequence of fermentation, toxin productions and the emergence of unfriendly microorganisms, such as yeast and undesirable bacteria. *Ama* is the Ayurvedic term for undigested food toxins, which are believed to cause many diseases in classical teaching of Ayurveda. Anti-ama diets are used to cleanse the body by depletion, but these diets are used in a tailored manner for the three *doshas,* or constitutions, of the human body (*Vata* or *Vayu, Pitta,* and *Kapha*).

In order to counteract Ama, the process of Pancha Karma is often used. Pancha Karma refers to a series of five or six therapies to cleanse or nourish (and tone) the body. The basic idea is to cause a cleansing and gentle detoxification of the body by natural means. Ayurveda has its own system of diagnosis that can be baffling for the uninitiated, especially when one considers many statements from classic Ayurvedic teachings, which deny a necessity for clear disease classification on grounds of causation. Classification of disease by cause is well recognized by modern scientific methods, but not by Ayurveda to the same degree, as illustrated in quotations from

Table 11.1: A synopsis of an Ayurvedic approach to therapy.

Note it is a difficult task to summarize the highly eclectic nature of Ayurveda and this table is an oversimplification.

INTERVENTION	COMMENT
Diet	A natural, balanced diet is tailored to suit a particular "constitution"
Herbals, botanicals, and nutritional supplements	More than 2000 herbs are used in Ayurveda, alone or in combination
Pancha Karma	Detoxification by cleansing
Physical methods	Massage, Yoga, exercise
Stress management	A holistic regimen of aromatherapy, sound therapy, relaxation, etc.
Daily routines	Acts of hygiene and cosmetic activity
Healthy lifestyle	Ayurveda teaches lifestyle medicine

Ashthanga Hridayam Su (chapter 12, verse 64): "Physicians shouldn't feel shy if they don't know the nomenclature of the disease, for there is no rule, custom, or state that every disease has a name."

Ayurvedic medicine repeatedly stresses a holistic approach that is customized according to the rules of classic Ayurvedic teaching. The characteristics of an Ayurvedic program are summarized in Table 11.1. Note the similarity in approach between this ancient medical discipline and modern alternative medical approaches (and some modern conventional medical approaches). However, Ayurveda contrasts sharply with conventional medicine on some of its approaches. This contrast is highlighted in Table 11.2.

This diversion in discussion is important in our approach to the issues of bowel cleansing and detoxification. Three thousand years of the successful practice of Ayurveda with its focus on colon cleansing and detoxification is a potential benefit that is hard to ignore—even by the most hide-bound medical thinker!

UNDERSTANDING LEAKY GUTS

The gut has to protect the body from unwanted intruders, but it also absorbs nutrients. Any circumstance that alters the permeability of the gut can have untoward consequences on health because a leaky gut can let in unwanted guests. Nutrients have several potential pathways or mechanisms of access across the walls of the gut. Much transport from the gut occurs in a relatively passive manner through spaces between cells that are normally kept closed by special (tight) junctions. Molecules can move through the lining cells of the gut, but many biomechanical factors restrict the cellular route of absorption for the active uptake of molecules, in general.

The tight junctions that exist between the lining cells of the intestines are fused together in a manner that closes the pathways between cells. These junctions vary in structure and number (density) throughout the gut, and they go through a dynamic process of change to allow molecules of different size to pass. In simple terms, they act like a sieve with an adjustable pore size. Disruption of tight junctions can occur for a variety of reasons including inflammation, toxic damage to the lining of the gut (e.g., by drugs such as NSAIDs), as a consequence of disease of the bowel (gluten enteropathy or Crohn's disease), or as a result of general disease affecting the body.

There is a host of diseases in which alterations of intestinal per-

Table 11.2: Contrasting some features found in holistic medicine (e.g., Ayurveda) with modern healthcare approaches—especially those of conventional medicine (e.g., the allopathic physician's practice).

CONVENTIONAL MEDICINE	HOLISTIC MEDICINE
Focus on disease treatment and prevention	Care of the well and sick, emphasizing prevention
Locked into scientific proof	Empiric, willing to try alternatives in the absence of emergency
Synthetic medicine	Naturopathic approach
Distinct from food	Part of diet is medicine
Focus on body	Body, mind, and spirit
Correcting symptoms	Going to the support of functions
External healing influence	External and internal healing system
Focus on disease treatment	Focus on health maintenance

meability have been described (Table 11.3), but in some cases, a chicken-and-egg argument rages as to whether the enhanced permeability of the bowel is the cause or the result of the disease in question.

Clinical observations have isolated several documented causes of increased mucosal permeability in the small intestine. Several of these causes of leaking gut are highlighted in Table 11.4.

NSAIDS: THE BIG CULPRIT

Of all drugs that insult the gastrointestinal tract, NSAIDs lead the way. They cause inflammation and lesions in the gut by several mechanisms in addition to their effects on the hormonelike substances known as prostaglandins (PG). The PG can protect the gut from damage, but NSAIDs block an enzyme (cyclooxygenase) that plays a role in PG production. Focused on the role of disturbed PG synthesis by NSAIDs, pharmaceutical companies have moved to the use of drugs that affect different areas of the PG production cycle. These new drugs are called COX-2 inhibitors (e.g., Viox, Celebrex). They may cause less gut damage, but they may not be entirely innocent. I

Table 11.3 Diseases linked with enhanced intestinal permeability.

Note that the association of these diseases with leaky guts does not necessarily mean that leaky guts caused the problem.

AUTOIMMUNE DISEASES
Ankylosing spondylitis, arthritis of diverse form (e.g., rheumatoid disease), and mixed connective tissue disease

GASTROINTESTINAL DISORDERS
Gastroenteritis, Yersinia infection, ulcerative colitis, pancreatic disease, cystic fibrosis

TRAUMA TO BODY
Shock, endotoxemia from sepsis, burns

SKIN DISEASE
Eczema, urticaria, psoriasis

MISCELLANEOUS
AIDS, some cases of asthma, food allergy, some cases of schizophrenia, malnutrition, and following surgery

Table 11.4 Some causes of increased intestinal permeability.

CAUSE	COMMENT
Drugs	NSAIDs are a common, dominant cause of leaky gut, but certain antibiotics, chemotherapy for cancer, gold compounds used in arthritis treatment, estrogen, and drugs of abuse such as cocaine and amphetamine are potential culprits. Alcohol "rots" the guts and disrupts tight junctions.
Gut infections	Bacterial and viral gastroenteritis can cause leaky gut, especially if food and water intake is limited. Some specific infections, like Yersinia, can lead to immune phenomena that result in arthritis and skin rashes.
Other medical interventions	Radiation therapy, surgical trauma (or burns and severe injury), and the institution of parenteral nutrition TPN can cause leaky guts

believe that COX-2 inhibitors may affect the gut lining and intestinal permeability—but more studies are required.

The common block in thinking of nutritional interventions in medicine to correct diseases is apparent by the general failure to recognize the damaging effect of NSAIDs on phospholipids. Phospholipids are the structural components of cell membranes in the gut and elsewhere. NSAIDs may bind to cell membrane phospholipids (especially dipalmitoylphosphatidylcholine, DPPC) and damage the cell barrier to the corrosive or hostile contents of the gut. The administration of phospholipids (in animal studies at least) in the form of soy lecithin (containing the phospholipid phosphatidylcholine) prevents this problem. Unfortunately, this nutritional approach to correcting NSAIDs damage is overshadowed in conventional medicine by a desire to give another drug (e.g., misoprostol, a prostaglandin) to prevent NSAID damage to the gut.

TESTING FOR ENHANCED INTESTINAL PERMEABILITY

Leaky guts can be detected by tests that measure the absorption of molecules that are not normally absorbed or broken up by the body.

A number of orally administered test substances can be used in this test, including mannitol, lactulose, rhamnose, polyethylene glycols, and radioisotopes (Chromium-51) attached to nonabsorbable markers such as EDTA. EDTA is used commonly by the intravenous route for chelation therapy in alternative medicine but it is not normally absorbed when given by the oral route. Routine testing for leaky gut has not percolated into the clinical practice of conventional medicine to any significant degree, but it is used increasingly in alternative medicine. Conventional medicine may doubt the cost effectiveness of this test—at least in part due to its denial of the importance of the leaky gut in disease, perhaps compounded by a lack of knowledge on how it should be managed. The greatest protagonists of leaky gut testing are naturopaths. This discipline of medicine firmly believes in the common occurrence of food allergy, antigenic transfer across the bowel, and invasion of pathogens as a ubiquitous cause of disease. The modern discipline of naturopathy is in line with the principal concepts of Ayurveda.

MANAGING LEAKY GUTS

The approach to leaky guts involves the removal of those factors that are known to cause the condition and attempts to prevent further damage to the intestinal lining. A number of natural agents that are available in dietary supplement format have been used to prevent damage by inhibiting the release of inflammatory substances from white blood cells in the bowel wall. These agents include *Gingko biloba* and flavonoids such as quercetin. Quercetin is believed to work like the synthetic drug disodium cromoglycate to stop the release of inflammatory peptides from white cells.

The next issue in correcting leaky guts involves the reestablishment of normal bacterial flora in the bowel. The presence of friendly microorganisms in the bowel is a circumstance of symbiosis. Symbiosis is where organisms live alongside each other to mutual benefit. When unwanted organisms appear (unfriendly bacteria or yeasts, e.g., *Candida albacans*), a status of "dysbiosis" is said to be present in the bowel.

DYSBIOSIS

The central theme of the work of Nobel prize winner Dr. Eli Metchnikoff was that states of optimum health and longevity are dependent on the type and function of gastrointestinal bacteria. Thus, good health requires good bacterial inhabitants of the bowel. The term *dysbiosis* refers to a state where the ecology of the gut (primarily the bowel) is disturbed by the presence of the wrong kind of gut bacteria or other microorganisms.

Several causes or precipitators of dysbiosis have been identified, including: stress, malnutrition, poor diet (laden with a high content of saturated fat and simple sugars), antibiotic treatments, defective immune function, poor digestive function, alterations of normal gut physiology, and environmental toxins. In chapter 10, we examined the impact of an appropriate flora (friendly bacteria) in the gut on human health. In states of dysbiosis, a number of organisms that may not be very aggressive in their ability to cause infections (e.g., protozoa, certain bacteria and yeasts) can cause disorders by altering the nutritional status of their host or adversely affecting immune competence in the body. Dysbiosis creates an environment where opportunistic organisms can cause infections.

The importance of dysbiosis in naturopathic and alternative medicine has led to the development of special batteries of comprehensive tests that are not familiar to the conventional internist or gastroenterologist. The diagnostic value and clinical value of several of these tests require further definition before they can be recommended for routine diagnosis. For individuals with a special interest in these tests, an overview of their application can be found in the two-volume *Textbook of Natural Medicine*, edited by J. E. Pizzorno, N.D. and Michael Murray, N.D., (Churchill Livingstone, 1999).

HEALING A LEAKY GUT

After taking steps to eliminate the offending agents in the cause of leaky guts and correcting dysbiosis with friendly bacteria, the healing of inflamed or damaged mucosa involves the use of the right kind of special nutrients.

Glutamine supplementation has been used with success in naturopathic practice to correct leaky gut. An amino acid, glutamine is a principal source of fuel for the lining cells of the small intestine (enterocytes) and, to a lesser degree, cells lining the colon (colonocytes). Glutamine is an important component of glucosamine, which is essential for the synthesis of protective mucin (found in mucus in the guts). Studies indicate that glutamine may be able to assist in the healing and regeneration of the gut lining by increasing mucosal thickness and increasing the secretion of antibodies in the gut (especially the antibody IgA). IgA functions to stop the adherence of bacteria to the gut wall and helps to block the passage of bacteria or yeasts into the body. Of particular relevance to the use of glutamine in healing or preventing damage to the gut lining are experiments in animals where glutamine has been shown to be protective against gut damage induced by radiation or toxic drug exposures.

The role of dietary fiber in gastrointestinal health is well documented. It functions largely as a consequence of its physical and chemical characteristics. However, soluble fiber is fermented in the bowel to produce short-chain fatty acids (e.g., butyrate, acetate, and proprionate) that have several beneficial effects on the bowel, including their use as a source of energy for colonocytes. The dietary fibers of choice are pectin, guar, psyllium, and oat bran.

Several agents are valuable in the therapy of leaky gut and Table 11.5 summarizes the use of several remedies of natural origin in the management of leaky guts.

DETOXIFICATION: THE CONCEPT

The process of body cleansing and removal of toxins is very popular in modern alternative medicine practice. This concept is at the root of the discipline of modern naturopathic medicine, and it is widely practiced. However, body cleansing is still largely ignored by the orthodox physician. Modern-day naturopathic medicine has learned its lessons from Ayurveda and other natural treatment disciplines (e.g., Paracelsus theory). Conventional medicine may even deny the presence of significant autointoxication of the body that results from

Table 11.5: Substances used in the management of leaky gut and dysbiosis.

TREATMENT AGENT	COMMENT
Glutamine	Energy for enterocyte and key mucin component
Soluble fiber	Produces short chain fatty acids
Fish oil Omega-3 fatty acids	Decrease intestinal inflammation, decrease leukotriene B4, thromboxane A2, tumor necrosis factor and inhibit the proinflammatory prostaglandins of type 2 series
Flavonoids	Gingko, quercetin, and other flavonoids pycnogenol. (OPCs) are antioxidants with anti-inflammatory effects
Probiotics	*Lactobacillus acidophilus*, *Bifidobacteria*, and *Saccharomyces boulardii* are valuable and versatile (see chapter 10)
FOS	Fructooligosaccharides help increase the growth of friendly bacteria

the action of microorganisms, or their products, in the bowel, whereas the more zealous alternative physician may regard it as a universal cause of many ills. I reiterate the belief that the problem lies somewhere between these two polar opinions. In some cases of disease autointoxication or toxin exposure are a key problem, whereas in others they may not figure. If body cleansing and detoxification are worthwhile processes, what are we trying to rid our bodies of?

BODY TOXINS

Toxins, in this discussion, are any agents (molecules or compounds) that can damage cellular, tissue, or organ function. In the days of the modern industrial revolution, they are ubiquitous. Table 11.6 summarizes the groups of some of the toxins that are of biggest concern to health practitioners of all kinds (conventional, complementary, integrated, pluralistic, alternative, environmental, naturopathic, and eclectic healers). Toxins come mostly from the environment (external contamination), but they can come from within (autointoxication).

Table 11.6: Toxins in our inner and external environment.

Note: This list is by no means complete.

CHEMICAL TOXINS: drugs, some toxic dietary supplements, alcohol, formaldehyde, food additives, pesticides, herbicides, cosmetics (many), hair dyes, cleaning materials, petrochemicals, etc., etc., etc.

COMPOUNDS FROM MICROORGANISMS: bacterial or yeast (Candida albicans) fragments, e.g., endotoxin (components of all microbial cell walls and proteins); or substances elaborated by microorganisms, e.g., exotoxins, toxic amines, carcinogenic byproducts of bacterial metabolism, and toxic transformation of bile acids in the gut

FERMENTATION AND BIOTRANSFORMATION OF PROTEIN IN THE GUT: ammonia, sulfur compounds, mercaptans, methyl derivatives (a result mainly of digestion and bacterial action), nitrosamines produced in the stomach from nitrites

HEAVY METALS: Lead, mercury, cadmium, aluminum, nickel, arsenic, beryllium (other metals are toxic in excess, e.g., iron, copper, chromium, etc.).

Table 11.7: Some simple tips on how to cut down on environmental toxins.

These tips are not complete but will assist in sleuthing for toxins.

- Learn about the damages of synthetic compounds in household cleaning agents, cosmetics and skin creams.
- Avoid self-medication with unnecessary drugs, both prescription and OTC.
- Read food labels—look for additives with strange complicated names—junk food tastes good often because of its additives.
- Examine your environment at home, in the bedroom, at work—avoid the obvious chemical exposures, e.g., smoke, vapors etc.
- Think about your water supply—wells and tapwater may be suspect in many urban locations - filters may not remove all toxins.
- Wash fruit and vegetables—pesticides, herbicides and chemicals sprayed on to fruit to make it look good are to be avoided. Shop for organic food.

It is widely accepted that many of the toxins mentioned in Table 11.6 can cause serious acute, subacute, or chronic disease. The key issue in avoiding toxic damage is to clean up our external environment and consider the management of our own body environments such as the ecology of the gut. An individual can do a great deal to achieve this important public health measure.

Contamination of our environment occurs from industrial pollution, and it has created powerful movements and expressions from environmentalists—ranging from those who boycott to those who engage in the folly of ecoterrorism. The simple fact is that many people can decrease their toxin load by altering their day-to-day selections and preferences. Some simple antitoxic maneuvers are shown in Table 11.7.

While we artificially separate toxins based on their source, externally or internally generated, a substance taken from outside can be transformed in the body to a toxic agent. The human body is a chemical factory, the hub of which is the liver, which can metabolize (transform) compounds for use by the body or as a prelude to their excretion by the body.

DETOXIFICATION SYSTEMS: THE GUT AS A MAIN SEWER

The body has an elaborate series of working systems that result in detoxification. The liver is the key detoxifying organ with its ability to filter blood, process or secrete chemicals, and excrete bile. Detoxification processes take place in a highly complex array of chemical reactions—chemicals are detoxified in certain phases (sulfation, acetylation, glucuronidation, sulfoxidation, conjugation, etc.). These are examples of some of the many chemical reactions in the liver. The skin can excrete compounds in sweat, and the kidneys are one of the main portals of excretion from the body. Every day the kidneys produce urine that rids the body of unwanted waste chemicals of normal metabolism (e.g., urea from protein) or toxins (e.g., drugs or herbal metabolites).

The lungs play a role in detoxification that is sometimes forgotten. Volatile chemicals can be released in expired air in large amounts in states of health and disease. The gut and its appendages (the gallbladder attached to the liver) play a pivotal role in toxin elimination. Bile containing unwanted chemicals drains into the gut, which acts like the main sewer. Compounds can be secreted into the gut and are eliminated in the stool, along with the primary "unwanted" or indigestible components of the diet. Aside from these actions, the intestines have enzyme systems and physical and immune functions that all result in the process of detoxification. Block the main sewer in any urban location and the results are catastrophic!

AUTOINTOXICATION

I reiterate that the idea that the gut plays a role in poisoning the body with toxins is highly controversial in modern medicine. Of course, the gut has elaborate defense mechanisms to prevent this occurrence in states of health, but it bewilders me why some practitioners of medicine cannot accept that these defenses are optimal only in states of prime health. To deny that the bowel can be loaded on occasion with toxins is like denying the odor of feces. Toxins derived from the gut, either ingested or produced within the gut, have been implicated in a wide variety of different diseases, disorders, and complaints. We have learned a great deal about the balance of digestion, immune defenses, and liver function in the warding off of bowel toxins.

The subject of gut toxins remains underexplored perhaps because of the inaccessibility of the bowel to toxicologists. There are very few gastroenterologists or gut surgeons who've made their career on combining their work with toxicology (the study of the effect of toxins on the body). Gut toxins are not a myth or fairy tale—they are measurable and can be demonstrated sometimes to be highly damaging . The debris, waste products, or substances elaborated by the gut flora can be absorbed when gut defenses are suboptimal (especially in the presence of leaky guts), and body functions can be adversely affected by these toxins.

Endotoxins, exotoxins, toxic amines, transformed bile acids, and a whole host of toxic chemicals have been isolated from the gut and defined chemically. We know that these chemicals can trigger immune responses in the body. Antibodies that are produced against bacterial antigens are known to crossreact with body tissues. This means that an antibody that is made by the body against a microorganism can react with body tissues as well as the organisms against which it was initially directed.

To look at this situation differently, microorganisms share antigens (that trigger antibodies) with normal tissues. Elegant research has shown this situation to be the case quite often. An example is the crossreaction between *E. coli* (a bacterium) and gut-wall tissues. This finding has been proposed as a potential cause of ulcerative colitis. Thus, an antibody aimed at a bug can attack the body itself. This self-attack is called autoimmunity and it helps to explain the alleged association of autoimmune diseases with gut toxins.

Toxins derived from the gut have been associated with ulcerative colitis, rheumatoid disease, pernicious anemia, autoimmune thyroid disease, systemic lupus erythematosis (SLE), myasthenia gravis, and skin disease. Note that these are the more classic types of autoimmune disease that are described in the medical literature. Thus, the phenomenon of autointoxication appears to be inextricably linked to the occurrence of autoimmune disease. It is not that this link should be questioned in medicine, it is more relevent to what degree this link operates in disease. This is where alternative and conventional medicine differ in opinion.

WHAT EVIDENCE EXISTS THAT THE GUT MAY BE LEAKY?

Whereas the global view of digestion can be depicted in a simple format, Table 11.8, regional functions of the gut have some crossover. Barriers to transfer of many substances are not always efficient, and big molecules do get into the body on a regular basis.

Table 11.8 refers to a few concepts that are somewhat controversial. The mouth, stomach, and colon are not viewed as absorptive organs, but it does not mean that they do not let small amounts of ingested material enter the body. Rocking teeth during chewing can lead to entry of bacteria from the oral cavity into the body, and simple drugs or alcohol can get into the body through the oral mucosa (lining of the mouth). The stomach is primarily a storage organ, but it initiates enzymatic digestion, and if its barrier is disrupted, unwanted molecules may enter the body. Again, I am not suggesting that the stomach is a primary organ of absorption, but experiments in animals where the exit of the stomach is obstructed show the almost complete absorption of small molecular-weight compounds into the body (e.g., alcohol and some drugs). Furthermore, the bac-

Table 11.8: The classic teaching of digestion is summarized.

The italicized statements are often forgotten or minimized in teachings of digestive physiology. A diseased bowel is often leaky, e.g., celiac disease and inflammatory bowel disease.

SITE IN GUT	DIGESTION	ABSORPTION
Mouth	Begins carbohydrate digestion	Simple diffusion or entry of very low molecular weight nutrients and antigens, especially if poor dental and oral hygiene
Stomach	Grinding, starting of protein digestion (pepsin)	Forward and back diffusion of only simple molecules and acid mixing
Small bowel	Principal site of all nutrient absorption	Free fatty acids, amino acids, monosaccharides, salts, and water efficiently absorbed, "variably leaky"
Colon	Fermentation and biotransformation	Sodium, electrolytes, water, trace nutrients, "rarely leaky"

terium *Helicobacter pylori* manages to elicit an antibody reaction that can be detected in blood samples—again showing communication at least through immune defenses associated with the gut.

When the stomach functions in a state of health, it secretes acid and forms a highly effective barrier to bacteria, viruses, and other pathogens (microorganisms that cause infection). When gastric acid is absent, different circumstances may arise. Several studies imply that there may be an increased growth of gram-positive bacteria (unwanted bugs) in the intestines and an increased incidence of sensitivity reactions to macromolecular antigens in the diet in the absence of gastric acid (achlorhydria). Other studies show that individuals are more susceptible to infections when gastric acid is absent. In general, the stomach, with its pepsin and acid, plays a role in degrading macromolecules and sterilizing food, thereby limiting the passage of microorganisms, some toxic components of food, and certain antigens into the small bowel.

These occurrences are often dismissed in conventional medicine and sometimes overreacted to in alternative medicine. However, they cannot be ignored, and studies of the potential benefits of systematic acidification of the stomach with dilute hydrochloric acid are begging to be done. After all, many grandmothers and housewives swear by the panacea health benefits of apple cider vinegar.

In order for us to buy into the idea of leaky guts, we need evidence. Certainly we have some compelling observations. Antibodies to food antigens are detectable in the blood, immune complexes (food antigens linked with antibodies) are detectable, and studies show us enhanced permeability of the bowel in several diseases, including disease in which the bowel is not overtly abnormal or diseased but is functionally abnormal and leaky.

RESTORING AND BUILDING MUCOSAL INTEGRITY: GLUTAMINE AND SAME

Earlier in this chapter, I made a cursory review of nutritional and botanical agents that assist in dealing with leaky gut. Two agents that are both derivatives of amino acids have emerged as potentially important. These agents, which seem to play a special role in supporting the structure and function of the gut are L-glutamine (LG) and S-adenosyl-methionine (SAMe).

Glutamine falls into the category of a nonessential amino acid that can be synthesized in the body. Glutamine is the precursor of glutamate. The main role of glutamine is as a "nitrogen shuttle." It mops up nitrogen (often in the form of ammonium ions, NH_4), and it can donate the nitrogen when required to form other essential compounds for use in body metabolism.

Glutamine is the most abundant amino acid in the circulating blood, and the biggest end user of glutamine is the gut. We learned that glutamine provides fuel for the enterocytes. The role of glutamine in the support of the lining and function of the small intestine is most apparent in scientific studies of glutamine deficiency. Animal studies show that the administration of glutaminase (an enzyme that coverts glutamine back to glutamate) results in diarrhea and severe changes in the integrity of the bowel. These changes include loss of the villi (fingerlike projections of the intestine), development of gaps and breaches in the lining of the intestines, and areas of ulceration (leaky guts).

In states of severe stress (burns and trauma), the secretion of steroids (cortisol) enhances the concentrations of glutaminase (the converting enzyme) and protein breakdown occurs. Evidence has now accumulated that the addition of glutamine (or dipeptides of glutamine, such as glutamine linked with alanine or glycine) can improve the "barrier defenses" of the small bowel.

When increased permeability of the bowel is induced in animals, the administration of glutamine can help reverse the leaky gut and improve immune functions of the gut at the same time. Depletion of glutamine also results in depletion of the key body antioxidant called glutathione, and this may contribute to tissue damage. Much of the work on glutamine has been in animals, but its value in the nutrient support of intestinal mucosal function is increasingly apparent. Recent studies of glutamine supplementation imply a potential for reversing leaky gut, but doses as high as 20 rams per day or more must be used to achieve a therapeutic effect.

SAMe is a compound that is formed from methionine, and it works in the body by playing a key part in the body's methylation systems (a chemical reaction necessary for many vital functions in the body). This versatile chemical has been found to be valuable in the management of several diseases, including depression, arthritis, liver cirrhosis, Alzheimer's disease, and abnormal gut dysfunction. The effects of SAMe on liver function appear to be particularly beneficial, including its ability to decrease the consequences of toxic insults to the liver, increase bile salt production, and generally improve liver function. Drug detoxification that occurs predominantly in the liver appears to be enhanced by SAMe.

SAMe seems to have an increasing role in supporting gut function, especially small intestinel structure and integrity. A recent study published in the British journal *Gut* in 1996 shows that SAMe may help diminish damage to the colon-lining cells by preventing changes induced by sulfides. These findings have implications for the treatment of inflammatory bowel disease and the support of gut integrity (Dr. W. E. Roediger et al, *Gut*, 39, 1:77–81, 1996). Given the current unsatisfactory nature of conventional therapies for ulcerative colitis, it is surprising that nutritional approaches to inflammatory bowel disease have been frequently ignored. A simple and succinct message for the effective management of inflammatory bowel disease using natural, effective, gentle therapies is fish oil, plus probiotics, plus SAMe!

GETTING NATURAL THERAPIES THROUGH THE GUT WALL

While naturopaths and practitioners of alternative medicine have been obsessed with sealing the leaky gut, the importance of getting natural treatments through the healthy gut has become a contemporary area of focused interest. Natural agents such as colostrum, extracts of shark cartilage, and chemicals that can chelate metals, for example, EDTA, just do not get through the gut wall readily enough to exert beneficial effects in the body. Currently, approximately $50 million worth of bovine colostrum is purchased in health food stores and pharmacies on an annual basis. Colostrum is referred to as "life's first food" and its role in infant health and subsequent health in adults is well established, but often overlooked in conventional medicine. There are adults who were bottle-fed as infants who think that they may recapture the advantages of the colostrum they missed by taking supplements of cow colostrum. In part this is wishful thinking.

It's not hard to conclude that many of the beneficial contents of colostrum cannot be absorbed by an adult—especially molecules of large size. This fact is based on an established knowledge of bowel closure to big molecules in the diet that occurs early in life. The advanced actions of the adult digestive process destroy much of the colostrum given to an adult—especially when it is given as a supplement in a capsule or powder. Despite these drawbacks, the value of colostrum is well described in several traditional medical practices. For example, in traditional Chinese medicine, the phenomenon of "filial piety" used to be common. In this practice, old people (revered in Chinese culture) would be breastfed intermittently by their female relatives in order to maintain health.

There are many beneficial natural agents in colostrum that promote health, including: antibodies, protein growth factors, and complexed nutrients. Therapy with colostrum has many possible applications in chronic diseases, immune deficiency, and even body building (an unlikely but plausible application).

To overcome the problems that adults have in harnessing the benefits of colostrum, the supplement must be protected from digestion and helped or assisted in its absorption. Any colostrum product without a delivery mechanism to facilitate its availability to the body has limited value. Attempts to overcome this problem with variable success are liposome encapsulation of colostrum using bubbles of essential fatty acids (liposomes). Colostrum with facilitated delivery, which itself may be variably successful, must be preferred. This technique is used in the administration of extracts of shark cartilage and has been alleged to be much more successful than "solid" dosing with shark cartilage—accepting the residual lack of evidence for the shark cartilage in antiangiogeric therapy.

Leaky guts are found in many states of ill health, such as AIDS, cancer, and systemic disease, and people with leaky guts may be able to utilize the macromolecules in natural therapies such as colostrum or shark cartilage to varying degrees. I have repeatedly stated, against criticism, that there are patients with cancer who have used shark cartilage and who may have improvements that cannot be explained by chance. In my book *The Power of Cartilage*, I describe a positive (but by no means complete) response of about one out of every five (or more) cancer patients using shark cartilage. I propose that these one in five or so partial responders is explainable by their leaky guts. In fact, the occurrence of leaky guts in cancer patients (or AIDS patients) is about one in five or so. Can those people who are unfortunate enough to have leaky guts be fortunate enough to respond to macromolecules in natural therapies like shark cartilage and colostrum? If this is the case, it is a very novel trick of nature! However, I must stress that I am *not* promoting shark cartilage as a cancer treatment—at least until we known more about its benefits—or lack thereof.

DETOXIFICATION AND THE LIVER

The subject of detoxification of chemicals by the liver is extraordinarily complex. For the less chemically minded, an excellent review of this subject is found in two books: *Total Wellness* by Joseph Pizzorno, N.D., (Prima Publishing, 1996) and *Textbook of Natural Medicine* second edition, edited by Joseph Pizzorno, N.D., and Michael Murray, N.D.

The liver acts like a complex processing factory. It takes nutrients, hormones, drugs and other chemicals from within and outside the body and processes them—transforming them for use by the body or for elimination or neutralization. All foods contain unwanted elements as well as vital or useful nutrients. The liver is kept busy filtering the blood, making bile for digestive processes in the intestines, and using its enzymes to assemble and break down chemicals. Our environment is loaded with toxins such as herbicides, pesticides, and industrial chemicals (e.g., DDT, PCB, and other hydrocarbons). Without the liver's ability to efficiently process chemicals, chronic disease of all types may occur more commonly than they do at present.

The mechanisms of detoxification in the liver have been described in phases. Each phase can be amplified or improved by a whole host of factors. A wide variety of nutrients are required for enzyme systems to work on the various chemicals (substrates) that are dealt with by the liver. Some drugs can interfere with phases of liver detoxification and others can enhance the process. The same applies to nutrients. Other tissues such as the kidney and the bowel have detoxifying mechanisms, but the liver generally dominates in this process.

In order to go about its important job of processing chemicals, the liver needs a variety of nutritional agents to work efficiently. A balanced supplementation of essential vitamins and minerals is required, with special emphasis on antioxidants (vitamins C, E, beta carotene, zinc, and the trace element selenium). A number of nutrients have been termed lipotropic agents by naturopathic physicians—largely based on an evolution of knowledge from Ayurveda.

The term *lipotropic* in this context refers to the ability of certain nutrients to regulate fat metabolism and facilitate the manufacture and flow of bile. Lipotropic agents are discussed in chapter 13 in some detail, but the principal lipotropes are betaine, choline, methionine, B vitamins (especially B6 and B12), and folic acid. Much recent interest has focused on the use of SAMe and glutathione, but the latter is not always available (absorbed) for use in significant amounts by the body when it is administered in a supplement format. The use of methionine and choline, and perhaps betaine, to make more SAMe available is an interesting option. This may assist in liver repair and regeneration. A great deal of further research is required to define the role of nutritional support for liver function and detoxification. One important issue is the clear evidence that vitamin A has a supportive role in liver function but in excess is quite toxic especially in circumstances of pre-existing liver damage (e.g., cirrhosis). Therapies of this kind are reserved for specialists in nutritional therapy in liver disease—a defined speciality of "hepatology" in medicine.

SILYMARIN—A SPECIAL GIFT OF NATURE

Certain chemicals (flavones) found in silymarin (*Silybum marianum*, common name—milk thistle) have been shown in several studies to assist in the process of detoxification in the liver and to exert a protective effect on the liver against damage from toxins. Some evidence suggests that silymarin has several ways in which it can exert this effect, ranging from enhancing the availability of glutathione (a key protective chemical in the liver) to assisting the liver in its constant process of regeneration and repair. Repair to the liver is ongoing, as this organ accepts the constant insult of toxins from within the body or the environment.

In order to examine the beneficial effects of silymarin, one has to recognize the function of the tripeptide (three amino acids) glutathione. Glutathione is not only an antioxidant (preventing free radical damage to the liver), it is attached (conjugated) with toxic chemicals to form molecules that can be readily excreted by the body—especially water-soluble compounds (mercaptates) that pass into the urine. If excessive amounts of certain toxins are presented to the liver, glutathione depletion can occur. In its absence, these toxins do more damage. Glutathione is synthesized from cysteine, glutamic acid, and glycine (amino acids), and cysteine is synthesized from methionine. This discussion indicates some of the interdependence of various nutrients. The story is unfortunately not simple.

Against this background, the ability of silymarin to prevent the depletion of glutathione is of obvious importance. Many studies have shown that silymarin can prevent the depletion of glutathione that occurs as a consequence of a variety of toxic compounds including alcohol, organic chemicals (e.g., carbon tetrachloride), mushroom or fungal toxins and others. Glutathione depletion has been associated with a variety of diseases; and this relationship may be a causal link in some diseases. Diseases in which glutathione depletion has been noted include HIV infection, liver cirrhosis or chronic hepatitis, and fibrotic types of lung disease.

The adequate availability of glutathione in the liver has far-reaching consequences. The liver detoxifies many chemicals in different phases, and glutathione works in the second phase (phase II) of liver detoxification. Phase I of liver detoxification can produce chemicals that are very damaging when they accumulate without the proper functioning of phase II reactions involving agents like glutathione. To reinforce this concept, it is apparent that toxins, processed in phase I, can accumulate if glutathione, a phase II agent, is depleted. These accumulated toxins could damage the liver, the body, and play a role in the causation of chronic disease, including cancers. It is a special note that glutathione levels in the liver of healthy people may rise by a factor of one-third, or more, after the use of silymarin.

Studies using silymarin as a treatment seem to be focused on potential benefits in people with liver disease, but its potential benefits are far ranging and still largely underexplored. Average doses of silymarin are of the order of 80–200 mg one to three times a day, and in general it appears quite safe. The optimum dose of silymarin defies definition.

DIRECT CLEANSING PROCEDURES

Fasting

Fasting has both medical and religious significance for many people worldwide. It can be both beneficial and dangerous. People with serious metabolic diseases such as diabetes mellitus are advised not to engage in fasts, but for the average healthy person, the act of giving the gut a rest may be desirable on occasion. Fasting as treatment is not practiced in orthodox medicine, but clinical studies have shown temporary benefit in many disorders, especially those with an allergic basis. After all, dietary excesses are more common in the United States than dietary deficiencies.

Fasts should not involve complete abstinence from food and fluid, and they are best used with supervision. Adequate fluid intake must be maintained during a fast. The concept of modified fasting with the use of carefully selected dietary supplements has become increasingly popular in alternative medicine. There are several negative consequences of a fast including the possibility that certain "toxins" may be mobilized by a fast, and substances that protect the body (e.g., glutathione) can be depleted.

The notion of fasting is closely linked with the idea of detoxification. A suitable fasting regimen for the healthy includes vital support with vitamins, minerals, and essential fatty acids combined with antioxidant administration (e.g., selenium, glutathione, methionine, green tea extract, curcumin, etc.) and the use of herbs that assist in detoxification, such as silymarin. Again, I stress that people with significant illnesses should seek a supervised fast if they elect for this intervention. There are very few clinical trials on the benefits of fasting for health, but its benefit in making people feel better when applied correctly is indisputable.

Saunas, Sweating, and Hydrotherapy

Popularized in modern times by the Scandinavians, the use of the sauna is an age-old panacea for many. This historic act of presumed detoxification by heat-induced sweating has been modified over the years. The experience of a sauna is quite refreshing—but is it therapeutic? Rolling in the snow after sauna whilst being beaten with twigs is a more extreme example of this intervention, but its values are not readily explained with our current level of medical knowledge!

Like fasting, saunas have to be used properly by the right people. One hypothesis is that saunas encourage the excretion of body toxins in sweat, and they may result in excretion of fatty acids that have latched on to fat-soluble toxins (e.g., DDT or PCBs—polychlorinated biphenyls). Several studies have drawn attention to the ability of a sauna to assist in increasing fat breakdown in the body, facilitating body cleansing (inner and outer). Sauna therapy may have beneficial effects on hormone secretion (e.g., growth hormone). Saunas do present dangers of dehydration, and they should never be used in pregnancy or by people with serious heart disease. Saunas are best enjoyed as a safe, shared experience in a good social setting that does not involve alcohol consumption.

Hydrotherapy

The term *hydrotherapy* refers to the use of water to heal. Water can be used in many ways in internal and external applications to the body. Table 11.9 summarizes a number of types of hydrotherapy, some of which have been in use from ancient times. In many cases, hydrotherapy is believed to have a basic cleansing property or it "exercises" the body for cleansing. Orthodox medicine often considers hydrotherapy to be of nebulous benefit, but it is widely practiced in modified formats—even in "high-powered" medical institutions.

The use of hot or cold water applied to body surfaces was made into a scientific endeavor by the Romans. Exquisitely decorated baths exist in several European countries—especially England—that still stand as a memorial to Roman hydrotherapists. The use of hydrotherapy is so popular in Germany that it is a reimbursable health treatment. The French are spa lovers, and hydrotherapy is used often in medical practice in France. In contrast, the British and Americans see hydrotherapy as pampering, and it is used more as a cosmetic treat than a treatment.

Some recent scientific studies on hydrotherapy are emerging, and one could anticipate that with the right kind of clinical-outcome questionnaire, benefit could be shown definitively. Sensations of well-being, reduction of stress, feelings of invigoration and refreshment—all score high after bathing. Whether or not hydrotherapy detoxifies the body is under study.

Dr. A. Heywood and his colleagues studied the use of bathing for body detoxification in the famous English city of Bath. These English researchers suggested that full body immersion at 35°C for at least one and one-half hours together with the drinking of mineral water in copious amounts resulted in improvement in individuals with lead (or heavy metal) poisoning. Changes in cardiac output (function of the heart) and excretion of urine were documented with an objective measure of increased lead excretion in the urine. It appears that real measurable benefits are possible with hydrotherapy.

Table 11.9: Types of hydrotherapy.

The science, if any, behind these therapies defies definition but many swear by hydrotherapy for healing.

TYPE OF HYDROTHERAPY	COMMENT
Drinking	The body has an essential need for clean, uncontaminated water—eight 8-ounce glasses per day is probably optimal for the average adult.
Pressure hosing	High pressure impact of water is tiring and refreshing.
Needle sprays	Very fine spray of water of different temperatures—an invigoration and example of unguided accupressure.
Whirlpools, bubble air baths	These are used for relaxation—soothing after exercise.
Sitz baths	A "potty" of water bathes the pelvis—the sitz bath can be warm and a foot bath can be added, warm or cold; used for pelvic disorders (piles, cramps) and to promote circulation in lower extremities.
Epsom salt bath	Usually hot with several pounds of Epsom Salts–(magnesium sulphate)—sweating is induced.
Salt rubs	Salt of various sources is rubbed on the body and the individual is hosed down with cold water—said to cause euphoria and well-being.
Polar bear therapy	Usually a social gathering at the coldest time of the year, a group bathes communally in the sea, river or lake—promotes bonding.
Underwater massage	Both therapuetic and erotic. The outcome may be more related to the person giving the massage.
Turkish baths	Hot dip, warm dip, body scrubs, and cool dip.
Nauli	A type of Yoga, an exercise where one squats in water and creates negative pressure in the abdominal activity to suck water in and then discharge it with a bowel movement. Monsieur Petit-Pas learned this well!
Holy water	The water has holy powers.
Charged water	An individual transfers energy to water that is used in healing (quackery?).
Colon irrigation	See text—an ancient art of medicine.

Colonic Irrigation

The idea that an enema is a last resort for the severely constipated individual is a thing of the past! More and more people are self-administering fluids and enemas containing different substances into the bowel with the belief that they can both cleanse the body and treat disease. The coffee enema seems very popular in alternative medicine, but its specific advantages are not defined.

Perceived as fashionable, healthy, and enjoyable in the nineteenth century, colon irrigation has tended to be viewed in orthodox medicine as unnecessary, perhaps a little perverted, and of no measurable health benefit in the twentieth century. The wheel turns, and the new millennium is ushered in with a renewed interest in colonic irrigation for health—a clear sign of the growth of alternative therapies!

Colon cleansing has been of interest in medicine for at least four thousand years. The precise art of colon cleansing has been traced to ancient Egyptian medical documents (1500 B.C.) that were probably based on the earlier spread of Ayurvedic philosophy. The great historical healers, Hippocrates and Galen, used purgation for a variety of diseases, especially fevers. These practices were common in medicine until the turn of the twentieth century, when proponents of colonic therapies and irrigation presented works that fell on the deaf ears of modern, twentieth-century medicine.

Currently, colonic irrigation has become a well-defined alternative medicine practice with its own automated instrumentation for colonic lavage (washing). Dedicated training courses have emerged for colon therapists. Parties interested in the recommendations for training of colon hydrotherapy and other techniques are referred to the work of the Nutrition Research Council (a small interest group) and the DoTolo Research Corporation, which have presented recommendations for independent learning for colon therapists.

Despite modern, reactivated interest in colon cleansing and colonic irrigation, scientific support for its application in many diseases does not exist. Proponents of colon irrigation rely heavily on theories of body autointoxication (described earlier) and parasitic infestations to support their treatments. Most parasites are not disturbed by colon irrigation, they may even enjoy it! While the colon is

a potential route of excretion of toxins, the process of body detoxification is much more related to enhancement of renal and liver function than colonic function.

There are several organizations for training and applications of
colon therapy (e.g., International Association for Colon Hydrotherapy) that have a self-declared accreditation process for trainees.
Overall, I am against the movement of taking the practice of colon
therapy out of the realm of a licensed, trained healthcare giver,
because safety is a key issue when it comes to invasive therapies such
as colonic irrigation. Instrumentation and instillation of anything
into the colon is not a treatment realm for amateurs.

The list of diseases alleged to respond to colon irrigation by proponents of this therapy is very long. Colon cleansing is mandatory
prior to diagnostic interventions in the lower bowel, such as barium
enema examinations (colon x-rays) or colonoscopy (passage of a lighted tube into the colon by a trained endoscopist). However, high-
colonic washouts and repeated enemas for this purpose have been
superseded in modern medicine by the use of carefully designed fluids that can cause diarrhea and flush out the bowel. A good example
is the use of an electrolyte and chemical mix that fills the colon with
fluid after it is taken in large amounts by mouth (e.g., Golytely,
Braintree Labs, Mass.). These types of solutions are very useful, and
more investigation of their role in natural colon cleansing in diseases
is required.

Overall, I believe that there are efficient ways of emptying the
colon without resorting to sophisticated techniques of colon irrigation—except under specific, serious circumstances such as fecal
impaction (absolute blockage of the bowel by stool). Colonic irrigation can result in perforation of the bowel, depletion of body chemicals, metabolic disturbances, and cross-infections. My interest in
alternative medicine does not extend to the rituals of colonic irrigation as a panacea therapy.

One important issue that seems to be forgotten in medical practice is that instrumentation of the bowel can be quite painful and distressing. While physicians cling to symptomatic therapies for bowel
disorders, they sometimes forget the discomfort caused by tests such
as barium enema or sigmoidoscopy (examination of the lower parts
of the bowel). Colonoscopy (more complete examination of the

colon) is usually done under anesthesia. A very useful natural option to alleviate discomfort during bowel testing or enema administration is to have the individual take enteric-coated peppermint oil an hour or two before the procedure (Pepogest). Peppermint oil relaxes the bowel and facilitates entry into the bowel by acting as a natural anti-spasmodic.

THE CONCEPT OF CDR: CLEANSING, DETOXIFICATION, REJUVENATION

I have used the acronym CDR to represent the following processes in the bowel and body: cleansing, detoxification, and rejuvenation. The CDR approach has to be classified as alternative as it is certainly not recognized by conventional medicine, even though each component may already be practiced in orthodox medicine in a modified manner.

In this chapter, we have reviewed the scientific basis, or lack thereof, to support the activities of body cleansing, detoxification, and rejuvenation. These three indistinct processes involve the basic removal of toxins from our environment (and the bowel), a replacement of nutrients and good types of flora (or encouragement of the growth of friendly bugs), and attempts to assist in bowel repair or regeneration that fall under the category of rejuvenation. I stress that these concepts are not novel. They form the basis of several ancient treatment systems (e.g., Ayurveda, Native North American medicine, Paracelsian theory, and traditional Chinese, Egyptian, Korean, and Japanese medicine). The large amount of information presented in the medical literature on CDR requires simplification in order to understand its potential applications for health.

Cleansing

Food, hygiene, and optimal diet are important interventions to avoid unwanted contents in the bowel, especially gut parasites and unfriendly bacteria. Foods to which individuals have intolerance or allergies are best avoided, and the diet must be balanced with adequate nutrients (low saturated fat, adequate omega-3 and omega-6 essential fats), high fiber (at least 30 gm/day), moderate protein (a balance of meat, dairy, and vegetable protein), healthy complex carbohydrates (limit simple sugar intake), and a good array of vitamins and essential micronutrients. Gluten (from wheat) and dairy products tend to have a high level of antigens, and alternatives such as rice (rice milk), soy (soy protein isolates), or modified dairy products (e.g., whey) can be considered desirable for some people.

Regulation of bowel habit is optimum but it should not be an obsession. Adequate fluid intake with a good amount of dietary fiber and good lifestyle habits (e.g., exercise) is a first-line, simple, natural method of bowel regulation. Purgation should be only occasional when required or perhaps intermittent with a CDR regimen. Simple osmotic purges by mouth are often safe, and herbal purgatives or drug purges are best used sparingly.

Detoxification

We have discussed this subject ad nauseum, because it is more important than currently recognized in conventional medicine. The avoidance of toxins or toxin buildup is recommended. Washing food (commercial, natural vegetable washes are safe), maintenance of bowel regularity, and education about environmental toxins are key issues.

Herbal adjuncts to detoxification, such as silymarin, may be very useful, and detoxification is closely linked with adequate nutritional supports (e.g., maintenance of glutathione, omega-3 fatty acids, vitamins, and other cofactors for body metabolism). Detoxification is synonymous with body cleansing in many areas of alternative medicine, such as hydrotherapy and bowel purges. Remember the bowel is but one portal of exit for toxins—the kidneys, lungs, and skin are also routes for the exodus of toxins.

Rejuvenation

Naturopathic medicine recommends replacement therapies for the gut with hydrochloric acid, digestive enzymes, bile salts, and probiotic therapy. Many but not all of these approaches are rooted in science. Repair of the gut requires nutrient support, a rest from gut insults (e.g., NSAID drugs), and some specific nutritional therapies, for example, glutamine, omega-3 fatty acids, antioxidants, glutathione, pantothenic acid, probiotic agents, and prebiotic agents (complex sugars that promote the growth of friendly bacteria, e.g., FOS or inulin). I believe that of these interventions, probiotic therapy is the most important.

SCIENTIFIC SUPPORT FOR CDR

Therapies in alternative medicine that involve detoxification should include initial cleansing, reduction of exposure to toxins (internal and external), together with a plan to support the body functions that result in detoxification. One of the pioneers in the concepts of detox-ification in modern alternative medicine practice is Jeffrey S. Bland, Ph.D. Dr. Bland has developed teaching manuals and supplement products to support detoxification with a focus on the gut. Several studies have been funded by Dr. Bland's corporation, Health Comm International, Inc. Preliminary data imply that the supplemental food programs proposed by Dr. Bland and his colleagues can provide important adjuncts in the management of a variety of illnesses.

Some studies of interest that support detoxification have sur-faced in recent times. Drs. K. H. Kilburn, R. Warsaw, and M. Shields described improvements in a fireman who had been exposed to PCBs (polychlorinated biphenyls) after a detoxification program involving nutritional supplementation and sauna therapy. Many reports of the successful use of detoxification programs have appeared in the non-peer-review literature and several papers in medical journals point to the dietary regulation of the liver detoxifying process. Drs. J. S. Bland and J. A. Bradley have published their experiences with the nutri-tional support of liver detoxification. These researchers have described beneficial outcome with medical, food–supplemented (dietary supplement), detoxification programs in several chronic health conditions (J. S. Bland et al. *Alternative Therapies*, 1, 5:62–71, 1995; J. S. Bland and J. A. Bradley, *Journal of Applied Nutrition*, 44:2–15, 1992). Concepts are many, science is appearing, but the bur-den of proof remains to be completely satisfied for interventions, with gut detoxification in some diseases.

CHAPTER SUMMARY

I support the CDR approach for health in selected people. In general, cleansing of the bowel and body are functions of good lifestyle habits—good nutrition, avoidance of substance abuse and toxins, and so on. Detoxification should be made less necessary by prevention—less toxin exposure. Preventive efforts include alternatives to NSAIDs, reduction of substance abuse, avoidance of potentially toxic foods and food additives, water filtering etc. I believe in the concepts of herbal support for detoxification, for example, silymarin, and the process of bowel (and body) rejuvenation is sound. Table 11.10 summarizes a very simplistic CDR approach.

Table 11.10: CDR approaches simplified and facilitated.

CDR APPROACH

Cleansing	High fiber, balanced diet, good fluid intake, exercise, osmotic laxative (e.g. magnesium sulphate) as required.
Detoxification	Silymarin, modified fasting, probiotic therapy, and other alternative approaches.
Rejuvention	Nutrient support for gut function and probiotics present a sound option.

FACILITATING THE CDR APPROACH

C	Magnesium sulphate orally and mixed fiber supplements in the absence of contraindications and used occasionally, e.g., epsom salts, milk of magnesia. If used intermittently, an herbal purgative is acceptable.
D	Silymarin 150 mg tid. Probiotic formula, enteric coated for viability, containing at least *Lactobacillus* with FOS.
R	Fiber supplements administered with glutamine, antioxidants, omega-3 fatty acids, glutathione, ginger, vitamins, trace minerals, and fermented soy.

CHAPTER TWELVE

EMERGING
ISSUES

FACT AND FICTION

Throughout this book, we have learned that medical opinion is fragmented when it comes to the management of certain gastrointestinal conditions. Alternative medicine has proposed hypotheses that make sense in many respects, but many alternatives have not satisfied the burden of proof for acceptance in modern, orthodox medicine. Opinions vary, and frank contention prevails in many segments of the study of gut diseases.

We have discussed the arguments that prevail in medicine concerning the presence of food allergies, detoxification, and probiotic therapy. The value of addressing these problems is often questioned by conventional medicine, which in some cases may even deny their existence. Among the most important emerging concepts in alternative medical thinking about gut health are the role of parasitic infections, the value of enzyme supplements, and the acceptance of yeast infection of the bowel as a common cause of ill health. Alternative therapies are being used to address these issues that have recently caught public attention.

PUSHING THE ENVELOPE

A by-product of the close link between medicine and commerce may lead to overenthusiastic support for new concepts in disease causation and treatment. We see examples of this phenomenon in both conventional and alternative medicine: pharmaceutical companies develop new drug therapies that address issues that are important for health with a view to serving large-scale needs. Anything needed on a large scale has great commercial prospects and serves important public health concerns. However, the issues can readily become overplayed or magnified. One example is the use of antisecretory (gastric-acid-suppressing) medications to treat peptic ulcer. When first launched, these drugs revolutionized the treatment of ulcer disease because of their ability to soothe ulcer symptoms in a safe and effective manner. It soon became apparent that an even greater area of potential application of these H_2-blocking drugs (antisecretory drugs) was nonulcer dyspepsia (functional dyspepsia). Physicians were encouraged to use these drugs for this disorder, but controlled clinical trials did not often support the use of H_2 receptor antagonists for these functional gut disorders.

The other side of the coin exists in theories of the practice of alternative medicine. Leaky guts, intestinal dysbiosis, and food allergies are very important issues in general health, but they are not all-encompassing explanations for many diseases. There is a tendency in alternative medicine literature to focus on one potential causative issue, for example, gastrointestinal Candidiasis (yeast infection), and implicate it as a cause of a vast array of medical disorders, even in circumstances where the evidence for a causal link is sometimes quite dubious.

I believe that the phenomenon of pushing the envelope in medicine causes confrontation between alternative and conventional medicine. Pushing the envelope in conventional medicine is the Achilles heal of orthodox medicine, according to the proponents of natural therapies. Pushing the envelope in alternative medicine leads to a quick label of quackery—a label that is not always justified. Time for balance now exists.

Taking these circumstances into account, it is important to analyze the way in which we may approach new theories in medicine (or reactivation of old ideas). After all, one cannot be too critical of the lateral thinker who wants to get a point across, no matter how tenuous the point of view. Debate and scientific study in medical practice leads to advances in diagnosis, prevention, and treatment of disease. Furthermore, it is fun for the intellectually inclined. Precedent shapes the evolution of law, but it does not exert the same influence in medicine. The emergence of natural medicine has created legal issues for which there is little precedent—at least in the eyes of doctor watchers.

UNWANTED GUESTS

Parasites are living organisms that nourish themselves at the expense of another organism. An intermediate type of existence occurs in some living systems, referred to as symbiosis, where two organisms (e.g., plants, friendly bacteria in the bowel, etc.) live together in mutual harmony. The word *parasite* has two roots. The first, *para*, means "beside," and the second, *sitos* refers to food. In literal terms, the parasite is one who eats beside one. In other words, parasites eat someone's food at that person's table.

Recent books defining the ubiquitous nature of parasites have appeared in the popular literature. They reinforce the important concept that parasites are much more common than often suspected, have a good way of hiding, cause a wide variety of debilitating symptoms, and are not at the forefront of the average physician's mind when it comes to diagnosis. Along with the discussion of parasites comes alternative plans to rid the body of parasites, sometimes using dubious or ineffective techniques. Many alternative approaches to the management of parasites have been superseded by modern advances in antimicrobial therapy.

The clever parasite does not kill its host, or cause too much trouble, otherwise it destroys its own advantageous lifestyle. However, the body's accommodation or resistance to parasites can change with age, waning immune function (e.g., HIV), and intercurrent illness. Our environment is loaded with parasites that can enter the body in a variety of ways. Often present in tainted food or water, parasites can enter the body via many routes (skin, lungs, urinary tract). It is an alarming estimate that more than one-half of the entire population of many Western countries may harbor at least one parasite. In many third world countries, carriage of parasites is often the norm.

There are many different types of gut parasites that have complicated names, life cycles and adverse health effects. Among the most common are amoebae, *Giardia*, cryptosporidia, pinworms, tapeworms, and whipworms. The earth is "shrinking" to a global village with increasing foreign travel, and certain parasites that are most often found in exotic places are starting to turn up in people on our own doorstep. Parasites hitch a ride on jets, cruise ships, and in cargo transport. The idea of parasites in the body gives many people a sense of intense fear, but many states of parasitosis may be quite innocuous, even though it is better to be without parasites! Parasitosis is mistakenly associated with dirt or lack of personal hygiene. While these factors can make parasitosis more prevalent, parasites know no social boundaries—especially among children in schools or day care centers.

SYMPTOMS AND SIGNS OF DISEASE FROM PARASITES

Parasites are great mimics of many specific diseases or nonspecific disorders of health. There are often no specific diagnostic signs, and symptoms of parasites and their detection often rest on careful investigations by laboratory tests. Table 12.1 lists a whole host of clinical features that can occur with parasites. It is notable that parasites often cause symptom complexes that are identical to functional gut disorders.

Table 12.1: An incomplete list of the clinical consequences of parasites.

GASTROINTESTINAL UPSET: almost any upset ranging from gas and bloating to mechanical obstruction of the bowels requiring surgery.

MUSCULOSKELETAL COMPLAINTS: a wide variety of muscle aches, joint pain, and arthritis.

ALLERGIC CONSEQUENCES: creeping sensations, itching, and a variety of skin rashes.

GENERAL PROBLEMS: sleep disturbances, chronic fatigue, metabolic upset, debility, nutritional deficiencies, mental problems, excessive hunger, and immune dysfunction.

GUT PARASITES

There are so many parasites that can freeload on humans that curiosity can be satisfied only by reference to large medical textbooks on the subject. Unwanted parasitic guests fall into the broad categories of protozoa (single-celled organisms) and worms or helminths. Worms and helminths are world citizens and common travelers. A variety of routes of transmission exist for parasites, including food and water contamination, insect or animal contacts, and sexual practices.

Giardia lamblia is a protozoan parasite that infects as many as 20 million people in the United States. *Giardia* is transmitted in its hardy cyst through food and water, and it is a frequent guest in human and animal stools. Infection with this organism can cause myriad gut symptoms, and its presence can be frequently overlooked. Diagnosis is not always easy because *Giardia* is present intermittently in the stool and, sometimes, it has to be located by diagnostic tests by direct sampling of its principal site of colonization, in the upper parts of the small bowel.

This organism is particularly common in the water supply of certain Rocky Mountain communities (e.g., Banff in Canada), and the chances are that a trip to St. Petersburg in Russia will result in infestation—at least at the time of writing this book—where outbreaks of giardiasis are continuous. You do not need to be a world traveler to encounter Giardia, it is present in urban areas and it seems to have found a well-suited home in children's day care centers. Alternative sexual activities (oral and anal sex) are identified as risky practices for the spread of *Giardia*, which is a member of several organisms that make up the infectious components of the "gay bowel syndrome." This syndrome has been described in male homosexuals (and more adventurous heterosexuals).

Tapeworms from dogs (*Diphylidium caninum*); from rats, mice and hamsters (*Hymenolepsis nana*); from cattle (*Taenia saginata*); from pigs (*Taenia solium*); and from fish (*Diphyllobothrium latum*), and roundworms from equivalent sources, are quite common. In general, food hygiene and good personal hygiene are important preventive measures, but the diagnosis and treatment of these parasites, and significant infection with other parasites, is not a job for self-medicators or the occasional medical "expert." A wide variety of effective drugs are available to treat parasites, but they are often toxic and the results of these treatments need to be monitored. Many other common parasites exist—some just live in harmony with humans. Perhaps the most common of all parasites, which occasionally causes serious problems, is the pinworm (*Enterobius vermicularis*). This worm is present in one of five adults, and infection rates are up to 80 percent in children below the age of eleven years.

NATURAL THERAPIES FOR PARASITIC INFECTION

Some natural therapies for parasites are to be recommended, but in general, remedies of natural origin are best used in the prevention of parasites with lifestyle changes or as adjuncts to specific medical treatments. Digestive enzymes, enemas, essential plant oils, laxatives, and changing diets to foods that are unfriendly to parasites are not ideal approaches to ridding the body of parasites. The concept of purging parasites is a modern myth. Parasites are clever organisms that are not easily fooled by a dose of salts!

Despite advances in antiparasitic drug therapy, a significant proportion of people in third world countries use herbal combinations to prevent or treat parasites. There is a reactivated interest in the use of herbals and botanicals to combat parasitosis, but this use of remedies of natural origin has not been fully researched and it cannot be considered reliable as sole or principal therapy. There may be an adjunctive role for herbs in the therapy of parasites, and a number of natural agents with potential value are summarized in Table 12.2.

THE CANDIDA CONTROVERSY

Medicine recognizes yeast, *Candida albicans*, as an opportunistic infection, but the disease of chronic yeast infection (candidiasis) of the bowel has precipitated all-out fights between orthodox and alternative physicians. Conventional medicine perceives *Candida* as a nor-

Table 12.2: Some natural agents used to treat parasites.

Note, these approaches are at best adjuncts, should not be used for self-therapy of parasites and their clinical value is sometimes dubious.

NATURAL AGENT	COMMENT
Garlic	Relatively large doses of garlic have antimicrobial properties and inhibit the growth of several worms and helminths—effects not reliable.
Angelica	Has been used to inhibit trichomonal infection with variable success—it has unpredictable toxicity.
Wormwood	Artemesia species are used to help expel round-worms, but they are toxic at even moderate doses.
Berberine-containing plants	Goldenseal (Hydrastis canadensis) and Berberis species contain berberine, which is an ancient antimicrobial and antiparasitic—it is rarely standardized in supplements and cannot be considered reliable treatment unless used by an expert.
Ipecac	Causes vomiting but it is toxic—a derivative, dehydroemetine, has been used for amoeba infestations, but its use has been superseded.
Turmeric	Contains powerful antioxidants, e.g., curcumin. In Ayurveda it is a "blood purifier." It may help expel worms.
Grapefruit seed extract	Relatively safe and it possesses a wide antimicrobial and antiparasite spectrum. Useful adjunctive therapy when used by an expert.
Holistic approaches	Intestinal cleansing, dietary modification, digestive enzymes, and probiotics are often used but clinical outcome studies are lacking.

mal and innocuous inhabitant of the gut except in cases of immunodeficiency (or severe body compromise), but alternative and naturopathic medicine sees *Candida* as a sinister, disease-causing agent. I believe that the real circumstance lies somewhere between these polar viewpoints.

Two books published in the early 1980s (C. Truss, *The Missing Diagnosis,* and W. G. Crook, *The Yeast Connection*) precipitated a heated medical debate that has gone on for two decades. These books highlighted gastrointestinal yeast infection with *Candida* (candidiasis) as a cause of much ill health and infection or general toxicity affecting the body. The publication of these books did not provide a new hypothesis, because a debate on the significance of gut candidiasis had "grumbled" on in medical circles since the 1950s. At present, conflicting publications are appearing that either question or reinforce the significance of gut infection with the yeast *Candida albicans*.

Is Candidiasis of the Gut a Real Disease?

The answer to this question is a qualified "yes." In states of weakened immune system (e.g., HIV), *Candida* can cause very severe infections with tissue inflammation, penetration of the gut wall by this yeast organism, and systemic spread of disease (e.g., esophageal candidiasis). Several convincing studies show that the gut is a reservoir of *Candida* infection, especially in females with vulval or vaginal yeast infections. If the source of *Candida* in the bowel in patients with vaginal thrush (candidiasis of vulva or vagina) is not treated, relapse of infection is common and cure is unlikely. *Candida* is, however, quite difficult to completely eradicate—it is a commensal organism often, that does little harm.

Beyond the presence of yeast alone at a site of infection, some scientific studies show the development of circulating antibodies to *Candida*. These antibodies can result in localized or more generalized hypersensitivity reactions. While these immune phenomena have been well-defined in vaginal candidiasis, fewer studies are available on patients with suspected gastrointestinal candidiasis. Studies in naturopathic medicine seem to imply a relationship between a number of troublesome symptoms (ill health) and both the presence and degree of *Candida* growth in the gut, as measured in yeast cultures from stool samples.

There is no doubt that *Candida* can enter the body readily through the gut. Events that are more likely to lead to this entry of *Candida* include antibiotic administration or severe coexisting illness. Antibiotic administration may suppress friendly bacteria (normal bowel microflora) and allow greater adhesion of the yeast to the gut wall. One compelling piece of evidence on the ease with which yeast enters the body from the gut comes from a brave experiment by Dr. W. Krause, published in 1969 (*Lancet*, 1:598–599). Dr. Krause, an otherwise healthy person, swallowed a large dose of *Candida*. Following this self-administration of yeast, Dr. Kause suffered headache, fever, and chills. Up to six hours after the ingestion of the *Candida*, the yeast organism (of the same specific type) was found in blood and urine samples taken from this self-experimenting scientist.

Candida Has Measurable Toxins

Careful microbiological studies demonstrate that *Candida* presents a variety of toxic components from its own structure (endotoxins) or as a consequence of its own chemistry producing toxins (exotoxins). One toxin of specific interest, called gliotoxin (an epipolythiodiox-piperazine compound), has measurable effects on immunity and white cell function. Gliotoxin from *Candida* can cause immune supression by reducing the number of lymphocytes in the bone marrow, the spleen, the thymus, and the lymphatic tissues of the gut. In addition, it can interfere with the ability of special white cells to engulf antigens (phagocytic inhibition). The controversy about the real significance of gut candidiasis involves complex arguments and some chicken-and-egg debates. These debates involve: Which came first, the immunosuppression followed by *Candida* infection, or *Candida* infection causing the immune deficiency?

One of the most questioning, but well-presented, points of view against the significance of chronic *candidiasis* syndrome was published by Dr. W. E. Dismukes and his colleagues in the *New England Journal of Medicine* in 1990 (*NEJ Med*, 323:1717–1723). In this randomized, double-blind trial of antiyeast therapy (nystatin) in women with vaginal candidiasis, the control group seemed to respond as well as the group receiving active treatment. Of course, this study is not adequate information to dismiss the occurrence of the chronic yeast syndrome due to gut candidiasis and clearly more work is required.

There are many credible reports of benefits of the treatment of chronic gut candidiasis in patients who are not significantly immuno-suppressed, and it appears that this disorder is a potential cause of digestive upset that may otherwise be labeled functional in nature. I am less convinced that chronic candidiasis in the gut is at the root of many diseases that are alleged to be closely or causatively linked to infection with this yeast. Gut candidiasis is notoriously difficult to detect with simple tests. On balance, the empiric treatment of yeast infection of the gut seems a reasonable option for carefully selected patients, because treatment of *Candida* is generally safe and several remedies of natural origin are beneficial. Perhaps eradication of *Candida* is not the key, but a reduction in the number of yeasts present in the gut that act to tip the balance. Nystatin is a safe drug to treat *Candida*. Ketoconazole is more effective, but it is not as safe as nystatin. Undecylenic and caprylic acids (fatty acids) inhibit yeast growth, as do essential oils of certain plants—especially peppermint, fennel, oregano, thyme, and cinnamon. A highly effective way of tipping the balance is to take enteric-coated peppermint oil, which is very unfriendly to yeast and other microorganisms. Probiotic supplements are quite valuable in restoring normal flora that compete to "knock out" excessive growth of the *Candida* yeast.

I believe sufficient evidence exists that chronic gut infection with *Candida* in people with intact immunity can cause ill health. Yeast may cross the gut barrier, and produce toxins that can damage gut function to a variable degree. The diagnosis of this entity requires the development of more stringent criteria, but cultures and special antibody testing may help. Since the treatment of this disorder is often safe and simple with selected drugs or natural remedies, empiric therapy may be justified in select cases of suspicion.

MIND-BODY MEDICINE

Traditional medicine has tended to stay away from faith, prayer, love, belief, and spirituality in healing. Physicians who dared to address these issues in the first half of the twentieth century often paid a heavy price for their proposals about the power of mind-body medicine. Things have changed greatly as we start the new millennium. Psychosocial issues and belief systems are being studied increasingly in disease treatment and prevention. Evidence has accumulated that attention to these more ethereal aspects of medical treatment is justified by their apparent effectiveness. This emerging situation provides great support for the art of holistic healing.

This book has tended to concentrate on functional gastrointestinal disorders with strong mind-body and body-mind links. The future of dealing with functional gastrointestinal disorders may rest in dealing with more holistic concepts. Unfortunately, training in behavioral sciences has not been emphasized in conventional medical training, but it forms the basis of modern alternative medical approaches. Modern alternative medicine has taken its cues from several ancient treatment disciplines. The notion that psychological well-being and faith are powerful healers is not a strange proposal, but conventional medicine appears to be somewhat reluctant to act in these areas.

There is quite convincing evidence that faith is linked to health. At least two dozen modern studies show a positive relation between faith (spiritual or religious commitments) and health or longevity. Individuals with spiritual (or religious) belief have been shown to have better outcomes in chronic disease treatments and cancer therapy. Depression, suicide and more destructive types of lifestyle habits are less common in the spiritually inclined. Of surprise to some physicians may be surveys which show that members of religious groups have lower disease rates and death rates than nonmembers. This health advantage appears to be present even when risk factors such as obesity, lack of exercise, smoking, and drinking alcohol are taken into account.

The roles of love, good interpersonal relationships, and sex in health and healing have caught much recent attention. In my book *The Sexual Revolution* (Wellness Publishing Inc., 1999), I review evidence for the role of close and optimal emotional ties as key determinants of health.

There are many disciplines of alternative medicine that are focused on mind-body healing. Biofeedback training has infiltrated modern gastroenterology practice. In this technique, the body's functions (e.g., defecation or gut pressures) can be monitored using specially designed equipment. The information derived from the monitoring process is given to the subject so that they can gain control over body functions. The simplistic notion that the organs of the body are controlled by only the voluntary and the autonomic nervous system is misleading. Groundbreaking work by Dr. Neal E. Miller in New York in the 1960s showed that rats who were paralyzed by curare (a relaxant poison) could be taught to control their autonomic nervous system responses. This work is well extended in human experiments that show that brain activity, and heart, and digestive function can be controlled by biofeedback training. This is visceral learning "from simple teaching."

A number of branches of alternative medicine that focus on the mind-body may have great use in the adjunctive management of gut disorders. Several excellent overviews of alternative medicine practice can be consulted for details about these treatments which include: Yoga, sound therapy, hypnosis, acupuncture, Ayurveda, and reflexology, with more controversial therapies such as pyramid healing, pattern therapy, radesthesia, and radionics. All of these therapies have a direct or an indirect mind-body approach.

Can Gut Contents "Talk" to the Brain?

At first sight, the idea that the gut contents can communicate with the brain seems too far-fetched to be worthy of consideration. Examples of this phenomenon exist, however. Under certain circumstances, such as liver disease, excessive protein in the gut can result in excessive production of ammonia produced by bacterial fermentation. Ammonia can enter the circulation, and it causes changes in personality, psychomotor function, and wakefulness—part of the syndrome of hepatic encephalopathy (brain upset).

The model of hepatic encephalopathy is a relatively crude example of how gut contents can communicate with the central nervous system. Let us hypothesize that there is an organism (a bacterium, protozoan, yeast, or parasite) in the bowel that elaborates a molecule or has a component part that can enter the body and cause a communication. It is known that receptors (targets) in the body tissues are activated by molecules. Then, why do we not have constant communications going on between gut contents and the tissues of the body? The answer is that we do, even if the gut contents (digesta) act by changing the gut itself, which then communicates!

In order to further consider these concepts, it is important to study the work and hypotheses of the psychoimmunologists who are perhaps better referred to as psychoneuroendocrinimmunologists. As I discussed earlier in this book, these new terms talk about the massive interconnecting highway of the molecules and receptors described by great lateral thinkers—most notably Candace Pert. I am scratching the surface of the concept of "Molecules of Emotion" described by Dr. Pert in her groundbreaking book.

I would like to extend and reiterate in this book some of Dr. Pert's observations on the "unity of life," which I have referred to earlier in this book by conceptualizing the Gaiaguts. Dr. Pert draws attention to the presence of many of the same body chemicals and messengers that are found in both primitive organisms and humans. In particular, she cites the single-celled tetrahymena, which has a variety of receptors on its cell surface, including those for insulin, endorphins, and opiates. Thus, humans share with primitive life forms the same types of molecules and receptor sites that can facilitate intercommunications (from organism to organism) and intracommunications (within the organism itself). Dr. Pert proposes that these shared biological and biochemical properties of organisms represent a clear example of the unity of life.

Obviously, science has a long way to go in understanding communication highways among organisms (and between live and inert objects in the universe). If we add to this scientific and philosophical soup the notion of unexplained life forces, such as those described by Rupert Sheldrake, Ph.D., and other scientists, we have a new horizon of potential understanding. Does it now seem so remote an idea that organisms within or outside our body can have a series of complex, yet-to-be-defined communications? One may dismiss these thoughts by pointing to the gut itself as the barrier to communication between the gut contents (digesta) and the body (or brain). However, the organisms may break down the communication barrier (cause leaky gut) or use the gut itself as the instrument of communication.

THE FOOD ENZYME CONCEPT

Enzymes are absolutely necessary for the normal absorption of nutrients from the diet. It has been suggested that "you are what you eat," but it is more accurate to say "you are what you absorb into your body" (a comment attributed to the naturopath and scientist Dr. Jeffrey Bland, Ph.D.). I add that you are also a function of your gut contents .

The idea of supplementing a diet with enzymes in order to improve digestion and health has become very popular. In part, this is a myth, related to a misguided notion that more is better. In states of enzyme deficiency, such as failure of the pancreas to secrete enzymes (e.g. chronic pancreatitis), the value of enzyme supplements is unquestionable. However, in states of health, there is still relatively little evidence that adding digestive enzymes is materially beneficial. Adding enzymes to the diet, for example, pancreatic enzymes, results in an inhibition of enzyme production (by the pancreas). Of course, we'll find that the story is not so simple as we examine the concept of food enzyme nutrition.

The most complete source of information on the food enzyme concept is the book *Enzyme Nutrition* by the late Dr. Edward Howell (Wayne, NJ: Avery Publishing 1985). Dr. Howell spent a lifetime dedicated to the study of food enzymes and human health. Enzyme supplementation has been considered a nature cure by many people. The basic series of ideas about this concept is that enzymes operate on chemical and biological levels, and at their core, they have a biological force. The hypotheses of Dr. Howell imply that everyone is given a finite supply of bodily enzyme energy at birth, and the faster one uses up the enzyme supply, the faster one ages. These concepts are interesting, difficult to study, controversial, but somewhat congruent with a few proposed models of aging.

Current biological theories of aging stress the repair budget that different species of animals possess. The repair budget refers to the body's investment in regeneration. Longevity is undoubtedly related to genetic factors (genes, DNA composition in chromosomes), and the expression of these factors is heavily influenced by environment. Many different biological experiments or experiences support this notion.

Mice and rats with a longer life span have been genetically engineered, and the same animals studied in different environments have different life spans. For example, the opossum living in the Midwest in a hostile environment does not live as long as the opossum living in a protected island environment off the east coast of America. The suggestion is that a safe environment permits the expression of genetic information that controls the body's repair budget. Thus, if enzymes have a finite supply and life, repair budgets are important in lifespan and health. The question remains whether or not there is a finite supply of enzymes or their biological core of "force."

This line of lateral thinking, however, is highly relevant if the elusive biological forces are accepted as being present in enzymes. In addition, the concept of a finite supply of enzymes requires acceptance, with the knowledge that the body can produce enzymes, even though the environment places a heavy burden on the body to manufacture enzymes. I have a difficult time swallowing these concepts of food enzyme nutrition, which require a belief system that transcends science. I stress, however, the limitations of our current level of scientific knowledge.

Howell's Axiom

Dr. Edward Howell proposed a concept that he referred to as the Enzyme Nutrition Axiom which reads: "The *length of life* is inversely proportional to the rate of exhaustion of the *enzyme potential* of an organism. The increased use of food enzymes promotes a *decreased* rate of exhaustion of the enzyme potential."

The axiom stresses the definition in biological rather than chemical terms, but orthodox science balks at proposals of unexplained forces in nature. The "vital energy factor" within enzymes that has been proposed by Dr. Howell defies any simple explanation. Dr. Howell emphasized that he believed that enzymes were not "mere chemical flunkies" that are "recklessly expendable." In brief, the concept of enzyme nutrition suggests that living organisms can endow enzymes with a "vital activity factor," and this factor can be used up over time. Unfortunately, the concept is not tenable for ye of little faith—including myself.

Using Food Enzyme Supplements

Having expressed my lack of faith for the food enzyme concept, I cannot ignore the repetitive claims that digestive enzyme supplements are useful for health purposes. I do not criticize the use of digestive enzymes if enzyme production is impaired in the digestive organs (e.g., pancreatic disease). I am very impressed by Dr. Howell's comparative anatomy studies of the digestive tracts of many animals, which he used in his efforts to explain the importance of the preservation of enzymes within food. The idea of preservation of enzymes in food is used in modern, alternative medicine theory to support the use of uncooked, raw, or "live food." The notion of "live food"—containing active enzymes—is of growing interest in naturopathic and alternative medicine.

This concept has led to the widespread sale of "green foods." These "green" products contain an array of vegetable and plant sources of enzymes that are considered very healthy and very versatile in their application. These greens are often sold in powders to make beverages with juice. While they are very healthful sources of vitanutrients, they have not been systematically studied for the vast number of health reasons for which they are sold. "Miracle greens" have flooded the supplement market with health claims that transcend any critical analysis or clinical studies.

A number of scientists of the New Age persuasion have expressed Old Age ideas. It is proposed in New Age medicine that the worst thing man ever did in his evolutionary process was to cook food. In modern times, a lobby existed for the inclusion of raw foods in the diet. These are often "live foods"—by virtue of their enzyme content. This approach sounds logical, but raw food comes with problems. Untreated milk, for example, is a great potential source of transmissible infection from cows (e.g., Brucellosis). In addition, raw foods like beans, nuts, and seeds contain enzyme inhibitors that may affect digestion. This is now recognized by food enzyme zealots who propose adding enzyme supplements to overcome the effects of naturally occurring enzyme inhibitors. This proposal seems absurd.

Enzyme inhibitors in certain foods have been called antinutrients as a consequence of their ability to impair protein absorption. A good example of a food of great medicinal interest is the soybean, which in its crude form is a rich source of trypsin inhibitors and other enzyme antagonists. Again, the situation is far from simple because these enzyme inhibitors in soybeans, which have received the bad label of "antinutrients," may be some of the most interesting naturally occurring medicinals. For example, the trypsin inhibitor known as the Bowman Birk Inhibitor has some exciting anticancer properties.

One solution is to focus on the use of germinated seeds in the diet (sprouts), where the presence of enzyme inhibitors is decreased. Soybean sprouts, barley sprouts, alfalfa sprouts, etc., are very healthy "live foods" with clear nutritional advantages for their phytochemical contents and arguable benefits because of their enzyme content.

To summarize, enzyme supplementation in the face of known enzyme deficiency is almost mandatory. The food enzyme concept is worthy of more research, and on an empiric basis, it may be valuable in selected people. Enzyme supplements from plants, e.g., papain and bromelain, have great use in alternative medicine—for reasons other than their reliability in assisting digestion. Bromelain is very useful in treating soft tissue bruising and joint injury.

Pancreatic enzyme supplements are reported in observational studies to improve a variety of diseases (e.g., cancer, diabetes, malnutrition), but hard scientific data on their benefit as additives to the diet, in the presence of adequate enzyme secretion, is lacking. Lipase has been proposed as beneficial for cardiovascular health, but its oral administration—like that of many other enzymes—is problematic because of its inactivation in the upper gut. Its actions are pH dependent. In conclusion, the jury remains out on digestive enzyme supplement use in the absence of enzyme deficiencies.

IT MAY BE YOUR DRUGS

The tail end of this century has seen an increasing scrutiny of iatrogenic diseases (doctor or treatment-induced disease). Nowhere is this more apparent than in the use of drug therapy. Side effects, illness, and deaths from prescription or OTC drug use are shockingly common and probably underestimated because of voluntary reporting systems of adverse drug effects. Recent studies place iatrogenic drug deaths as one of the leading causes of death in the United States.

The alternative medical profession has seized the opportunity to claim that remedies of natural origin are safer than drugs and cite the few reports of problems with herbs, botanicals ,and nutritionals in dietary supplement format. Again, balance is required in our approach to these polar viewpoints—there are problems on both sides of the fence!

Who said dietary supplements are safe? The biggest message on the safety of supplements comes from the people who sell them; they are often right, but they are sometimes wrong. The underreporting of adverse effects of supplements is a greater potential problem for herbals and botanicals than it is for drugs. This is largely because there is less research with less safety monitoring of dietary supplements, even in short-term studies or clinical experiences. The dietary supplement industry has not been given a responsibility to do any postmarketing surveillance studies. Herbals and botanicals, however, often have a leg up on drugs because of the frequently quoted precedent—based over centuries of use of herbs and botanicals in some circumstances in traditional medical disciplines.

The issue of drug safety is a mounting public health concern, and it is a principal disincentive to drug use that precipitates many people to question traditional (conventional) approaches. This argument is balanced by the uncertainty about the safety of some remedies of natural origin and a relative lack of scientific support for treatment claims of dietary supplements in some circumstances.

Adverse drug reactions can mimic many different types of gastrointestinal disease or upset. This issue has been the subject of several books that explain the complexity of the circumstances. Table 12.3 lists some examples of drugs that cause gastrointestinal side effects, but one should be aware that a similar—perhaps less extensive list of adverse events—can be constructed for herbs and botanicals. Some of these are addressed in Table 12.3.

Table 12.3: Drugs with gastrointestinal side effects.

This table provides an important but incomplete overview of how many drugs and certain dietary supplements can cause gut symptoms or serious gastrointestinal disease. Information on all drug and supplement toxicities on the gut is rarely carried around in the head of a physician or a pharmacist, and computer data or reference books may have to be consulted to link a side effect with a drug or supplement—especially when the adverse effect is not common. Doctors and pharmacists are encouraged by the government to report side effects so that our knowledge can approve. Note: not all side effects of dietary supplements or drugs are known when they are first released.

GUT PROBLEM	EXAMPLE
Esophagus	Tetracycline, aspirin, NSAIDs, potassium chloride, and irritant herbs may cause strictures; death from NSAIDs and cancer chemotherapy, e.g., 5 fluorouracid have been described.

GUT PROBLEM	EXAMPLE
Non-specific abdominal symptoms	Loss of appetite is common with several "mimics of functional disease," cardiovascular drugs (e.g., quinidine, digoxin), and antimicrobials (e.g., ketoconazole, rifampicin). A whole host of drugs or dietary supplements cause nausea or vomiting (e.g., NSAIDs, zinc lozenges). Abdominal pain is frequent with NSAID usage.
Pancreas	Azathioprine, chlorothiazide, methyl dopa, and tetracycline have been definitely associated with pancreatitis, a number of others may be, e.g., cimelidine, metronidazole, phenformin, NSAIDs and corticosteroids.
Stomach	Aspirin and NSAIDs are common causes of stomach damage and peptic ulcer; damage can occur from erythromycin, steroids, potassium, and iron salts. Supplements containing similar chemicals could have similar actions.
Intestines	A variety of drugs can cause small bowel or malabsorption damage, leaky gut, or malabsorption. Direct toxic effects on the gut lining are caused by colchicine, methotrexate, antibiotics (neomycin and tetracycline). Some drugs or agents cause enzyme inhibition, e.g., soluble fiber, chloramphenicol. Folate malabsorption caused by sulphasalazine (a sulphonamide), phenytoin, trimethoprim, triamterene. Binding agents, e.g. , cholestyramine, antacids, and raw plants or herbs can stop absorption of certain nutrients.
Diarrhea or constipation	Changes in motility (gut movements) and absorption processes and mucosal (lining) damage by drugs can lead to diarrhea or constipation. Hundreds of drugs and supplements can cause these problems, ranging from calcium supplements (constipation) to magnesium (diarrhea) through to sulphonamides, aspirin, hormones, cholesterol-lowering drugs, etc.
Liver	Many drugs and compounds in dietary supplements can affect liver function. The changes in the liver range from simple chemical interference through to severe liver damage (even causing death). Common toxins are acetaminophen (in excess), tetracycline, NSAIDs etc. Cholestasis (stagnation of bile) is caused often by sex hormones (oral contraceptives, hormone replacement), anabolic steroids, major sedatives, antibiotics, erythromycin, cephalosporins, etc. Fatty liver is seen with corticosteroids, tetracycline, and several anticancer drugs. Liver tumors are caused by anabolic-androgenic steroids—a real reason to avoid self-medication with hormones.

Safety of Dietary Supplements

Drug developments have often come from the study of active components of plants or herbs. In fact, hundreds of synthetic drugs can be considered variations on naturally occurring compounds. The study of the development of medicines from plants is called pharmacognosy. Over the past fifty years or so, the importance of pharmacognosy in medical science has been overshadowed by synthetic drug development strategies. Given the widespread availability of remedies of natural origin, more emphasis has to be placed on pharmacognosy. This important pharmacy discipline was until recently a subject that was dropped in many pharmacy and medical curriculae at universities.

I am a strong proponent of remedies of natural origin, but the chronic use of some herbs poses uncertain safety concerns. The whole situation has been compounded by the disappearance of descriptions of many herbal and botanical agents from treatment pharmacopoeias (books that describe herbal, drug, and botanical treatments). This trend started in the 1950s when the postwar advance in pharmaceutical science occurred.

Attempts are being made to piece this knowledge back together by creating revised pharmacopoeias of knowledge. Not enough is being done by governments in this important area. For example, the British Herbal Pharmacopea relies on the voluntary support of many experts with little—if any significant—government funding. The United States has not done a better job, but Germany, through its E-Commission, has produced valuable monographs on herbal use and safety. The E-Commission series of documents on herbals and botanicals takes the lead as a good source of information. The same effort must occur in other Western communities—even if it only involves "borrowing" German science.

Drug Depletion of Nutrients

While attention has focused on drug side effects, a new, important area of concern is emerging in natural medicine. Taking drug therapy is associated with many less obtrusive problems for health. An obvious example is the use of NSAIDs, which has been discussed extensively in this book. It is recognized that NSAIDs do their damage largely by interfering with the protective effects of the prostaglandins (chemicals made in the body). However, NSAIDs will deplete cell membranes of essential fatty ingredients such as phospholipids. Therefore, one approach to the problems is to give the phospholipids that are depleted by the administration of the NSAID. This concept is at the basis of a variety of drug-depletion formulas that have started to appear in retail pharmacy practice. (See www.drugdepletion.com)

This approach in preventive medicine is a good example of how dietary supplements can be used in a well-planned scientific approach in medicine. Hypothetical and substantive problems can exist with this approach of presenting drug depletion formulas of supplements. This is apparent when the components of the formula may interfere with the action of the drug. Concerns have been expressed about this circumstance in chemotherapy for cancer or other diseases, but recent data seem to dispell many of these worries.

A simple example is that if an antagonist to a vitamin is used as a drug, such as a folic acid antagonist, then giving folic acid may interfere with the treatment process. Extending this situation to the treatment of cancer, it has been suggested that there are circumstances where giving vitamins or nutrients to a patient with cancer may encourage the cancer to grow. Thus, another classic double-edged sword emerges, and we have to explore these circumstances with more scientific studies.

Examples of several of my drug-depletion formulas that use dietary supplements are to be found on the Internet (see www.drugdepletion.com). Dietary supplements can be used to support body functions that can be altered adversely by drug administration, as a consequence of specific nutrient depletion.

SUPPLEMENTS: FROM BRICK-AND-MORTAR TO E-COMMERCE

Pharmacists have always been in a unique position to contribute to prescribing decisions and provide counseling services on drug therapy to patients. Somehow, this important role of the pharmacist has never been realized fully in clinical practice. Things are changing dramatically as many ethical pharmaceuticals have become available OTC, and consumers of healthcare demonstrate an increasing self-reliance to self-diagnose and self-medicate.

There is an increasing need for pharmacists to provide information on natural therapies, remedies of natural origin, herbals, botanicals, nutritionals and nutriceuticals – call them what one will. Many "green pharmacies" (pharmacies selling supplements) have popped up in the past two years, where varying amounts of floor space are set aside for the sale of dietary supplements. In independent and chain pharmacies in Europe, as much as 50 percent of the floor space has been turned over to natural products, and these alternatives sometimes stand alongside branded OTC drugs.

These days, we contend with new developments in information technology, where consumers have mounting exposure to advertising, marketing, and educational material on an ever-increasing array of drugs and natural agents. One area of particular importance is the Internet or World Wide Web. Perhaps as many as 30 million people will be using the internet by the turn of the year 2001 and a large proportion of these users (percentage yet to be defined) seek healthcare information and engage in direct purchases from online drugstores, cyberpharmacies, and Web purveyors of dietary supplements.

Pharmacies are moving increasingly from retail locations (bricks) to online sales (e-commerce). In many respects, switching from bricks to e-commerce has greater social, medical, political, and legal implications than switching ethical drugs to OTC status. The 1990s will be recognized as the decade of the pharmaceutical switch. It is perhaps interesting that this switching has occurred simultaneously with a more widespread availability of remedies of natural origin, in dietary supplement format, largely as a consequence of the Dietary Supplement and Health Education Act of 1994.

For pharmacists to fulfill their role as counselors on drug and supplement use, they must now be represented on the Net. It is not unlikely that up to 10 percent of all drug sales could occur via the Internet within the next three years or so, (by the year 2003), and 20 percent of all nutriceutical sales could occur on the Net in the same time frame. That is why it is so gratifying to see emerging Web sites with significant educational content on nutriceuticals that are run by pharmacists, for example, www.arrowrx.com, www.familymeds.com, www.merckmedco.com, etc. We do live with an enigma when it comes to dietary supplement use. U.S. law does not permit dietary supplements to be used to diagnose, prevent, or treat disease, but consumer surveys imply that supplements are most often used for the latter two purposes.

Regardless of prevailing opinions on who should advise individuals about the use of dietary supplements, the Internet shows signs of taking over as a primary information source on healthcare and, in particular, the use of nutriceuticals (see www.enaturalhealth.com). The pundits in the health food industry tend to concentrate their attention on dietary supplements, but we now have to face even more complex issues with food products. The neologism *Frugs* is emerging in the language of regulatory affairs. A frug is food that is being misrepresented and sold with a drug claim. Frugs could breed new regulators who practice "frugology."

Even more confusing are many new terms applied to foods that have little or no regulatory meaning (in the United States at least), including: nutriceutical meals, functional foods, engineered foods, foods for special nutritional purpose, etc. Regulators are focusing increasing interest on distinctions between food, dietary supplements, and drugs. Precedent is sadly lacking to define many of the gray areas between these categories.

There is a growth of misleading (or frankly deceptive) information on the Web. Industry giants like Merck-Medco Inc., CVS Inc., Drugstore.com, PlanetRX, Soma.com, and MotherNature.com are tackling the issues of valid educational information for consumers. MotherNature.com is information intensive, and it has a prestigious advisory panel that reviews the content of the Web site.

In addition to consumers, physicians, pharmacists, and an eclectic group of healthcare givers are using the Internet increasingly to find condition-specific, drug-specific, and dietary supplement–specific information that is credible. Deciding on what information is credible in alternative therapeutics is very problematic. It is proposed that the sponsorship of the site give a clue to believability of its content. One point of view directs surfers on the Net to Web sites controlled by the government (suffix .gov), not-for-profit organizations (suffix .org), or higher learning institutions (suffix .edu). This is not the entire solution, because many commercial sites with the .com suffix contain valid scientific information. Government Web sites are often quite conservative in their content on health claims for natural products, and higher learning institutions (bearing the suffix .edu) may range from accredited institutions to nonaccredited and highly unconventional centers of higher education. It is very difficult to sort the wheat from the chaff on the Net!

The newfound process of Internet counseling, drug prescribing, and supplement recommendations confuses matters. Pages may solicit consumer questions to be answered by "experts." Whatever the level of expertise of the Net respondent, virtual diagnosis is fraught with problems. It may even be frankly dangerous in some circumstances. We live in fast-moving and exciting times in healthcare.

NEW TESTING FOR GUT DISORDERS

A revolutionary approach to testing gut function, screening for disease, and monitoring alternative or nutritional therapies is emerging. This new type of testing is in many circumstances based on "good science," but its value has not often been adequately defined. In some circumstances, the testing is performed with certain assumptions, e.g., *Candida* overgrowth is a common cause of disease, or oxidative stress is a principal factor in the causation of chronic disease, or leaky guts need detecting and treating?

While a scientific rationale may exist for using some of these new approaches in laboratory diagnosis, the test panels are expensive and they are not always approved by regulatory affair bureaus. Without a clear examination of the sensitivity or specificity of these newly proposed tests, their cost-benefit cannot be assessed. In this newfound area of elaborate testing, there are examples of alternative medical thinking engaged in leaps of faith, sometimes resulting in the confusion of faith or belief with science.

Testing Examples and Concepts

One commercial laboratory that specialized in "alternative diagnostics" alleges that there is a single test for the assessment of intestinal-barrier function using sensitive detections of serum IgA, IgG, and IgM antibodies to purified proteins from different dietary proteins. These proteins are listed as components of "three aerobic" bacteria (oxygen requiring), "two anaerobic" bacteria (nonoxygen requiring), and three strains of *Candida*. The reasoning behind the use of this test contains assumptions that alterations in immune responses to microflora can be considered a reliable measure of a leaky gut. I doubt the validity of this assumption that involves naïve thinking. The naïveté is that one test could measure a process subject to many complex variables, using only a small number of examples of immune reactions.

Another test of increasing popularity in alternative gastroen-terology is the detection of toxic products in stool samples. In this type of testing, it is alleged that the detection of chemicals or metals in the stool can provide a comprehensive evaluation of environmen-tal exposure to toxins, accumulation of toxins, and signs of detoxifi-cation by the body. While the detection of heavy metals and other poi-sons is important, fecal-toxin testing tells one only what is present at the time of testing and little else.

There are many more different types of new and expensive exam-ples of alternative testing that often emanates from the lateral thoughts of alternative or environmental medicine. It remains quite possible that some of these new approaches to testing may be help-ful in selected cases, but until they can be accepted as a routine part of clinical practice, a lot more research is required to determine their value.

One of the best overviews of new types of approaches to gas-trointestinal testing has been provided by Dr. Jeffrey Bland, Ph.D. Table 12.4 summarizes proposed approaches, but I recommend cau-tion about their validity, diagnostic accuracy, and overall management value.

HOMEOPATHY

There has been an exponential increase in the use of homeopathic remedies in a variety of diseases. Homeopathic medicine is based on "contrarian" principles—contrarian only to orthodox thought in med-

Table 12.4: Examples of some functional testing approaches in several diseases that link concepts of "alternative gastroenterology" to testing.

The author does not entirely endorse this approach but acknowledges some of its values in future research. The data are modified from the work of Dr. Jeffrey Bland and colleagues.

Indications	Functional assessment options
• Impaired detoxification	Functional liver detoxification
• Exotoxicity (e.g., chemical exposure, environmental sensitivity, alcohol and chemical dependency)	Elemental hair analysis Provocative heavy metal analysis Urinary markers of dysbiosis
• Endotoxicity (e.g., food allergies, dysbiosis)	
• Fatigue-related disorder (e.g., fibromyalgia)	
• Neurocognitive support (e.g., Parkinson's disease)	
• Imbalanced detoxification (e.g., im balanced phase I/phase II activity)	Functional liver detoxification Elemental hair analysis
• Multiple chemical sensitivities (e.g., environmental hypersensitivity)	Medical Symptoms Questionnaire
• Fatigue-related disorders (e.g., fibromyalgia)	
• Functional GI disorder	Digestive stool analysis
• Gastrointestinal lining integrity (leaky gut)	Intestinal permeability Parasitology
• Imbalanced gut flora (dysbiosis)	Urinary markers of dysbiosis
• Candida with gastrointestinal symptoms.	Medical Symptoms Questionnaire

icine. The major concept of homeopathy involves the recognition that agents that cause certain signs and symptoms in states of health can ameliorate the same signs and symptoms that occur in disease. It is believed by some that the more the homeopathic treatment agent is diluted, the more potent it may become, and by others, vice versa! I have oversimplified the principles of homeopathy in order to try to explain its basis. Of course, there is a great deal of theory behind the practice of homeopathic medicine.

The medical discipline of homeopathy was proposed as an alter-

Indications	Functional assessment options
• Chronic inflammation • Bronchial asthma • Rheumatoid arthritis • Psoriatic arthritis • Ulcerative colitis • Crohn's disease	C-reactive protein Sedimentation rate Functional liver detoxification Intestinal permeability Digestive stool analysis Essential fatty acid analysis Medical Symptoms Questionnaire
• Allergy management • Atopic disorders (e.g., eczema, psoriasis, dermatitis, asthma, serous otitis media) • Postantibiotic support	Digestive stool analysis Essential fatty acids analysis Urine/serum amino acids Food allergy testing Weekly Symptom Inventory Checklist for Children
• Energy-related disorders (e.g., postexercise fatigue, fibromyalgia)	Serum lipid peroxides Urine/serum amino acids Functional liver detoxification Medical Symptoms Questionnaire
• Glycemic balancing • Low-allergy, high-quality protein • Weight management/maintenance • Protein rebalancing	Glucose-insulin tolerance evaluation Body composition analysis
• Poor digestive elimination • Lipid management • Appetite control • Glycemic management	Digestive stool analysis Intestinal permeability
• Bowel irregularity (e.g., bloating, cramping, constipation) • Lipid imbalance • Glycemic management	Digestive stool analysis Intestinal permeability

native to conventional medicine by Dr. Samuel Hahnemann (a German physician) at the start of the nineteenth century. Dr. Hahnemann had many of the opinions of modern alternative physicians. He believed that conventional medical treatments of his era were dangerous and crude. This opinion was understandable at the time when medicine was still quite empiric. Medicine at this time was quite apt to resort to the use of purgatives and bloodletting. Homeopathy was introduced as a safe and gentle alternative type of medical treatment. Dr. Hahnemann experienced great opposition to his therapy, but homeopathy has survived for two centuries, and it is now an increasingly popular type of therapy.

Homeopathic medicine uses natural substances of plant, animal, and mineral origin that are believed to have the property of being able to stimulate the body's own response to healing or well-being. The potential of the body to heal itself has been reemphasized in contemporary writings by Andrew Weil, M.D. The principles of homeopathic medicine are sometimes referred to by the Latin phrase *similia, similius, curentur,* which can be translated as "let like substances be used to treat diseases."

In general, homeopathic remedies are made by preparing serial dilutions of the natural substances that are recognized as stimulating a beneficial effect on the symptoms of the disease under treatment. It is the power of the remedy to stimulate a favorable healing response in the body that is important in the practice of homeopathy.

Homeopathy has been studied in comparative clinical trials, and there is increasing evidence that it can be effective in the treatment of many diseases. About three thousand homeopathic substances are used in variable combinations as therapy, and many books have appeared on the subject. I recommend two books. The first is entitled *Discovering Homeopathy,* by Dana Ullman. This book presents a good general overview. The second book has a much more specific approach to treatment recommendations because it was written for healthcare practitioners. This book is titled *Homeopathic Medicine: A Doctor's Guide to Remedies for Common Ailments.* It is written by Dr. Trevor Smith, a renowned homeopath.

The use of homeopathic remedies is an art that takes many years of training and apprenticeship to learn. The practitioner recognizes symptoms and signs, but he or she also matches treatments to characteristics of the patient such as personality, attitude, and so on. Homeopathy affords great promise as a treatment discipline, and it has become very popular in Western Europe. However, I believe that homeopathy is not very suitable for general use as self-medication. For homeopathy to be used successfully, it has to be applied by a knowledgeable individual with experience and expertise. One exception may be the use of tried and trusted formulas that are applied to problems that can be readily self-identified.

OTC ADVICE AND UNDER-THE-TABLE CLAIMS

These days, as patients seem increasingly willing to self-diagnose and selfmedicate, they forget their responsibility of self-education in healthcare. The vast aray of OTC drugs and dietary supplements tests the knowledge of the healthcare practitioner and sometimes presents confusing options for consumers. The revolution in green pharmacy (the sale of natural products, notably dietary supplements) has swept America in the past decade. OTC drugs often stand next to dietary supplements. To most people, supplements present alternatives to drugs, even though by law dietary supplements are not to be used to diagnose, prevent, or treat disease. Consumer surveys indicate that most people take supplements to treat or prevent illness. This is the principal enigma of natural pharmacy that I need to reiterate and revisit.

Allowable claims on dietary supplements involve a body structure/function statement, e.g., "glucosamine is nutritional support for joint function" not "glucosamine treats arthritis." This latter statement is a drug claim, not a supplement claim. Healthcare professionals may express concern that they do not wish to make disease treatment or prevention claims for dietary supplements, but discussions about the promotion or maintenance of body structure and function cannot be easily divorced from considerations of disease states. As more research becomes available, that shows altered clinical outcome as a consequence of supplement use, healthcare practitioners will tend to feel more relaxed about linking disease treatment with natural therapies. Of course, many followers of the natural healthcare movement feel strongly that legal controls that limit the discussion of disease and alternative medicine should be abolished.

The real question remains: Who should be giving advice about supplements? Opinions vary but realities surface when this question is addressed. Perhaps a natural selection for advice is a physician. However, physicians with significant knowledge about natural medicine are among the minority, and they have no presence at the point of purchase of the remedies. Pharmacists are the ideal professionals to provide this advice to consumers, but the validity of the research (if any) that supports supplement claims and a lack of an agreed-upon source of information on herbals, botanicals, and nutrients make the pharmacist's delivery of "value-added counseling services" quite difficult. While pharmacists hold back on advice, consumers are enticed by the relaxed atmosphere of a health food store where open, unencumbered dialogue is normal. I am very supportive of new pharmacopea, for example *The Physician's Guide to Nutriceuticals*, which tries to make sense of supplement use.

Many health food stores have in-house consultants. These consultants vary in their educational background from registered dieticians or naturopaths (N.D.) through to individuals with no biomedical training. The proponents of natural medicine protest that the realm of herbal, botanical, and nutritional product use for wellness is not a domain of healthcare "owned" by the person with traditional credentials. The education of consumers in dietary supplements using reliable information is a key public health initiative for the next millennium. Education on natural remedies is an absolute prerequisite for public safety.

An argument exists on how a person with no biomedical training—who derives his or her knowledge often from marketing information created by dietary supplement manufacturers—can give advice that may sometimes be tantamount to treatment or disease-prevention recommendations. These debates must continue.

CHAPTER SUMMARY

There are many emerging issues in alternative medicine. Diagnostic approaches are often different than those applied in orthodox medicine and "natural medicines" figure strongly. We are learning about the limitations of legislating the practice of medicine—it often conflicts with patients' desires for natural options.

CHAPTER THIRTEEN

GALLBLADDERS,
GALLSTONES, AND
ATTACHMENTS

GALLSTONES ARE COMMON—
TREATMENT IS PROBLEMATIC

Gallstones occur in up to 20 percent of the population of several Western communities. About three-quarters of all gallstones are composed of cholesterol, while the remainder are formed of pigment or variable mixtures of pigment with cholesterol and/or calcium salts. The identification of the composition of gallstones has become an important issue in current medical practice, because only cholesterol stones are generally amenable to medical dissolution therapy (medical treatment designed to dissolve gallstones). This therapy is possible with the increasingly unpopular use of prescription preparations of bile acids, such as ursodeoxycholic (UDC) and/or chenodeoxycholic (CDC) acid, alone or in combination. Most gallstones are radiolucent on a plain abdominal x-ray (do not cast an x-ray shadow) because they are composed largely of cholesterol. A radio-opaque gallstone (one that can be seen on an x-ray) cannot be effectively treated by dissolution therapy.

There has been explosive interest in gallstone dissolution therapy in the past two decades. This approach to treatment is not novel. The feeding of bile has been used in ancient, traditional medical disciplines. Naturopathic medicine and complementary medical practices have attempted gallstone dissolution with natural agents, but controlled clinical trial data are not often available. Gallstones cannot be considered "functional" because they occupy valuable anatomic space and alter the architecture of the gallbladder and bile ducts, which is carefully constructed to ensure good flow of bile into the upper parts of the intestines (duodenum). It is pertinent to review natural therapies that may be of value to the management of gallstone disease. My proposals are common to my earlier approaches to gut disorders. They involve a pluralistic medical approach with the selection of treatment interventions from conventional and alternative/complementary medical options. Gallbladder disease should not be self-managed.

ARE ALTERNATIVES TO CONVENTIONAL MEDICAL THERAPY REQUIRED?

The common approaches of conventional medical practice to the treatment of gallstone disease are summarized in Table 13.1, together with general comments about the upside and downside of each approach. The avoidance of surgery is a frequent quest in medical practice, but medical therapy of gallstones with pharmaceuticals has been somewhat disappointing. Conventional medical treatment often produces short-term benefit on the clinical course of cholelithiasis (gallstones), but long-term benefits have not been shown in a consistent manner. Innovative methods of treatment such as extracorporeal biliary lithotripsy (using shock waves to fragment gallstones) have not been found to be worthwhile, even after a large financial investment in this treatment technique. There is no question that the prevention of gallstone disease is easier than its therapy. Despite the common occurrence of cholelithiasis, preventive strategies have not been applied frequently in medical practice. Prevention of gallstones is a prime target for alternative medical strategies.

GETTING TO THE CAUSE OF STONES

A great deal of research has been performed on factors that cause bile to become lithogenic (stone forming), but the precise patho-

Table 13.1: Principal conventional medical approaches to gall-stone therapy, some upsides and downsides.

TREATMENT	COMMENT
Cholecystectomy	Suitable for acute cholecystitis, occlusion of cystic duct. Laparoscopic approach preferred with mortality from surgery. < 1% under age of 50 y, but 2–10% over 70 y. Post surgical syndromes in up to 3%.
Medical dissolution therapy (UDC and CDC)	Long-term, expensive therapy for radiolucent, small (< 20mm) cholesterol stones only, recurrence when treatment stops. Side effects diarrhea and liver toxicity.
Endoscopic or invasive dissolution, interventional radiology	Methyl-tert-butyl ether and monooctanoin solvents. Invasive, serious problems occasionally, residual fragments left.
Extracorporeal shock wave Lithotripsy	An expensive fad that faded.
Watchful waiting	See text—an approach for the silent or minor symptomatic disorders. Conventional medicine often denies the value of complementary regimens, lifestyle changes, etc. in this context.
Endoscopic techniques	Papillotomy (endoscopic) can be used in some high-risk elderly people as an alternative to surgery, and it permits stone retrieval from the common bile duct

physiology (disease mechanism) of gallstone formation remains to be completely defined. The main factors that cause gallstones include metabolic derangements (e.g., excessive pigment production from hemolysis, which is breakdown of red blood cells), abnormal liver function and dietary or intrinsic causes of lithogenic bile, infection (e.g., ascending bacterial infections, clonorchiasis in S.E. Asia, a kind of parasite of the gallbladder and bile ducts), and the many causes of stasis of bile (e.g., poor gallbladder function, partial blockage etc.). Different types of gallstones have different causes. The causative factors require definition in order to apply the correct preventive or therapeutic interventions.

The relative inaccessibility of gallstones in the body makes a definition of their composition and inferences about their cause difficult in clinical practice. Noninvasive techniques such as ultrasound and oral cholecystography (gall bladder x-rays, using dyes) may help identify and characterize different types of stones. Medical imaging techniques have led to noninvasive means of defining gallstone composition with reasonable accuracy. These techniques should be applied in clinical practice if dissolution (dissolving) therapy is contemplated.

GALLSTONES OF DIFFERENT TYPES

The importance of the differentiation between cholesterol and pigment stones in the planning of therapy has led to intensive research to improve diagnostic acumen. Gallstones have many different causes and composition, and therefore they have a variable response to therapy. I am very concerned about some of the literature in alternative medicine, including textbooks and teaching material, that makes statements about potential natural therapies for gallstones without distinguishing the types of stones. Naturopathic physicians and alternative medical practitioners are apt to discuss and propose possible stone dissolution or nutritional or herbal therapy for cholelithiasis, without attempting to make the important differentiation of the type of stone.

CRITERIA TO SELECT GALLSTONE THERAPY

Table13.1 draws approaches that can be applied in the management of gallbladder disease. When gallstones block the cystic or common bile ducts, problems arise that require surgery. Obstructive jaundice (obstruction and damming up of bile flow), ascending cholangitis (infection that goes up the biliary tree), and acute pancreatitis (inflammation of the pancreas) are some of the serious sequelae. Under these circumstances, surgical intervention or, on occasion, specialized endoscopic therapy (e.g., with a lighted tube through which a gastroenterologist can access the biliary tree), is mandatory.

Patients with mild to moderate or infrequent symptoms may be candidates for medical dissolution therapy with UDC or CDC. General guidelines for the selection of individuals for this type of dissolution therapy include the presence of radiolucent, noncalcified (less than 3 mm of center of calcification), small (< 20 mm diameter) stones in patients who have been informed of all available treatment options and their risks or benefits. Many patients can be selected for this type of therapy, because about 85 percent of gallstones that are detected by ultrasound (use of a sound wave machine used to create images of the body) are less than 20 mm in diameter.

Medical dissolution therapy with UDC and CDC takes between one and two years of continuous therapy in many patients. These treatment agents are expensive and difficult to take. Common side effects of dyspepsia and altered bowel habit occur, and occasional serious liver toxicity is encountered. Cessation of dissolution therapy leads to recurrence in about 50 percent of patients within five years. The limitations of current conventional medical therapies have led many patients and some physicians to seek more gentle and natural treatment alternatives.

A great deal is to be learned from failed conventional medical approaches. Alternative and complementary medicine can draw upon this experience so that natural options can be applied in a manner that is most appropriate and likely to succeed. To emphasize this point by example, a natural agent that may work by assisting in the dissolution of cholesterol stones cannot be expected to work in dissolving pigment stones. Unfortunately, far less research exists on natural therapies in comparison to conventional options of treatment.

MANAGEMENT OF "SILENT" GALLSTONES

For many years, there was a tendency for medical practitioners to recommend prophylactic (doing something in advance to prevent later problems) cholecystectomy (gallbladder removal) for asymptomatic (silent) gallstones. This practice was based on the poorly founded notion that complications of gallstones are inevitable. Stones that cause recurrent symptoms, acute cholecystitis (an acute often painful inflammation of the gallbladder), and gallstone-associated pancreatitis (dangerous inflammation of the pancreas gland) almost always require removal and cholecystectomy (surgical removal of the gallbladder).

However, in some patients with coexisting disease, such as coronary heart disease or diabetes mellitus, a high risk exists for surgical interventions (surgery is dangerous when people have other serious diseases present). This situation has led to the emergence of less invasive endoscopic interventions (using the endoscope, a lighted tube that is put through the mouth to access the biliary tree in a backwards manner), but their value in the long term remains relatively underexplored.

Some important differences in the occurrence and severity of gallstone pancreatitis are apparent between genders, with a tendency for the sequelae (outcomes) of gallstones to be more severe in the male than in the female. The reasons for this are not clear, but this situation has been documented and discussed in detail in papers written by my colleagues and I. It may be related to anatomic variations in the biliary tree between males and females. There is an unpredictable idiopathic disorder (something of unknown cause) of acute acalculous cholesystitis (inflammation of the gallbladder without the presence of stones), which tends to occur in association with a variety of severe, acute illnesses. However, gallstones occur most often without symptoms (they are silent).

There are several studies that support a nonsurgical approach to silent gallstones and conclude that "watchful waiting" may be the most prudent option for asymptomatic (silent) gallstones. This is a situation in conventional medicine where proactive natural therapy, in terms of lifestyle adjustment and natural options, is overlooked as potentially effective therapy. Watchful waiting without some form of natural intervention or preventive strategy may be more likely to result in the conversion of the asymptomatic to the symptomatic (causes overt discomfort) status. The control or reduction of factors that promote gallstone formation by natural means is one of the greatest potential contributions that can be made by alternative, complementary, or naturopathic medicine.

CIRCUMSTANCES THAT SUPPORT NATURAL APPROACHES

Large population studies in the United States and Italy imply that there is a low incidence of symptoms in individuals with detectable gallstones (stones found by testing). Italian investigators undertook ultrasonographic (used the diagnostic sound wave machine) studies in two geographic areas of Italy and reported that 65 percent and 78 percent, respectively, of all people with gallstones were asymptomatic. Some of the most compelling evidence that supports a nonsurgical approach to silent gallstone emanates from a follow-up study of 123 members of the faculty of the University of Michigan with asymptomatic gallstones. The cumulative probability (chance of something occurring) of developing biliary pain in this group of subjects was 18 percent after twenty years. Furthermore, the risk diminished with an increasing time of follow up, and the incidence of biliary complications was only about 10 percent. These complications were heralded invariably by premonitory biliary pain (pain that occurred before full blown attacks of inflammation of the gallbladder).

These studies and others support a noninvasive approach to the management of silent stones. Decision-tree analysis (a type of mathematics that predicts the occurrence of something) projects that life expectancy may be higher with expectant (doing nothing) management, and health costs of the approach are claimed to be about one-quarter that of prophylactic surgery (removing the gallbladder that contains silent stones to prevent future problems). These data support my proposal that a large number of patients with gallstones or a tendency to develop gallstones may benefit from medical and, in particular, natural therapies.

A CLOSER LOOK AT SYMPTOMS IN CHOLELITHIASIS

There is sometimes great difficulty at the clinical level in directly associating digestive symptoms or other complaints with the presence of gallstones. It is unwise to ascribe digestive complaints to gallstones in an indiscriminate manner, because of the coexistence of other gastrointestinal disorders with gallstones. Dyspepsia in the presence of gallstones can often be due to gastroesophageal reflux disease, peptic ulcer, *Helicobacter* infection, therapy with NSAIDs, or functional gastrointestinal disease. In classical, surgical writings, the disorder of Saint's triad (the coexistence of biliary disease, diverticular disease

301

[outpouchings of the bowel], and hiatal hernia [a bulge through the diaphragm involving the stomach and lower esophagus] has been proposed and some evidence exists that these disorders may go hand in hand, especially in the "fat, flatulent [gassy], fifty-year-old female."

Physicians of the conventional or alternative persuasion must be careful that they do not hoodwink themselves into the assumption that all digestive symptoms are due to gallbladder problems or gallstones, even when stones have been demonstrated to be present. There is a group of patients, however, that has vague, nondyspeptic symptoms of suboptimal health that appear to resolve with the treatment of gallstones. The diagnostic dilemmas presented by gallstones can result in a conundrum. These circumstances and the benign natural history of asymptomatic stones may make natural therapies an appealing first-line option in many cases, providing an acute problem does not exist.

GENERAL PRINCIPLES OF NATURAL THERAPIES FOR GALLSTONES

Gallstone formation occurs most often as a consequence of lithogenic bile, and a rational approach to the understanding of natural or complementary therapies involves an understanding of how these interventions may affect this process. Lithogenicity of bile is related most often to metabolic events, stasis (standstill) of bile, and infection. Remedies of natural origin exist to counter these pathophysiological (disease-causing) factors. In general, natural therapies can be used to alter metabolic events, such as excessive biliary cholesterol excretion or circumstances that precipitate insolubility (precipitation of stones) of cholesterol in bile (e.g. nutrient elimination or addition). In addition, lipotropic (reduction of fat deposition in the liver) or choleretic (causing bile flow) initiatives that improve bile flow can be applied with certain botanicals or herbs.

DIETARY CONSIDERATIONS

The typical Western diet is high in saturated fat and refined carbohydrates, and low in fiber, fruit and vegetables. Diet seems to be important in the causation of gallstones. Dietary fiber is an important and often overlooked therapy for gallstones. Both soluble and insoluble fiber may prevent gallstones by reducing the absorption of deoxycholic acid (a bile acid), and fiber produces a favorable shift in the triad of factors that controls cholesterol's solubility in bile (makes cholesterol stay dissolved in bile and stopping stone formation). Soluble fibers such as guar gum and pectin are effective, as are other classes of fiber that are present in many fruits and vegetables (e.g., oat bran, wheat bran and soy fiber).

The beneficial role of fruit and vegetable intake is apparent in studies where vegetarians are found to have a lower incidence of gallstones compared with omnivorous (eats meat and veggies) individuals. This lower prevalence of gallstones in vegetarians is due to several factors, including dietary fiber intake, alteration of the bacterial flora (bugs in the guts) in the colon, and a positive benefit of certain phytochemicals. Lithogenic factors such as excessive intake of simple sugars and animal proteins (e.g., casein from milk) may be associated with gallstone formation. Thus, a general switch in dietary preferences is a major factor in gallstone prevention and treatment.

A strong relationship exists between gallstones and abnormalitites of blood lipids. The ability of soy protein–containing isoflavones (genistein, daidzein, and glyceitin) to normalize blood lipids could be of value in gallstone prevention or therapy. The protein in soy is necessary to alter blood lipid profile, and this has led to the widespread popularity of soy protein isolates containing isoflavones, such as Genista, or similar products.

ERRONEOUS RECOMMENDATIONS CONCERNING LEGUME INTAKE

Certain studies suggest that diets rich in legumes (peas and beans) may be a risk for gallstone development. While it can be shown that certain types of saponins (specific chemicals in some plants), present in several legumes, may promote the saturation of cholesterol in bile, the evidence to support the recommendation for the restriction of legume intake in individuals with gallstones can be questioned. It has been reported that legume-rich diets are associated with gallstone formation, but the populations in which this has been studied include a preponderance of individuals with an ethnic origin that is highly associated with the occurrence of gallstone disease (e.g., Pima Indians, Chileans, and North American Indians). Cholelithiasis is common in this group of people regardless of their legume intake. Studies of the effect of diets containing soybeans (legumes) on gallstone formation show a preventive benefit for soy in gallstones. These results are the complete opposite of those studies that may have led to the erroneous recommendation to reduce legume intake in order to avoid gallstone formation.

The role of food allergies in the causation of gallstones remains arguable. It is reported that elimination diets may benefit some patients with gallstones, but it is hard to separate out the presumed benefit of the elimination of a putative, offending food allergen from the beneficial effect of the dietary substitutions. For example, the use of an elimination diet (removing offending types of foods from the diet) in some studies claims benefits in gallstone patients, but the substitution diet contained agents such as soy and fiber that could have accounted for the benefit.

In general, individuals with defined food allergies should avoid the offending agents. There may be a tendency for an overdiagnosis of food intolerance as a cause of gastrointestinal symptoms in alternative and complementary medical practice. In contrast, there may be inadequate attention paid to food intolerance by conventional medicine. Expensive testing using serological tests for food allergies is not often justifiable, because these tests are often not as cost effective, or any more accurate, than a well-taken medical history and a trial of specific food eliminations.

Certain dietary exclusions and inclusions have been proposed as beneficial in the management of gallstones. Carbohydrate in complex sources (starches not simple sugars) is preferred because of the associated health benefit of fiber intake and the knowledge that a high intake of refined sugar may contribute to gallstone formation. Some studies support the use of unrefined vegetable oils or fish oil in the prevention or treatment of gallstones. The real benefit of these oils is probably related to their content of essential fatty acids of the omega-6 (predominantly plant or vegetable) and the omega-3 types (predominantly fish oil or precursor format in flax seeds or soybeans). The alleged beneficial effects of polyunsaturated fats (lots of hydrogen bonds in the molecule that are incomplete) do not match observations of the reports of enhanced lithogenicity of bile after the institution of certain polyunsaturated fats in the diet.

The idea of the "olive-oil flush" (giving a high dose of olive oil by mouth) of the gallbladder in patients with gallstones is obsolete and unsafe. Olive oil (or any fatty substance) in large doses causes sudden gallbladder contraction, which in the presence of cholelithiasis may precipitate biliary pain or stone dislodgment. Furthermore, not all oils are ideal for people with gallstones because they may contain fatty acids, such as oleic acid, that have been shown in animal studies to contribute to gallstone formation. A general recommendation for gallstone patients is fat elimination, but the type of elimination should be a reduction of saturated fat intake with the inclusion of normal intake of essential super-polyunsaturated fats (e.g., fish-oil-type fatty acids). The blanket recommendation of the fat-free diet for gallstones in conventional medicine is not healthy because of the potential occurrence of essential-fatty-acid deficiency (certain fats are as essential as vitamins because the body cannot make them). Essential fatty acid deficiency (especially of omega-3 fats) may aggravate or contribute to cholelithiasis.

THE OBESITY DILEMMA

There is a strong relationship (mathematical association) between obesity and the presence of gallstones. This results in the frequent recommendation of weight loss by calorie restriction in patients with cholelithiasis. This situation creates a double-edged sword because calorie restriction, weight loss, and fasting can increase the risk of gallstone formation. Gallstone formation can occur frequently during accelerated periods of weight loss, especially if a very low calorie diet is used. Fat people who lose weight often develop gallstones.

There are many proponents of the simple theory of thermodynamics (energy into the body and energy out of the body) in weight loss. This approach assumes that people who are fat have excessive calorie intake, whereas people who are thin have low calorie intake. Modern research implies that this is not the whole answer, but restriction of calorie intake is important for short-term weight loss. There are many types of dietary regimens that can be successful in short-term weight loss management, but not enough emphasis has been placed on healthy types of weight-loss regimens.

Lifestyle adjustments, sustained and decreased calorie intake, together with behavioral modification (learning to stick to diets or retraining in healthy lifestyle habits) are good approaches to weight loss, but the substitution of healthy foods in weight-loss diets is an underestimated intervention. Of relevance to weight loss in the obese individual with gallstones is the inclusion of soy protein containing isoflavones, dietary fiber, and fish oil. Soy food is relatively low in calories, and it has low glycemic index (does not cause big swings in blood sugar). Evidence exists that soy is preventive against gallstones. Furthermore, patients who develop gallstones during calorie restriction tend to have higher blood cholesterol and serum triglycerides (fats in the blood). This gives soy protein an added advantage for use in weight loss regimens because of the unequivocal evidence that soy protein containing isoflavones can lower blood cholesterol and serum triglycerides, thereby decreasing the risk of cardiovascular disease and affording potential, simultaneous treatment for the gallstone diathesis (overall gallstone problem).

A ROLE FOR SPECIFIC NUTRIENTS

The deficiency of vitamins C and E is associated with gallstone formation in animal studies. This has led to suggestions that megadose (very high doses) therapy with vitamin C (more than 2 gm/day) may decrease the lithogenicity of bile by enhancing the solubility of cholesterol. The role of bioflavonoids (special plant chemicals that are antioxidants and vitamin C "helpers") such as proanthocyanidins and isoflavones remains underexplored, but anecdotal observations of benefit appear promising. In general, nutrients that are vitamin C helpers, such as pycnogenol or grape seed extract, could be anticipated to be beneficial in the nutritional management of gallstones.

A number of scientists have proposed the value of lecithin (phosphatidylcholine) in enhancing the solubility of cholesterol in bile. Regular supplementation with lecithin can result in measurable increase in lecithin excretion in the bile, but the use of lecithin alone has not been reported to result in successful dissolution of gallstones. However, lecithin is a useful dietary adjunct for the management of cholesterol gallstones, and its presence in soybeans may explain, in part, the known benefit of soy in gallstone prevention and perhaps therapy.

LIFESTYLE ADJUSTMENTS

Gallstones can be regarded as a disease of adverse lifestyle. There is no doubt that dietary interventions can be beneficial, but exercise and the avoidance of substance abuse are important and often overlooked interventions. The drinking of coffee, whether or not it is decaffeinated, can produce gallbladder contractions, and alcohol is a potent hepatotoxin (toxic to the liver). The incidence of gallstones is higher in patients with alcoholic liver disease, and abstention or moderation of ethanol intake is important advice for the individual with cholelithiasis.

There are no specific studies of the role of exercise in the management of gallstones in contemporary literature. However, exercise promotes weight loss, improves general metabolism, reduces cholesterol levels, and therefore could be anticipated to exert a favorable effect on gallstone disease. One study has suggested that exposure to ultraviolet light (sunlight) may contribute to gallstones, but this notion may be a little far fetched. Further studies on lifestyle and gallstone management are required.

FISH OIL

Considerable evidence from animal experiments suggests that fish oil may be of value in the management of cholelithiasis. To date, there have been few studies in humans to define the benefit of fish oils in gallstones, but epidemiological studies of chronic disorders, including gallbladder disease, imply a benefit of omega-3 fatty acid intake as preventive against cholelithiasis. In addition, studies in primates (monkeys) show evidence that fish-oil intake results in a much lower incidence of gallstones compared with the occurrence of stones in monkeys fed a saturated-fat diet (threefold difference). In this latter study, a high concentration of lecithin was found in the bile of the fish-oil-fed primates. Studies in prairie dogs with fish oil supplementation have revealed similar results, and researchers have concluded that fish-oil feeding may result in a stabilization of vesicles (little blobs) of phospholipids (types of fats in bile, containing cholesterol) in bile.

The precise amount of fish oil required for gallstone management is not known, but it seems to be quite high. When fish oil is used as treatment, it is seldom possible to deliver enough oil in liquid or standard capsule format because of gastrointestinal upset, halitosis and expense. Enteric-coated capsules of fish oil are the preferred type of supplement to assure compliance (sticking with treatment) and enhanced bioavailability (how much gets into the body) of the important omega-3 fatty acids, including docosahexanoic acid (DHA) and eicosapentanoic acid (health-giving types of fatty acids in fish oil).

The only delayed-release, enteric product available in the U.S. dietary supplement market, at the time of writing, is Fisol (BioTherapies Inc., Fairfield, NJ, and Natures Way, Springville, Utah). Although fish oil has found its greatest use in cardiovascular health, the versatility of DHA and EPA as potential treatment for inflammatory disorders (e.g., Crohn's disease and rheumatoid arthritis), immune dysfunction, breast cancer, and bipolar disorders (depression with mania) is being actively investigated at several centers of medical excellence.

GALLSTONE DISSOLUTION

Conventional medical therapy has formerly focused a great deal of attention on medical dissolution therapy with CDC and UDC. The safety and cost effectiveness of this intervention has been questioned, and other ways of dissolving gallstones by natural therapies remain underexplored.

The most promising alternative approach to gallstone dissolution involves the use of plant essential oils such as peppermint and fennel oil. These plant essential oils contain terpenes (cyclic monoter-penes) that have potent and versatile biological effects (special com-pounds in plant oils). Examples of terpenes in essential oils include menthol, menthone, pinene, cineole, borneol, etc. Monoterpenes have been used effectively in the therapy of IBS, when used in a delayed-release format. This treatment has been discussed in detail in earlier chapters of this book. These compounds are smooth-mus-cle relaxants that act in a similar manner to calcium channel antago-nist drugs (drugs that block the entry of calcium into cells).

In a number of studies, terpenes have been shown to be effective in gallstone dissolution. Two natural agents appear valuable in this situation. Rowachol is a mixture of plant terpenes in which menthol is a prominent component, but Rowachol is not available is the United States. Many physicians have elected to use enteric-coated peppermint oil (Pepogest). While UDC and CDC therapy can dissolve small, cholesterol stones, its effects are amplified by adding plant ter-penes. Combing CDC or UDC with plant essential oils or other sources of terpenes is an effective and frequently forgotten option in gallstone dissolution therapy.

Several gallstone-dissolving formulas have been proposed in naturopathic medicine. These formulas may be more effective if used with UDC or CDC. An example of such formulas includes menthol, menthone, pinene, borneol, comphene, cineole, and citral in variable amounts and combinations.

CHOLERETICS, CHOLAGOGUES, AND LIPOTROPICS

The use of agents that promote the flow of bile (cholagogues), increase bile secretion (choleretics), or decrease the deposition of fat in the liver (lipotropics) are favorite interventions in naturopathic medical practice. Whilst the use of botanical agents with choleretic or lipotropic properties seems to offer much promise, a need exists to demonstrate the value of these types of therapy in well-conducted clinical studies.

Commonly used lipotropic agents include choline, methionine, folic acid, vitamin B12, and betaine. It is popular to combine these putative, lipotropic agents with choleretics (or cholagogues). Several choleretics have been proposed (e.g., dandelion, milk thistle, artichoke, turmeric, and boldo), but most evidence supports the use of silymarin (milk thistle extract). Silymarin appears to cause measurable increases of the solubility of cholesterol, and it decreases the sequestration (hanging around) of cholesterol in bile. The precise mode of action of silymarin is not completely understood. Choleretic agents that provide liver support are available in many formats. Among the most desirable include Artichoke Extract and Super Thistle X. Super Thistle X is a very interesting patented form of milk thistle extract that is bound to phosphatidylcholine to provide stability and enhance the absorption of the active components of the extract.

TRADITIONAL CHINESE MEDICINE

The treatment of gallstones in traditional Chinese medical practice is quite complex. It is proposed that the free flow of Liver-Qi is important in maintaining the normal composition of bile acids. A stagnation of Liver-Qi may lead to the accumulation of "damp heat," which is said to cause gallstones. Chinese diagnostic methodology differentiates stagnation of Liver-Qi from damp heat in the liver and gallbladder. The application of appropriate therapy with acupuncture or herbs demands that the treating physician be able to differentiate these disorders. Chinese medicine is not for self-treatment.

Stagnation of Liver-Qi involves specific acupuncture point therapy on certain meridians, and herbal therapy is available in several formats including Chai Hu Su Gan Tang and Shu Gan wan. Jin Qian Cao and Hai Jin Sha (*herba desmodii styracifolii*) are believed to be capable of dissolving gallstones. In contrast, damp heat in the liver and gallbladder is reported to be amenable to an herbal prescription of Da Chai Hu Tang or the patent remedy of Li Gan Pan. Acupuncture has been reported to be of use in the control of biliary pain and the facilitation of expulsion of gallstones (according to classic theory).

The treatment of liver and gallbladder dysfunction is based on the philosophy of balanced yin and yang. Specific herbal agents that have been used as choleretics or hepatoprotectives in traditional Chinese medicine include Yu Jin (containing a variety of essential oils) Dong

Yao (containing mixed glucosides), Wu Wei Zi (containing mixed lydrocarbons), Zhi Zi (containing garderin, shanzhiside and crocin), Yin Chen (containing chlorogenic and caffeic acids with essential oils), Chu Pen Cao (containing alkaloids), and Shui Fei Ji (silymarin). For a more complete account of the treatment of liver and gallbladder dysfunction in cholelithiasis, readers are referred to standard textbooks on the subject of Chinese medicine or herbal pharmacopoeia (books that explain herbs and their actions in detail).

CLUES FROM PREDISPOSING FACTORS

There is a general impression in medicine that gallstones are a familial trait. Genetic predispositions (hereditary tendencies) are often investigated by studying disease occurrences in twins. Forty years ago, a very important, prospective study (forward planned) of the genetics of gallstones in Danish twins failed to show a simple inheritance pattern. The tendency of gallstone disease to be more common among relatives of individuals with gallstones or certain ethnic groups may be determined to a significant extent by environmental issues, in particular diet. The acceptance of this discordance in observations in genetic studies helps to underscore my proposals about lifestyle factors in the causation of gallstones. This argument is contrary to the limited observation that the pathogenesis of gallstones may be similar in certain ethnic groups (e.g., Pima Indians or Chileans) and Caucasians.

Important lessons on lifestyle and chronic disease are being learned from studies of Pima Indians in North America and Mexico. The Pima Indians are a nation in crisis in America (especially Arizona), because they have the highest incidence of obesity, heart disease, and gallstones of any ethnic group. However, Pima Indians who live in the northern mountain regions of Mexico have little obesity, good cardiovascular health, and less problems with cholelithiasis. While some studies imply that the genetic programming of this ethnic group predisposes them to chronic disease, current studies point to lifestyle issues as being of overriding importance for their health.

DIET IS THE KEY

Conventional medicine continues to lack a clear definition of the importance of diet in the formation of cholesterol gallstones. Diet is perceived as one factor alone, but its contribution to gallstone formation is probably highly complex and multifactorial. For example, it is known that a high intake of cholesterol in the diet produces saturated bile (a condition where cholesterol cannot be maintained in solution in bile), but decreased cholesterol intake or enhancement of polyunsaturated fat intake in the diet cannot be easily shown to reduce gallstone formation. In fact, enhanced intake of certain types of unsaturated fat may act to enhance gallstone formation, perhaps by mobilizing tissue stores of cholesterol and increasing the fecal excretion of neutral steroids (molecules related to bile chemicals). The answer to these apparently incongruous findings may reside in a consideration of multiple factors that contribute to gallstone disease, including, but not limited to, obesity, diet, ethnic factors, genetics, environmental pollution, gender differences, metabolic disorders, etc. A simple positive correlation exists between age and gallstone formation. Therefore, it appears that many years are required for the evolution of gallstone diathesis. This reinforces the need for preventive strategies by lifestyle adjustments that are applied in a timely manner.

The common occurrence of gallstones reinforces the constant concern that is expressed by practitioners of natural medicine that drug therapies predispose to a number of chronic diseases such as gallstones. Oral contraceptives and estrogen replacement therapy (ERT) lead to lithogenic bile and gallstones. The widespread use of ERT for menopause is being reexamined in conventional medicine and questioned by alternative medicine. The risks of uterine cancer, peripheral venous thrombosis, breast cancer, and a multitude of troublesome symptoms are apparent with ERT, but relatively few studies have examined the gallstone diathesis in the mature female in relationship to ERT. It is known that soyfoods and fractions of soy contain isoflavones. Soy isoflavones may be a viable alternative to ERT, and coincidentally soy is preventive against gallstones.

The widespread interest in conventional medicine in the lowering of blood cholesterol with drugs to promote cardiovascular wellness may be a negative event in relation to gallstone disease. Little is known about the long-term consequences of taking some cholesterol-lowering drugs, but it is known that the use of cholestyramine (a drug poised for OTC use) may predispose to gallstone formation. Cholestyramine is an anion exchange resin (picks up and binds certain charged molecules) that binds bile acids and decreases the bile acid pool, resulting in lithogenic bile. In addition, clofibrate (an inhibitor of cholesterol synthesis) causes increased biliary secretion of cholesterol with consequential increases in cholesterol excretion, and it decreases bile acid synthesis and pool size. Again, a circumstance of preference for natural options emerges. Soy-protein-containing isoflavones lower blood cholesterol, and soy may prevent or treat gallstones. This situation of substituting a natural therapy (soy) for a drug (clofibrate) seems preferable to the twofold increase in gallstone disease that is reported with clofibrate use.

GUT ECOLOGY AND PROBIOTIC THERAPY

If ever there was a key to the treatment of gallstones, I believe it lies in an understanding of the internal milieu of the gastrointestinal tract. There are no great profits to be made in balancing the function of the gastrointestinal tract, and drugs that will control the microenvironment of the guts will never exist. Few physicians or scientists would argue that alterations of the bile acid pool are at the root of the basic pathophysiology (causation) of gallstones, but studies of the manipulation of the gut flora and fauna in the management of gallstone disease are begging to be performed.

Bile acids (cholic and chenodeoxycholic acid) are secreted into the small bowel in a conjugated form (linked together) with glycine and taurine. Under normal circumstances, about 80 percent of the bile salts are reabsorbed (get back into the body) and returned to the liver, whereas about 20 percent are metabolized in the colon. These bile acids undergo a series of chemical transformations including: deconjugation, oxido-reduction, and dehydroxylation in the colon (chemical transformation). The participants in this series of reactions are many different types of colonic bacteria, including: *Bacteroides*, *Eubacteria*, *Lactobacilli*, *Clostridia*, and *Veillonella*. The dehydroxylation (remove OH groups from molecules) of the unconjugated forms of chenodeoxycholic and cholic acid to deoxycholic and lithocholic acids, respectively, is undertaken principally by *Bacteroides, Bifidobacteria,* and *Clostridia.*

The interactions between the bile acid pool and bacteria are extraordinarily complex. While bacteria metabolize (chemically alter) bile acids, the concentration of fecal bile acids alters the growth and survival of the colonic bacteria that are involved in their metabolism. To add to this complexity, the amount of bile acids present in feces is influenced by the amount of fat in the diet. These variables are particularly important for the survival and function of the friendly gut bacteria of the *Bifidobacteria* family.

Bifidobacteria, and other organisms, when present in the colon, contribute to general health including: general body metabolism, immune function, and cancer prevention, and they confer antimicrobial benefits (kill bacteria or stop their growth). The presence of *Bifidobacteria* has been associated with health and longevity in certain Japanese communities. If one examines the lifestyle of *Bifidobacteria,* it is known that these bacteria are sensitive to alterations in the level of fecal bile acids. In addition, an increase in the dietary intake of fat increases fecal bile acids and exerts an inhibitory effect on *Bifidobacteria.* The growth of *Bifidobacteria* in the colon is also altered by factors in the diet such as indigestible carbohydrates. For example, the nonabsorbable carbohydrates stacchyose and raffinose that are present in soybeans will promote the growth of *Bifidobacteria.*

Alternative and complementary medicine is faced with a surge of interest in the use of friendly bacteria such as *Bifidobacteria* and *Lactobacilli* as probiotic therapy. The rational for probiotic therapy in the management of gallstones seems quite plausible, but arguments prevail about the effectiveness of the treatment technique in general. Unfortunately, as is often the case in alternative medicine, hyperbolic claims of efficacy of probiotic therapy can create polar viewpoints. I propose that the correct use of prebiotic and probiotic therapy may have a lot to offer in the prevention or treatment of cholelithiasis, but further research is required to define its precise role.

CHAPTER SUMMARY

There is a rational basis for the use of natural medical interventions as important in the management of gallstones in a large proportion

Table 13.2: A summary of some natural approaches to the prevention or treatment of gallstones.

OPTION	COMMENT
Balanced diet and weight control	Very viable options. Dietary changes with enhanced fiber intake and reduced cholesterol and saturated fat intake. Avoidance of precipitous weight loss, substance abuse, and sedentary life
Detoxification and probiotic therapy	A logical approach that requires considerable further research.
Soy-based diets and supplements	Processed soy food is often not healthy. Well-designed soy supplements can be used to provide a continuous intake of the desired soy fractions. Soy is underexplored as a gallstone remedy.
Choleretics, lipotropics, and cholagogues	Herbal and botanical agents applied but more research is required.
Plant essential oils	Relatively high doses required with minor safety issues. Enteric-coated oils preferable.
Fish oil	Large doses required. Best taken in palatable, well absorbed format (e.g., Fisol).
Proactive natural therapy	Natural therapies may play a major role in watchful waiting for asymptomatic stones.
Treatment of food allergies	Elimination of dietary allergens is required for general health.
Vitamin supplements	At least the RDA of vitamins C and E is required. Bioflavonoids may assist.
Lecithin	May play an adjunctive role
Chinese medicine	Not to be used by the untrained.
Natural options for cholesterol lowering, hormone replacement	Estrogen replacement therapy with hormones and certain cholesterol-lowering drugs cause gallstones. Soy isoflavones are a viable alternative.

of patients with this disorder. Of all natural options, nutritional interventions, dietary changes, and lifestyle adjustment appear to offer great promise. Natural adjuncts in the prevention and treatment of gallstone are summarized in Table 13.2. Medical and surgical therapy of gallstones occurs often in conventional medical practice at the expense of considering gentler, safer and more cost-effective remedies of natural origin. These natural therapies may have a lot to offer in the management of cholelithiasis. Natural therapies for gallstones deserve more research and greater empiric use, in the face of some failures of conventional medical approaches.

CONCLUSION

The increasing emergence of alternative and complementary medicine in the twenty-first century has more to do with healthcare consumers than with any revolution in thought among physicians. While alternative medicine remains somewhat lacking in research and development strategies, a practicing physician can expect that about two thirds of their clientele will have used or sought nonconventional medical therapies. Given our increasing knowledge about the potential interactions between alternative and conventional medicine, a major dilemma presents itself in modern medicine.

There has been a massive increase in the use of vitamins, herbs, and botanicals by healthcare consumers. However, much of the medical profession remains poorly educated about their value, or lack thereof. Even greater ignorance exists about more specialized forms of alternative therapies—there is no defined curriculum for the teaching of alternative medicine. In the case of "nutraceuticals," information is sometimes misleading and sometimes hyped to a level that transcends any reasonable knowledge of science; but it is occasionally accurate. The U.S. Dietary Supplement and Health Education Act of 1994 permits the sale of dietary supplements with limited claims of their benefit for body structure and function. In a somewhat schizophrenic manner, the same legislation prevents the sale of natural "therapies" for the prevention or treatment of disease—the very reason why people take supplements! After all, disease is invariably associated with alterations of normal body structure and function. This enigma of modern medicine must be rationalized one day.

Conventional medicine has changed its approach to functional gastrointestinal disease and we see a glimpse of the benefit of alternative medical practices creeping into the peer-reviewed medical literature. In this book, I adopt the philosophy of pluralistic medicine, with its many confusing definitions, and integrate it into "disease" concepts and treatment options. I have only been able to scratch the surface. While I'd like to give you just the straight facts, much interpretation and even opinion clouds the issues of the safety or efficacy of both conventional and alternative medical interventions.

Even the term "alternative" can be misleading. For example, the use of hypnosis or behavior modification for functional gut disorders is arguably "alternative" if it is embraced, even in part, by orthodox opinion. Modern physicians have a hard job when patients' demands lead them to apply therapies about which they have little knowledge or experience. I reinforce my preferred use of the term "medical pluralism." The increasing willingness to acknowledge or accept "biopsychosocial" models of diease must follow with pluralistic approaches to the mixed bag of tricks that many diseases present. Once considered a flash in the pan, alternative treatments appear to be here to stay. The age of pluralistic medicine has dawned, and nowhere is this more apparent than in the management of gastrointestinal disorders.

BOOKS

Fugh-Berman, A. *Alternative Medicine: What Works*. Tucson, Ariz.: Odonian Press, 1996.

Gershon, M. D. *The Second Brain*. New York: HarperCollins, 1998.

Griggs, B. *Green Pharmacy*. Rochester, N.Y.: Healing Arts Press, 1991.

Herbal Drugs and Phytopharmaceuticals. N. G. Bisset, editor. Boca Raton, Fla.: CRC Press, 1989.

Holt, S. *The Soy Revolution*. New York: Dell, 2000.

Holt, S. *The Natural Way to a Healthy Heart*. New York: M. Evans and Company, Inc., 1999.

Holt, S., and L. Comac. *Miracle Herbs*. New York: Kensington Books, 1997.

Holt, S., and J. Barilla. *The Power of Cartilage*. New York: Kensington Books, 1998.

Nutrition and Health. F. Bonner, editor. New York: CRC Press, 1995.

Pert, C. B. *Molecules of Emotion*. New York: Scribner, 1997.

Present Knowledge in Nutrition, 7th ed. E. E. Ziegler and L. J. Filer, editors. Washington, D.C.: ILSI Press, 1996.

Smith, T. *Homeopathic Medicine*. London: Thorsons, 1982.

Textbook of Natural Medicine, 2nd ed. J. E. Pizzorno and M. T. Murray, editors. New York: Churchill Livingstone, 1999.

EDUCATIONAL WEB SITES

www.wellnesspublishing.com
www.drugdepletion.com
www.biotherapies.net

COMMERCIAL WEB SITES

www.naturesway.com
www.biotherapies.com
www.naturesbenefit.com